The Easy Way to
GOOD LOOKS

SHIRLEY LORD

The Easy Way to
GOOD LOOKS

Drawings by Martha Voutas

THOMAS Y. CROWELL COMPANY
Established 1834   New York

On pages 9 and 30, photos courtesy of Redken Laboratories; on pages 25, 70, 71, and 165, photos courtesy of Helena Rubinstein; on pages 33, 34, 64, 75, and 128, photos by William Silano, courtesy of the Revlon Public Relations Department for whom they were taken; on pages 38, 80, and 108, photos by Sarah Moon, makeup by Carita; on pages 42, 63, and 199, photos courtesy La Costa Resort Hotel and Spa; on page 57, photo courtesy Palm-Aire Spa; on page 60, photo courtesy of Elizabeth Arden; on page 103, photo courtesy Vidal Sassoon; on pages 107 and 151, Dior woman created by Serge Lutens, photo and makeup designed by Serge Lutens for Parfums Christian Dior; on page 109, Elura wig by Brentwood, photo courtesy of Monsanto; on page 115, A La Contessa wig, photo courtesy of Monsanto; on page 122, photo by John Cole, color and hairstyle by Derek Roe of London; on pages 133 and 216, photos by Neal Barr; on pages 176 and 177, photos courtesy of Clairol Loving Care Color-Lotion; on page 202, photo by Elisabetta Catalano.

Copyright © 1976 by Shirley Lord

All rights reserved. Except for use in a review, the reproduction or utilization of this work in any form or by any electronic, mechanical, or other means, now known or hereafter invented, including xerography, photocopying, and recording, and in any information storage and retrieval system is forbidden without the written permission of the publisher. Published simultaneously in Canada by Fitzhenry & Whiteside Limited, Toronto.

Designed by Abigail Moseley

Manufactured in the United States of America

Library of Congress Cataloging in Publication Data

Lord, Shirley.
   The easy way to good looks

  Includes index.
  1. Beauty, Personal. I. Title.
RA778.L866   646.7'02'4042   75-20216
ISBN 0-690-00763-9
       1 2 3 4 5 6 7 8 9 10

To David

Contents

	Introduction	1
1	**The Basis of Good Looks** *A Good Skin: How to Achieve It as Your First Goal*	5
2	**Dressing the Skin** *From the Deodorant to the Bath and What Each Can Do for You*	43
3	**Your Makeup** *Tyranny or Therapy?*	65
4	**Hair** *Our Best Asset with a Little Care*	85
5	**The Dieting Game** *Played by Martyrs (165 Pounds Trying to Be Size 10) and Missionaries (the Size-8 Girl Friends)*	129
6	**How to Fall in Love with Exercise** *And Everything You Ever Wanted to Know About the Subject*	163
7	**Has She or Hasn't She . . .** *Had her Face/Bosom/Thighs Lifted?* *Had a Nose/Stomach/Chin Job?*	203
8	**Scent and Its many Implications** *There's Much More to It than Meets the Nose*	217
	Index	226

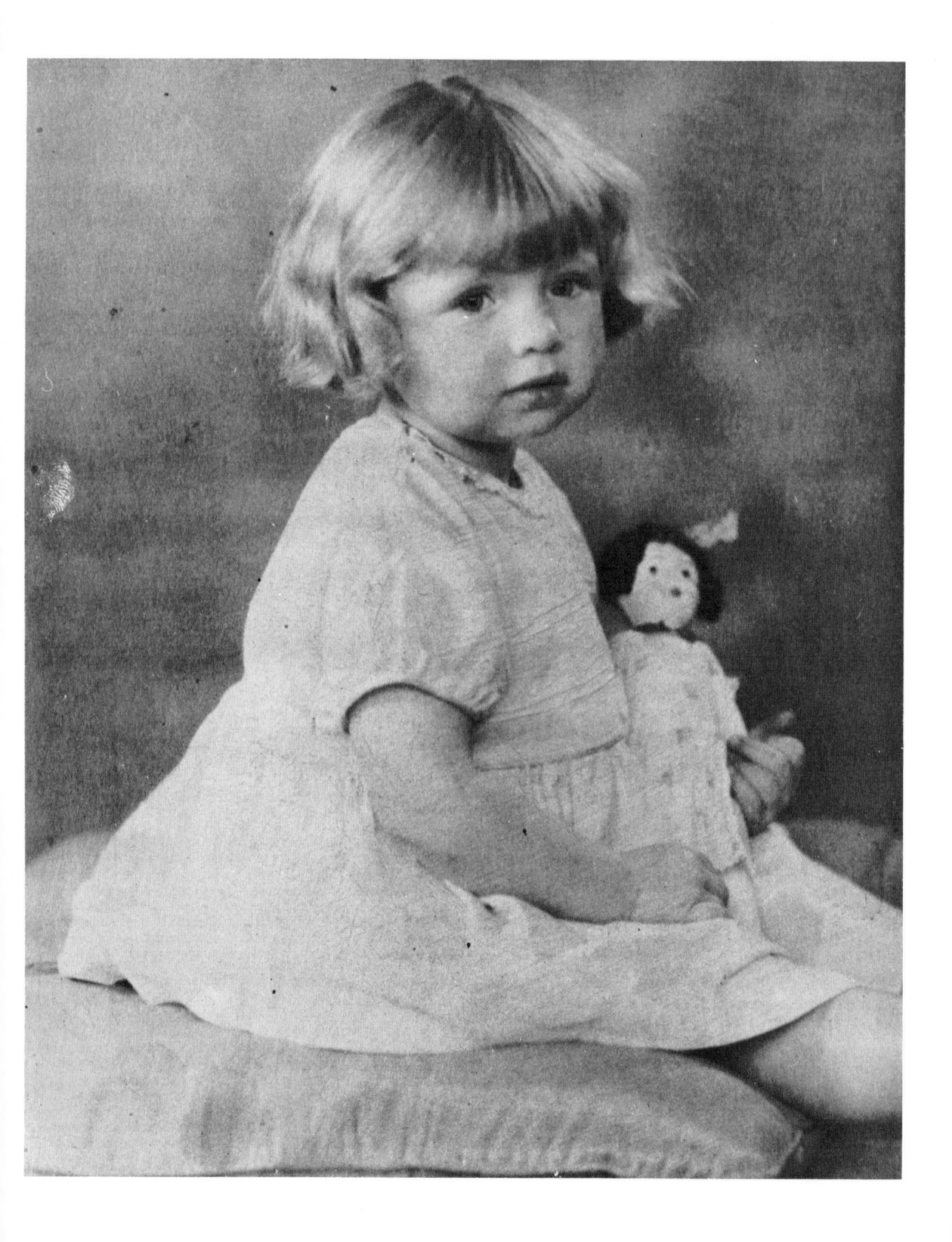

Introduction

As Beauty and Health Editor of *Vogue*, I covered the hottest subject on earth as far as women are concerned—beauty, an out-of-date word for an up-to-date subject. Today the word beauty means a woman's *looks*, which may have nothing or little to do with being born beautiful. My job now with Helena Rubinstein—as one of the few female vice-presidents in the cosmetic industry—is still to find out how a woman can best improve what she's got as quickly and as easily as possible. Nobody has the time or inclination to devote hours to any regime, and "good looks can be had for the asking" is my attitude.

I've been quoted more than once on my chance remark at a party that "one day I believe we'll have a wrinkleless society—though I'm not sure we'll really like it. Human beings could look pretty dreary and monotonous without their character lines." Today, whether we like it or not, expensive technology is working toward making us wrinkleless, first by taking the "wrinkles" out of the many thousands of beauty products available. Scientists with impressive degrees are no longer magisterial about the cosmetic industry; they spend their lives improving the gloss and durability of our lipsticks, the moisture in our moisturizers, the benefits of our masks, and—above all—making products look as natural as possible on the skin. The "natural look" isn't a passing gimmick. Every woman wants to look as terrific as possible, doesn't mind wearing a lot of makeup to get there, but doesn't want to look *made up*—and that will never change.

Did You Know . . .

Did you know that under today's kind of microscope you can clearly see wrinkles on a two-week old baby's skin, wrinkles that are programed genetically, passed on from one generation to another? I didn't, until I met Dr. John A. Cella, the chemist in charge of research and development at a huge cosmetic company with a huge Big Daddy pharmaceutical company behind it. He's working on ways to make sure we can cope with those wrinkles, however many we inherit. In

FACING PAGE
The author—preparing to be a beautiful lady.

INTRODUCTION this book I tell you what we can do to ensure they have no depth, and so no visibility, when we're far beyond the baby stage. (Read what to do and how to do it on pages 5–22.)

Did you know that hair at growth (root) level can change from breakfast to lunch, from lunch to dinner, depending on the kind of day you've had? I didn't, until I spent a day in a multimillion-dollar lab with a whiz kid of the hair industry. How you can improve your own hair with very little effort is all here, too (on pages 85–127).

Did you know that the body gets bored doing the same exercises every day and can block shape-up progress if it doesn't get a break or a change . . . that the same diet day in, day out, can ruin all chances of getting and staying slim? I didn't, until I warmed up myself with the man responsible for many of the most beautiful bodies in the world. He told me and I'll tell you (on pages 163–201) how he helps stars like Cher, Raquel Welch, Barbra Streisand, and Burt Reynolds streamline their bodies with exercises everyone can do. The diet story is an incredibly complex one—but there are diets for every mentality and every shape on pages 129–161.

Self-Doubt Destroys

What really matters is what you *do* with what you *have*. Good looks, or the lack of them, may start the day you're conceived—when you inherit the frame on which your skin is going to live, your coloring, and your characteristics—but real beauty in the genes can be snuffed out by the time your teens are over. Poor nutrition can kill it (too much of the wrong food is as bad as too little of the right), so can poor health, poor habits, and—often forgotten as the biggest killer of all—an upbringing that neglects to build up self-confidence, that invaluable asset.

Self-doubt is the weevil that can destroy any look. Doubt *shows* and *spoils*, while self-confidence *shows* and *enhances* when it's built on the self-knowledge that you've made the best of the raw material that's you.

The girl with glossy, tumbling, luxuriant hair and piano legs will soon learn in the barbaric teen years how well she's using the advantage of her beautiful hair over the disadvantage of her thick legs. Taught to maximize the effect of an asset (while trying to improve, but not dwell on, a drawback) means that what could be a disastrous hang-up just fades from view—literally.

On the other hand, the girl most "unlikely to succeed" in her teens, the one who's a constant wallflower with a gap in her front teeth, big feet, and mousey hair, can emerge as a startling and successful beauty in her twenties. Ask top model Lauren Hutton or actress Lois Chiles, both of whom at twenty felt their chances for any success, personal or professional, were zero.

Lois Chiles told me in an interview for *Vogue* that even at twenty-two she felt a complete failure: "I came to New York from the University of Texas where everybody was into petite blonde cheerleader types and where I was pretty much of a permanent wallflower. I was sure I was fat and ugly and decided to bury myself in my studies until I found out what to do with my life." She was spotted at a drugstore counter by a photographer—and after a few months, modeling became her career and she never looked back. Now she says she feels her looks have improved: "I never felt attractive in Houston and perhaps I wasn't. Now I *feel* more attractive, and people say I am, so perhaps it is just a matter of believing in yourself."

This is the key, for believing in yourself and liking yourself is all a part of good looks—and I've said so in print and in speeches hundreds of times. After the uncertainties of teen-age, there's no excuse for not taking a good hard look at yourself to see the woman you've become and to analyze whether you'd like to make any changes.

Help Yourself

Most of us would like to make changes, but many don't know how or where to begin . . . which is what this book is all about—how to, where to, what to—but not *why*. Here every woman has a chance not only to take stock, but to take note and to act upon it.

Helping ourselves means thinking the right way—and that doesn't mean being able to evaluate the differences between two nail enamels, but being able to give *love* and receive it, equating with emotional security, tranquility, trust. How we feel emotionally shows right up on our faces, even if we think we're the inscrutable kind. As you'll read on pages 6–10, the amount of love or hate we feel or have experienced affects our looks more than we'll ever know. If we think of hate as stress and tension, it all becomes much more obvious.

Health doesn't come next on the looks agenda—it's right up there with love, for without health no amount of makeup or beauty treatments can be effective.

A healthy approach means the *right nutrition* for the sake of *skin* and *hair* as well as vital statistics. It means *exercise* as a *natural part of life,* not as an act of martyrdom or a twice-weekly crusade.

Cleanliness is next to *healthiness,* and that means a clear, sparkling skin that can only improve makeup's effect.

The woman who never seems to look any older is the one who *is* thinking the right way—who perhaps through trial and error has worked out the right rhythm for herself—sleeping enough, making love enough (regular sex is important for a woman's good looks), breathing clean air—plus the three big musts: nutrition, exercise, skin care. As the Hungarian cosmetician, the late Dr. Erno Laszlo, said loudly and often, "It's never too late to improve—even though it may be too late to retrieve everything."

I've said it before on the pages of *Vogue,* I'll say it again: every woman alive can be better looking. This book will show you how. . . .

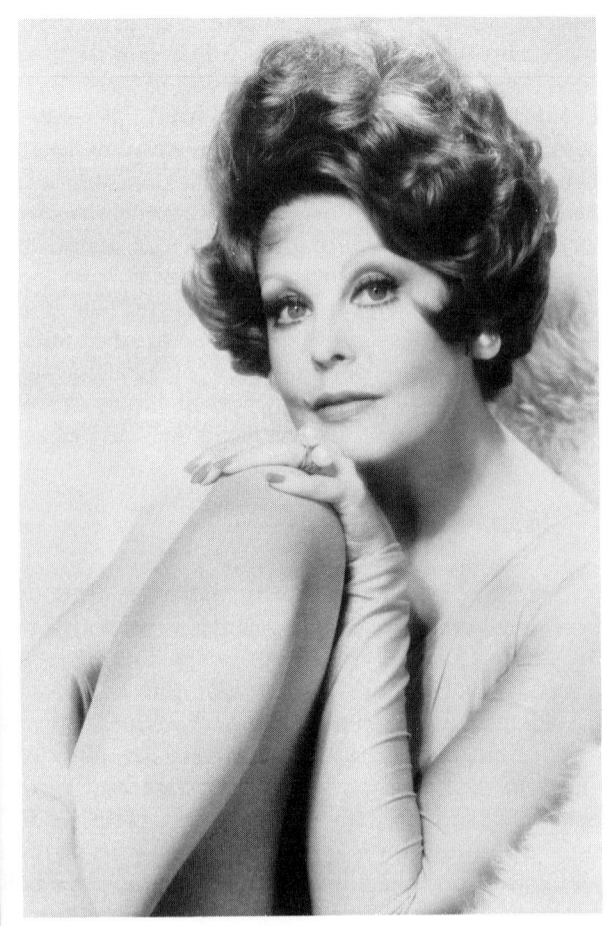

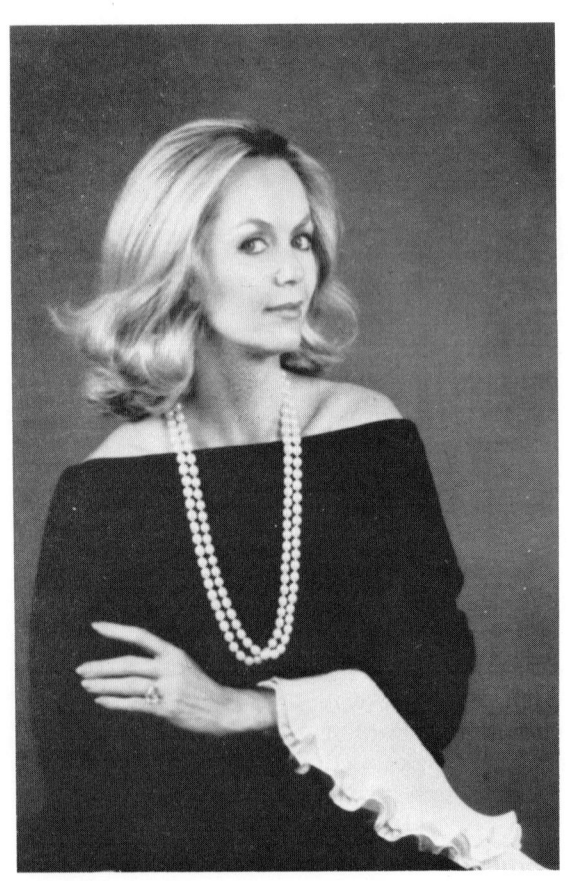

1

The Basis of Good Looks

A Good Skin

How to Achieve It as Your First Goal

We all know them, women who never seem to get any older, whose looks don't seem to change—or age. What is the common denominator linking these women who apparently defy the passing of time? One may be thin, another fat, one active, another lethargic—but they all have one thing in common: beautiful, glorious UNLINED SKIN.

Our features—eyes, nose, mouth—don't age and give our birthdays away. *Our skin does,* usually too soon. Aging skin is entirely responsible for those extra looks in the mirror—those extra minutes spent on cover-up makeup—sometimes too much in the wrong places at the wrong time of day.

Whatever any beautician or cosmetic manufacturer says—and I

FACING PAGE
Great skin . . . who has it? Arlene Dahl and Mrs. Guilford Dudley.

know hundreds of them all over the world—the sort of beautiful skin I'm talking about, the sort other women sigh over, is a gift from the genes, not the genie, inherited but more important MAINTAINED during life with as much care as an owner gives his vintage car.

The Most Beautiful Skin in the World

Who has it? The Baroness de Rothschild for one. Living between schlosses in Austria and apartments and yachts in Monte Carlo, Jeanne de Rothschild is certainly over fifty and under seventy, but her skin is the skin of a girl of twenty-two, truly translucent, pink and white. Arlene Dahl possesses glorious skin—unlined, with the bloom of a peach. Models Betsy Theodoracopulos and Mrs. Leo Kelmenson; the Begum Aga Khan; Mrs. Guilford Dudley, wife of the diplomat and businessman from Tennessee—all these have been born with stunning skin, and they've kept it that way easily. How? They all stay out of the sun, knowing what every dermatologist knows, that *exposure to the sun is skin damaging,* aging it to look like old leather, if not producing more serious skin problems such as carcinoma.

None of the women just mentioned has ever *had a deliberate sunbath in her life.* Further, to ensure good skin stays in the family, where there are daughters, as in the case of Arlene Dahl, Jane Dudley, and Sally Khan, they have been telling "Don't-Sunbathe-Darling" stories to their daughters since they were old enough to listen.

Losing Your Temper Can Age You, Too

There are other factors to aging, not the least being the way you cope with life—your temperament and whether you can handle your problems or not. As Dr. Joseph Hoffman wrote in his tome, *The Life and Death of the Cell,* ". . . if one went to the trouble, it would be feasible to measure the degree of love, hate, and anxiety experienced by a human being by the rate of his or her cellular destruction." You have only to look in the mirror after a row, tears or no tears, to see its effect on your looks, and what you *see* is your skin *disturbed* by the signals sent from your brain.

The late cosmetic scientist Marguerite Maury elaborated on Hoffman's theme when she pointed out in *The Secret of Life and Youth:* "The sexual life of the woman is of the greatest importance to her appearance. Whereas the functions of the man are exogenous and extroverted and he will suffer most from premature old age by abuse of these functions, the woman—being introverted and indigenous—will grow older swifter by *deficiency.*"

How does this relate directly to your skin—dry, oily, spotty, smooth, whatever it may be? Easily. Skin isn't just a convenient covering for all our component parts. It's as vital to life as the heart, lungs, or brain. IT ISN'T ONLY ANOTHER ORGAN—IT'S THE LARGEST ORGAN OF THE BODY, wrapping us up in almost 15,000 square inches.

At the embryo stage of life, there are the ectoderm and the endoderm. The ectoderm becomes the skin *and* the brain; the endoderm becomes our insides—which shows us clearly why the link between the brain and the skin is far more intimate than that between the brain and other organs of the body.

Your Skin Picture

Your skin consists of three main layers: the epidermis at the top that the world sees; the dermis beneath, that provides nutrition and oxygen; the subdermis, the lowest layer. Distributed among these three layers are cells, glands, blood vessels, nerves, hairs, hair follicles.

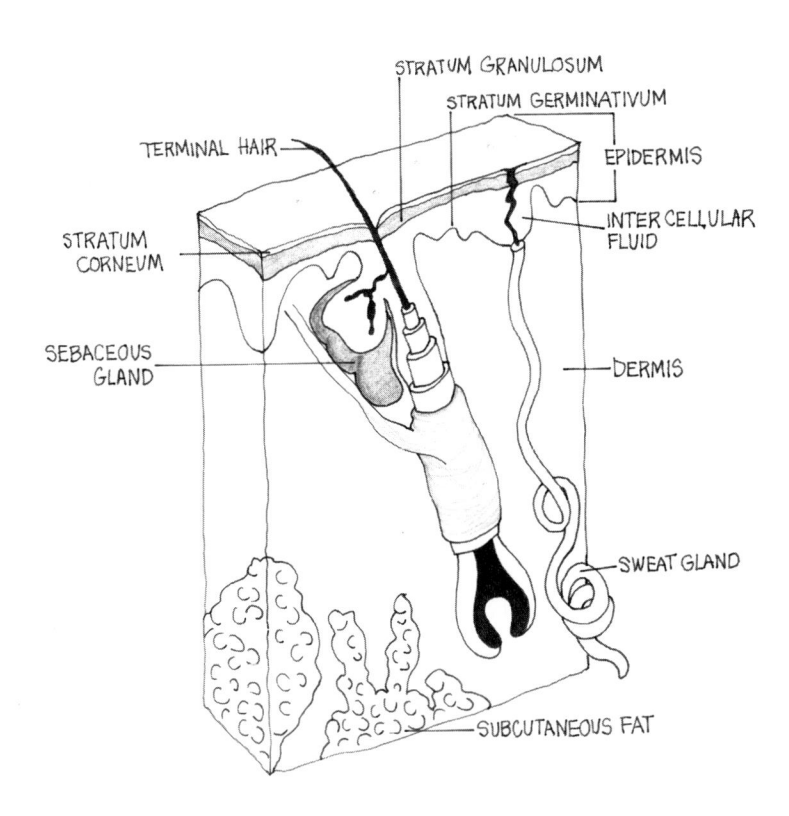

Skin Jobs

1. Skin acts as the body's thermostat, regulating body heat as much as it can to protect the body from destruction whenever there are dramatic swings in temperature.

2. Skin excretes waste the body doesn't need.

3. It keeps in vital fluids the body does need.

4. It keeps out unwanted external fluids, and that means these days it acts as a first line of defense against pollution.

5. Skin acts as a control station for sensation, relaying messages to and from the brain faster than the speed of sound—of temperature, touch, pain, and pleasure. This is where Madame Maury and Dr. Hoffman's words become appropriate. Think of the skin of the people you love—it's special, whether it's your baby's, your husband's, or your lover's. It reflects inner chemistry, and you would know that particular skin anywhere, even in the dark when—particularly between lovers—skin can act as a supercharged antennae.

How Does Skin Work?

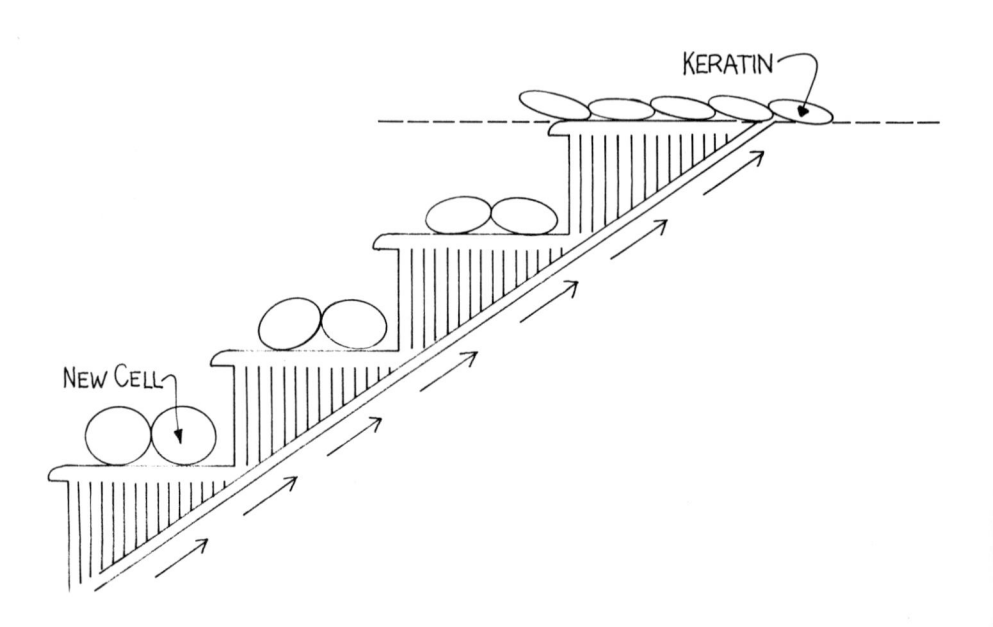

Think of your skin working the way an escalator does. On the "bottom step" are fresh new cells created deep down in the subdermis. As they rise to work their way up through the middle layer—the dermis—to the epidermis on top, another layer is forming right behind them, and another and another, just like the steps of the escalator—never ceasing and always moving upward on the same route.

When the cells arrive in the epidermis area, they begin to die. They become flat bits of keratin, for living cells can't survive exposure to air or water. Adhering to each other, the keratin bits form the strong shield of dead tissue we see that protects all the skin-making machinery and body tissues from the outside world.

Tough protein, keratin is as resistant as it can be to the changes it has to face, but it still needs all the help it can get to fight the elements and look its best. Dead cells that stay around too long make skin look dingy, dull. That skin needs a mask or exfoliating cream to whip dead cells away.

Don't Blame a Cell Slowdown for the Aging Process

There's never a slowdown of the rate of cell production—often erroneously blamed for signs of old age.

There is a slowdown or weakening of other parts of the skin-making machinery. The sebaceous glands, for instance, excrete less sebum, the skin's chief lubricant. As the amount of sebum in skin's repository makes all the difference between an oily- or dry-disposed surface, the

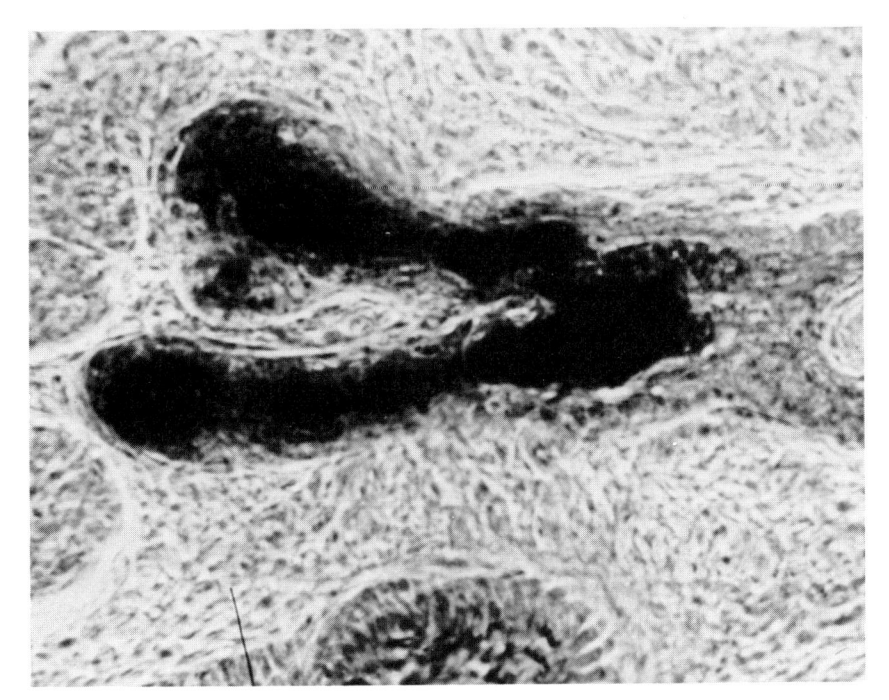

Don't blame a cell slowdown for the aging process . . . it's our sebaceous glands (one is seen here in this skin biopsy) that let us down.

skin becomes drier, and a dry surface "creases," wrinkles, much more easily than a moist one.

The dermis—the depot in the middle layer—is mostly made up of collagen, the protein fiber responsible for skin's elasticity. It's collagen that allows a smile or an expression to flit on and off a young face leaving no evidence behind. Around forty, when a woman complains she's starting to wrinkle and has to do something about it, she isn't *just* starting to wrinkle. It's been going on for at least twenty years, but her collagen support meant her many expressions left behind no visible trace. Suddenly collagen starts to sag—and so does her face.

Start as Young as You Can

At twenty your skin fits your face like a new girdle. It's firm, gives plenty of control, snapping easily back into place after a yawn, a grimace, a big hello. After a lot of wear (just think how many expressions cross *your* face in one day) and little care, the skin acts like a worn girdle. It's looser, thinner, the elasticity is weakened. You can replace your girdle. You can't replace skin elasticity overnight. It takes time unless the plastic surgeon is called in to take in a few tucks and darts to restore a tauter surface. That's another story (see pages 203–212).

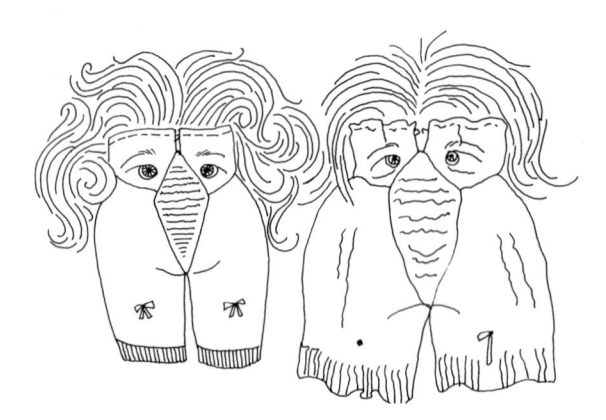

Recognize Your Type

First, get to know your skin type. Touch your skin. Get to know its *feel* as well as its look. Your skin has to fall into one of the following types. Choose the one that's most applicable:

1. *Dry.* The most common state of skin in the United States (90 percent of women here have been statistically labeled as having skin

that is too dry). If you're in the majority, your skin is obviously lacking in oils. It *feels* "fragile." It can look "transparent." It's subject to blotches, little red patches with *dry* skin in the center.

2. *Dehydrated*. This skin is worse than dry. It lacks moisture to a painful extent, wrinkles easily, is scaly, so that you can see bits of skin flaking—just as if you were peeling after a sunburn.

3. *Mixed or "Normal."* This means you have a "combination type skin." At its best it's slightly oily down the center panel from forehead to chin with drier sides. At its worst the oily patch develops into large pores on the center panel with even dehydrated sides.

4. *Oily*. This skin has overactive sebaceous glands that excrete too much sebum causing pores to dilate. Skin looks slightly to very coarse, and the general complexion tone is poor, smeary, never quite clear.

5. *Hydrated*. If your skin contains *too much sebum*—oil—it's hydrated. It looks and feels swollen, even congested.

On top of the kind of skin you have, what is known as "the acid mantle" plays a vital part in good skin.

To determine skin health, dermatologists use the pH (hydrogen potential) scale, which ranges from 0 to 14. A pH of 7 is neutral—anything below is acid, anything over is alkaline.

The most healthy skin (i.e., "normal") will be between 5.4 and 6.2 . . . acid (hence "acid mantle"—*the description inferring protection*—for bacteria, forever settling on our skin cannot thrive on an acid surface!)

Below 5.4 will be a skin that is too acid, usually extremely sensitive, in need of special products and/or treatment.

From 6.2 to 7 and over will be a skin with insufficient acid, therefore a skin that is alkaline (which it should *not* be) also needing a skin-balancing treatment to bring it back to its correct slightly acid state.

Skin Can Change Its Type

The leopard may not change its spots, but a skin can change its character. It has a lot to do with where you live.

When I first came to live in New York from London, with a stopover in Barbados, I was constantly flattered with that old cliché, "You have that great English complexion, lucky girl." I took it for granted, just as I'd taken it for granted all my life—a good skin that never let me down, no spots, no blotches, just smooth and reliable through thick and thin. In Barbados my skin had thrived, not surprisingly, because I was living in the best possible atmosphere—slightly humid, light, clean air, air-conditioned only by soft Atlantic breezes. As I'd learned from early fry-ups to stay out of the sun, the Barbados sun as reliable as clockwork didn't bother my skin. It was really peachy.

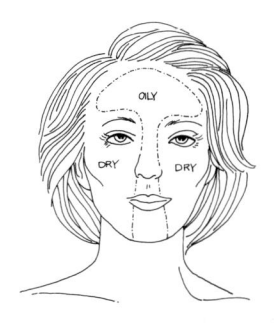

After three months of living in New York, I no longer received any "English skin" compliments, for the simple reason I didn't have that celebrated type of complexion any more. My skin was dry, hard, even painful on occasion. It didn't respond to superficial moisturizing with a variety of products. It needed a lot more than that, but I didn't realize it at the time. My skin was telling me it wasn't used to living in what I now consider to be the most punishing environment for skin in the world—the supercontrolled atmosphere of overheating and over air-conditioning. Where air is dehumidified, moisture is obviously extracted, but I didn't think about that for a time. When I finally followed a new pattern of supercleansing (with a gentle liquid cleanser and moisturized toner), and extramoisturizing with a regular moisturizer, then in winter an under-makeup moisturizer, too, my skin started rewarding me with an occasional trace of bloom. This proved to me more than any textbook that skin *can* and *will* change. It isn't only emotional. It's elementary in its approach to weather and environment. All this to point out that if you've spotted your skin type from the list just given, it doesn't mean you're that type for life. It all depends on where you go to live and the treatment you think corresponds to the geography.

Still on the Dry Side . . .

You can be born with very dry skin, which is usually a situation needing medical help. More often you can inflict dry skin on yourself by washing too much with the wrong soap, robbing the skin of its acid mantle, leaving it exposed for the elements to strip it further of any natural moisture supply. If you are over twenty-five and have a tendency toward dry skin, you should leave soap alone—unless it's very, very mild, nonalkaline, and even specially devised for sensitive dry skins. A liquid cleanser is the best bet. Not only prolonged exposure to air-conditioning and steam heat hurts. Wind velocity and dry air—riding in a fast open car, for instance—can sap skin (and hair, too).

Diuretic cures that dehydrate the body of liquid content in a "quick diet" (there's really no such thing—see pages 135–137) can also dehydrate the skin. Then, as I never tire of pointing out, the radiation of the sun speeds up oxidation in the cells—drying skin out just like old leather. Look on Miami Beach to see I'm speaking the truth. You can polish up old leather to look beautiful. Leathery skin is *never* beautiful, however hard you polish.

How to Help Dry Skin

Now you know that the predominant skin type in the United States is dry and that our man-made environment is mostly at fault, for skin has to negotiate rapid changes of temperature and humidity wherever it goes these days—in offices, planes, cars, not to mention homes. The experts say man has been slow to adapt to changes in his environment, even though he created them himself. It's said it will take generations to build up skin's resistance to the deteriorating effects of constant air-conditioning and central heating.

So the sooner a dry or dehydrated skin starts looking for outside help the better. The help is pretty simple, and summed up in one magical word, now part of the language—the MOISTURIZER.

Dr. Erno Laszlo, the Hungarian cosmetician, whose beauty principles are still followed slavishly by many of the world's renowned beauties, used to reiterate, *"If you want skin beauty after forty, you should begin to work at it when you are twenty."* Luckily for those who didn't know at the time he also said, *"It's never too early or too late to cultivate a beautiful complexion, because the skin has tremendous powers of self-regeneration when properly cared for."*

Helena Rubinstein told me the same thing herself, but everything really changed for the better when an unassuming chemist with the even more unassuming name of Dr. Irwin Blank from the University of Massachusetts discovered in 1931 that to transmit *moisture to the skin,* it was necessary to create an oil-in-water emulsion, even then described as a moisturizer. What else could you call it?

"Moisturizers have changed everything." Over the last twenty years a variety of people, from Gloria Swanson to the Queen to England have told me this, and nobody can refute it. The right moisturizer used *regularly* on a dry skin can change even the most arid state of affairs.

How does it work? It increases the water content of the outer layer of the skin, so just as a plant revives with a drink, so does skin, part of the human plant. It blooms, softens, even has a moist, melting look.

Contemporary moisturizers have now advanced to the point that they don't only *add* extra moisture; they *prevent* any existing moisture escaping. This double dose of treatment is what any dry condition needs to ward off early wrinkling, for skin to look prettier. When dermatologists refer to the "natural moisture," they mean exactly that—it's water from the intercellular fluids of the skin's lower layers, which in cold weather easily evaporates in the atmosphere. This means the "barrier" part of a moisturizer's work is as essential as anything extra it may add.

There's just no excuse for not combating dry skin, whether you inherited it or brought it on yourself from any of the reasons mentioned.

To maintain skin's natural humidity and prevent further dehydration, a moisturizer is the answer, forming an occlusive film on the skin's surface.

There Are Many Ways to Wear a Moisturizer

If you have very dry skin, you can start the day's cleansing with a cleanser that has a moisturizer built into its formula.

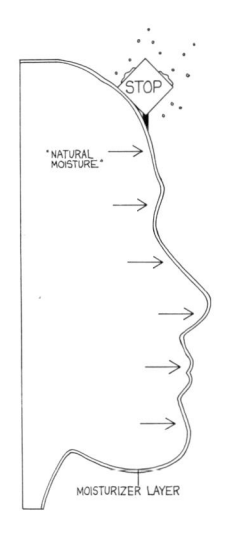

As your body retains some moisture after a bath or shower, even after you've towel-dried, this is the best time to apply a straightforward moisturizer or one that's been formulated especially to wear beneath makeup (usually labeled as such: an undermakeup moisturizer). This type of product increases the affinity of the skin's surface to makeup, so that it glides on more easily, stays longer.

Most makeup comes moisturized now, if you want it that way—a positive answer to the consumer's recent command for *skin benefit* along with *makeup color*.

At the end of the day a mask is the latest and most effective way to give the skin a "drink." *Make sure it's a moisturizing mask.* Read the labels; that's what they're there for.

The reason a mask is such a good—and quick—way to moisturize an overly dry or dehydrated skin is that the skin is a *captive* audience beneath its film.

The skin takes from the mask whatever benefits it has to give, while any moisture present can't escape.

You can help dry skin a lot *in* the bath, too, when bath oil or an emollient type of bath product should *always* be used. If you're a shower girl, smother yourself in bath oil or gel before you turn on the faucet. In winter extra moisturizing this way should be a MUST.

Can the regular use of a moisturizer prevent wrinkles—which appear so easily on dry skin? The superficial kind, yes, especially those tiny sun lines that look so unattractive out of the sun. If you start at twenty, *regular*—with emphasis on the word—moisturizing can delay age's insignia.

Remember to study labels for a moisturizer is different from a product labeled as an emollient. While *a moisturizer* adds moisture, it doesn't necessarily prevent *natural moisture* escaping. An *emollient*, however, both *lubricates* and *traps moisture* in the skin. For instance, water is a moisturizer, but can't help your skin keep its own supply. Petroleum jelly and olive oil are emollients with no trace of water, but they both add moisture and prevent its loss.

Does Normal Skin Need Care?

Every skin needs care, and in any case, "normal" skin, as I've already described from my own experience, doesn't necessarily stay normal. It all depends on who owns it and where it goes.

First, it has to be kept clean—wherever it lives because every day skin collects on the surface waste matter thrown out by the body—gland secretion, cellular debris, dead-skin cells. That garbage all has to be collected and removed for skin to stay looking great, whether it's normal or not.

Soap is the most efficient collector. It's also the most drying (except the transparent and/or the especially mild kind) so it shouldn't be a three-times-a-day way of cleaning up. *Over twenty-five the less soap on the face the better.*

What you eat makes a big contribution toward maintaining a good skin, and what you drink does, too. Nobody has proved yet that alcohol harms the skin, but they're working on it. WATER is the drink skin likes best, and we don't drink enough say most nutritionists. Eight full glasses a day is the recommended dose for a better digestion, better "flushing" out, and so better unblemished skin.

It isn't only oily skins that need astringents—now called anything from toners to rinsers to scrubs and clean-ups. This type of product does a great tidy-up job following the first cleanse, collecting any debris left over, while the alcohol content (often menthol) cools the skin, makes it feel fresh and ready for business—which means makeup.

Astringents, by the way, don't reduce pore size. *Pores cannot be changed in size* with beauty products. They can be "tightened."

Oil Heiress

You need a lot of moisture. You don't need a lot of oil, and the only oil heiress happy to lose her oil deposits is, of course, the girl with oily skin. As she gets older, her skin gets better and easier to cope with, for the simple reason that the excessive sebum flow—that probably made her teens and twenties miserable—starts to diminish around twenty-five. At forty her oily skin may have been replaced with a great skin—if she takes care.

Oily skin can be accompanied by acne, a scourge at any time, but particularly in adolescence.

But acne or not, an anti-acne regime can't hurt, which means a low-fat, high-fruit diet, plenty of sleep and exercise, and—difficult to prescribe, but *always* prescribed for acne sufferers—as little tension and/or anxiety as possible.

You have to wage war on oily skin—it can't just be ignored or forgotten. The best way to fight it is with vigilant cleansing, using a medicated or soapless cleanser and cleansing up to six times a day with *lavish* rinsings. Astringents should follow every cleanse, not only because they "tidy" up the debris, but because they give skin a good send-off for makeup, essential for looks—and morale. The trick is to look for *water-based foundations and medicated makeups* formulated to cut through oil deposits. Some bases contain powders made to absorb oil all day long.

If your face isn't oily all over, but only in patches, don't forget to use a moisturizer on the drier spots! They need help, too. A cleansing mask with moisturizing properties is a help for the patchy skin, fast removing excess oil, trapping moisture skin always needs. Never forget oil is *not* moisture. Never forget that when others are bewailing their early wrinkling, oily skins can be coming into their prime.

Help for the Hydrated

Hydrated skin is congested skin—needing help from an experienced facialist to reactivate poor circulation, responsible for skin becoming clogged with waste matter that the veins should have carried away. This isn't a time for do-it-yourself techniques. Professional help should be sought, and then products chosen with extreme care. This condition rarely occurs in the young. It's more often the result of skin machinery slowing down, cells not being properly nourished, so skin becomes clogged just like a blocked-up drain with toxins and waste matters. It shows up through the face being puffy, bloated.

Acne and What Can Be Done About It—if Anything

At one end of the age scale is often the hydrated state just mentioned. At the other, acne, puberty's scourge, often inherited, triggered off by a hormonal imbalance that can cause huge hang-ups right out of proportion to its medical status—all because it generally hits at the time when self-confidence is at its lowest ebb: teen-age.

Doctors agree on what affects acne most—*emotional stress,* causing skin to flare up and look disfigured even overnight.

Diet is controversial. Some doctors think diet has no adverse or advantageous effect, while others ban chocolates (particularly), fried food, nuts, and soft drinks.

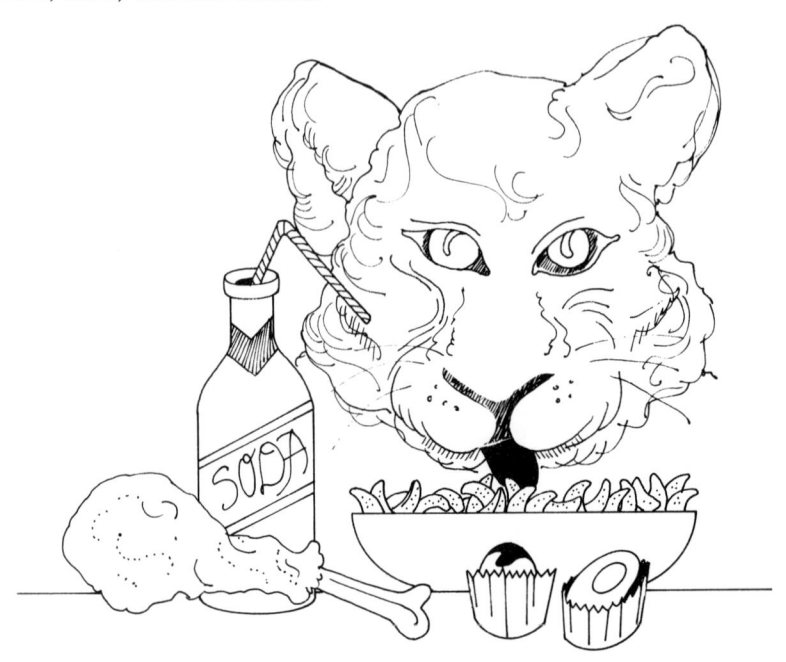

Unfortunately acne is like the common cold, much discussed, highly publicized, but still with no real cure, although certain antibiotic treatments have produced remarkable results in the last two years.

The main stumbling block is the inability to induce acne in any animal for lab tests. We don't need to wonder why there are no human volunteers.

In short, as with an oily skin, acne means too much sebum is produced at too rapid a rate. Pores become clogged, but with acne the sebum production never ceases. Infection sets in; the result is ugly pimples and spots.

It isn't contagious, and contrary to what many think, dirt is not the cause—although obviously a *lack of proper cleansing* aggravates it. Acne sufferers just can't wash enough—for the more they wash or scrub with medicated soap, the more sebum is removed, reducing bacteria on skin's surface, producing a drying and peeling effect.

The New Solutions

Although antibiotics are increasingly being tested on acne patients across the country, each case has to be treated independently, because patients respond so differently to the same treatment.

The latest *control* methods (but not cures) are medicated soaps, lotions, and creams containing sulphur, resorcinol, alcohol, salicylic acid, benzoyl peroxide. Because the male hormone, testosterone, is partly responsible for the trouble, careful doses of female hormone are used to *decrease* the size of the sebaceous glands, on the theory that the smaller the gland, the less sebum gets out. This method is restricted to severe cases—and because of possible feminizing side effects, only to females.

Ultraviolet light is used to peel and clear up the skin's outer layer, while natural sunlight—providing the atmosphere is not humid—can help, too.

Vitamin-A supplements are frequently prescribed, the "good skin" vitamin, and vitamin-A acid is sometimes used to clear up the infected areas.

"No more acne" isn't a shadowy pipedream. That day is drawing nearer as research progresses to control excessive sebum, to inhibit the bacteria, and to produce a *topical estrogen* that works without feminizing or other side effects.

The Pill—Does It Affect Our Skin?

Yes, it does. Some of us. I first learned this one summer a few years ago when a gorgeous model friend and neighbor showed me with alarm little patches of brown pigment that had suddenly turned up on her otherwise flawless, lightly tanned skin.

There was a patch about the size of an olive above her eyebrow, two more—like odd-size patches on a pair of denims—on both cheeks. They had appeared faintly the past week, then deepened after gardening in the sun one afternoon. I suggested she see a dermatologist, who told her that her patchy problem wasn't unusual, but an increasing phenomenon among women on the Pill. Our melanin (pigment) supply is controlled by the pituitary and adrenal functions; which are also in charge of ovulation. As the Pill suppresses ovulation, it can also in an excess of zeal trigger off extra supplies of melanin. Then sunlight literally *sets* the patches in place, as my friend had unwittingly set hers, making them far more visible by spending too much time outdoors. In winter, the doctor told her, the patches would fade, and in time, providing she avoided sunlight, they could become invisible. Meanwhile, he told her to use a depigmenting bleaching-type cream and a cover-up base on top.

It was also suggested she switch to another form of the Pill or stop taking it altogether, but as she told her doctor and me, "I'd rather be blotchy than pregnant."

My friend was unfortunate, but statistics prove about 25 percent of women on the Pill can experience the same problem.

On the other hand, another 25 percent state their skins have improved after being on the Pill for a few months. Not surprisingly, most of these were acne sufferers who received the benefit of the estrogen, the female hormone, in the Pill, used as already described in acne treatments to combat the harmful effects of too much male hormone, testosterone.

Many dermatologists believe the Pill's best advantage is a psychological one. When a woman's outlook is more relaxed, and she is less fearful of unwanted pregnancies, her skin is more "relaxed," too, and even blooms. Never forget skin *is* emotional. It reacts to how you feel and think.

Allergies and What to Do About Them

The term *allergy* comes from two Greek words meaning "changed work." To develop a reaction to a substance your system has to take so violent a dislike to it that it creates an antibody ready to fight if and when the substance next appears in the bloodstream. This is when those well-known rashes or patches or red streaks emerge.

Unfortunately, allergic reaction to anything can be as sudden as a bolt of lightning. Thin-skinned people are the unlucky ones, for the protective barrier formed by the skin's layers is just that more easily penetrated, allowing unwanted substances to enter the bloodstream. The body reacts and rebels as you'd expect it to when irritating materials are forced or injected under the skin.

The thin-skinned know from experience they have to be extra

careful about products. With sense they'll choose a product distinctly labeled as "pure—for the delicate, sensitive skin" or "dermatologically tested." Hypoallergenic, once a familiar adjective on labels (which translated literally means "less likely to cause allergy"), is a word that the Food and Drug Administration has helped to phase out in the last few years.

If the sensitive-skin type doesn't use sense and chooses indiscriminately, she can be in for a lot of trouble. Fragrance, for instance, has long been known as a troublemaker when included in product formulas. The thin skin should *never* wear scented products, because fragrance itself is composed of so many ingredients, including, of course, pollens and flower extracts, the number-one and -two triggers of sneezing bouts and rash attacks.

Some companies have gone the completely "pure" route, ignoring fragrance in practically every case whenever a product is formulated. As a spokesman for this part of the industry says, "We do not feel fragrance adds to a product's cosmetic effectiveness, so we generally leave it out. Only in a few cases do we use a totally *synthetic* fragrance, where the addition makes sense as in a bath line."

Allergic reaction can happen to anyone, thin- or thick-skinned, and while the thin-skinned should *know* what and what not to use (allergy or reaction may only be one smear away), the thick-skinned can be hit with force, often leaving no clues as to what caused it.

The most frustrating fact about allergies is that you can suddenly become allergic to something you've used for years without any problem . . . not only products but food, a clothes' cleaner, the smell of your husband's pipe. Strange but true—and so far there isn't a general solution.

Dr. Earle Brauer, dermatologist for one of the leading cosmetic companies in the world, knows a lot about allergies and points out there's a big difference between an irritant and an allergen. "An irritant causes reaction in at least 80 percent of the people who use it, and it's dose-related—a lot will irritate more than a little. An allergen, however, might cause reaction in only one person in a million and is not dose-related. The most minute amount is enough to cause a huge allergy."

When you reflect that every time you use your fingers to put some cream on your face, you leave behind in the jar some new bacteria—present on everybody's skin—you begin to appreciate the huge task these cosmetic companies tackle, delivering products that not only do the job they're supposed to do, but products that eliminate as much as possible any chance of triggering off something as unpleasant as an allergy.

A product marked as "pure" goes through laborious tests. Every compound is lab-tested in conditions that look like a space station—stark white, technicians wearing masks, special clothes including boots—all to ensure absolute purity. Even if a shade of lipstick is changed, it's tested in the same long laborious way, then finally tested the human way. There are always plenty of volunteers for lipstick testing.

The temperature in the room where formulation takes place is just as important as the cleanliness of its walls—a difference up or down can dramatically alter what comes out of the test tubes.

To preserve all that purity after you buy, keep products in a cool dark place, even the fridge although it's not necessary. Don't buy large sizes unless you use them voraciously.

It's obvious that once a product produces reaction, you must stop using it. Let the manufacturer know about it, though. He wants to safeguard *you* as much as *you* want to be safeguarded. For this he needs to know the end result—how the cream or lotion behaves on *your* skin.

Natural Products: What Do They Mean and Do They Work?

During the past few years anything "natural," as opposed to synthetic, has been enjoying a popularity as sweet as mother earth. As far as beauty products are concerned, without a synthetic fixative "shelf life" can be doubtful, and who wants to fill up the freezer with moisturizing gels and lotions?

Natural or organic products (the latter refers to anything grown in earth never exposed to fertilizer or chemical) are formulated from things you'd expect to find in nature—fruits, vegetables, herbs.

Where a large company is involved, there may be plenty of peaches in the peach night oil, but there's sure to be plenty of methyl paraben and propyl paraben, too—both preservatives to give a cream long life without having to resort to the freezer. If it says avocado on the label and a reputable company's behind it, avocados will have been plucked from the trees in bushels to serve the needs of mass production. But if it's a moisturizer, it's certain a synthetic like isopropyl myristate will be part of the process, all helping the avocados to moisturize you more efficiently. My point is that going the *natural* route can be fine—but it doesn't mean you should turn your back on the companies that know best how to utilize nature's goodies, using them in conjunction with tried-and-true cosmetic ingredients. The bloom on your cheeks will be better and last longer that way.

Pow—It's a Vitamin

Tests have long ago proved that skin *can absorb pure nutrients and vitamins.* Victims of malnutrition, for instance, unable to assimilate food through the mouth have received the necessary life-saving food through nutrients being rubbed on their skin.

As Adelle Davis, the noted health-food spokeswoman, used to say, "When skin is 'starving' it can be *fed* with fruits, herbs, nuts, and minerals." To this end, she recommended face packs of papaya, avocado, and apricots. For very dry skin, soaks in oil from sunflower seeds, sesame, safflower, olives and castor beans, almonds and peanuts. From the sea she believed in treatments from plankton, seaweed, and kelp, all packed with minerals, nutritive salts, and trace elements.

If you're all for doing-it-yourself, remember your skin type matters just as much when you're dealing with the natural remedies as when you check in at your favorite cosmetic counter.

If you're too oily, you can use a mixture of honey, egg white, and ground oatmeal for a homemade cleanser that has powerful pulling power (from the honey), attracting blood swiftly to the surface, stimulating circulation; abrasive power (from the oatmeal), clearing up the oil with ease; and finally a bundle of benefits from the egg white to keep skin better balanced between dry and greasy.

Egg white is a beauty armory—it has protein, iron, vitamin A (the beauty vitamin), and methionine, well documented as a valuable asset to healthy skin.

Mashed papaya acts as a natural enzyme on the skin, has the ability to draw out any oxidized, hardened grit or pollutants from the pores, is antibacterial and tightening.

Old black magic is a combination of mashed bananas and peaches worked together in olive oil to deliver plenty of moisture and to keep in what you've got. Use this as a mask, then rinse off with tepid water after fifteen minutes.

No treatment cream need stay on the face longer than fifteen to twenty minutes—in that time it accomplishes the maximum it can do. A longer stay just isn't necessary, but it doesn't do any harm, either!

Some models make a kind of mayonnaise for a "skin snack" whenever their skin looks dreary. They use egg white, unsaturated oil, apple cider vinegar, water, and lecithin (which isn't cheating). Then when they're sure the doorbell won't ring, they cover their skin with this mixture (never forgetting the neck), and the skin seems to drink it up. After only a few moments, texture and elasticity seem improved. They "tone" or zip up circulation with cider vinegar, too, using one part vinegar to eight parts water, plus fresh grapefruit juice. The cider vinegar keeps in natural moisture content, while the grapefruit juice—lemon and watermelon would do as well—contains between 5 to 8 percent citric acid, a good pH balancer. This recipe, my model informants tell me, fades blotches and reduces the chance of blemishes.

Milk, an emulsion of 3.8 percent butterfat in water, stabilized by the additional presence of about 3 percent casein protein, is helpful as the big boys in the cosmetic business know. There was even a "milk war" sometime back when two of the biggest companies launched a skim-milk treatment and a whole-milk line at the same time—we lapped them both up!

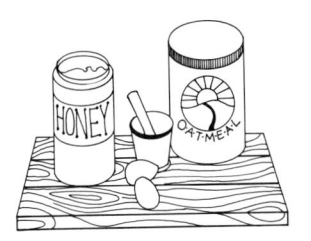

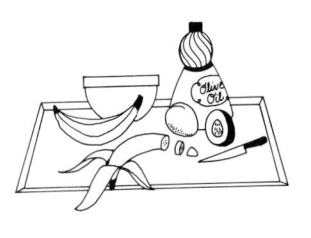

Whatever "food" we use on our skin, we have to realize that just like the food we eat, there's a time factor involved in its purity. Let's face it, if the do-it-yourself remedies were as efficacious as the products evolving from the laboratories and top research stations of the world, we would have never deviated from the potions handed down from our grandmothers.

Aromatherapy—Hokum or Helpful?

One step further on from fruity face packs and milky cleansers is *aromatherapy*, a normal part of beauty care in Europe—where it's literally as old as the hills, arriving there from the East hundreds of years ago—a newer, more unexplored therapy here.

Based on the knowledge of the regenerative powers of certain natural oils, aromatherapy is best explained as the *application or massage of those oils* on the nerve centers of the face and body, the object being to *stimulate* the reproductive action of the skin cells and thus to speed up the renewal process, and recapture a younger rhythm.

Rhythm is a key word here. As dedicated cosmetic scientist the late Marguerite Maury often reiterated: "*Aging is independent of time.* It is our physical and psychological pattern which determines the *real age of our body.*"

She believed that it is possible to remain "ageless" if women discover and maintain their own rhythm "which should stay with them until they die."

The rhythm she described means getting enough sleep, making enough love, eating and drinking the right amount—in fact, leading a perfectly balanced life for *oneself*—the rhythm differing from person to person.

Once we find the right rhythm for ourselves, she said, we could then find what she called "the gift of relaxation" for without relaxation "no rejuvenation or regeneration can take place."

True relaxation is a major object of aromatherapy, practiced for many years by Madame Maury in Paris and London, carried out today by cosmeticians all over the world. Specific massage with a variety of different natural oils induces total relaxation, *not* inertia but a state in which energy being freed, one's whole concentration can be directed onto a perceptive plane. *A truly relaxed person is an extremely alert and conscious one.* The natural oil plays its part in treating whatever skin problem exists.

The art of the aromatherapist is to know which oil for which skin, for just as with fingerprints and personality, skin differs from woman to woman, and there are hundreds of different oils imported from all parts of the world to choose from. Camomile, mint, and lavender are often used to treat sensitive, delicate skin; essence of rose to heal wounds and fade scars; Indian verbena and sandalwood to tighten open pores; geranium oil to stimulate circulation. Even oil from pulverized tree bark and linseed is used for special problems, while rose water is a must for broken capillaries.

The qualified aromatherapist will start the treatment by noting down all details of medical history, followed by a general examination—blood pressure, heart, lungs—then a blood test. Often highly magnified photographs are taken of the skin for later comparison.

In Europe and in the East, where it came from, aromatherapy is used medically to strengthen skin tissue and muscle before operations, and in the case of severe burns, to reactivate tissue so that scars are minimized.

For beauty's sake we have only to look at the Oriental skin to know that their strict program of care, which includes aromatherapy, shows results. From childhood the Oriental alternates "active" days of nourishing and feeding the skin (with many of the oils described) with "rest" days when the skin is kept scrupulously clean but free of any cosmetic or treatment.

It brings us right back to the main point of this chapter on skin: the earlier you learn about your skin (and how to treat it), the more the question of rejuvenation and retrieving looks won't be one you'll have to answer.

Masks—One for Every Skin

While aromatherapy is a treatment from the past, little changed in its application over the years, the mask—used by the Egyptians more than two thousand years ago—has been transformed with scientific know-how into one of the most contemporary skin-care products now available.

Aida Grey, an outstanding beautician in California, believes in masks for every skin, and she isn't the only one. Today many cosmetic chemists believe the mask to be the product that will produce a beauty breakthrough. Remember that wrinkleless society I mentioned?

Aida Grey says, "*After twenty every third cell is a poor one*. Skin can't be nourished from the outside alone. It needs *inside* help to throw off impurities." The best way for this to happen she maintains, is to *activate* circulation with masks or massage, "the only two ways a face can *really* exercise its *skin*, not to be confused with exercising the facial muscles."

A stimulated circulation brings fresh blood coursing to the surface, which reconditions poor cells and sweeps away toxic matters that cause dull skin tone and spots, brings nourishment to the tissues, cleansing, whitening, softening, refining pores.

The first mask we know of—centuries old—was invented by slave women. Washing clothes at the river's edge, they found that their feet, immersed in mud, became soft and white. The smart ones used the mud on their faces, and so the mud pack was born, followed later by packs or masks made out of a number of things from narcissus bulbs to butter and grain. Years later Madame de Pompadour used best sirloin to make protein packs for her delicate skin, catching on to the fact that the meat had an ingredient that helped her skin—protein—plumping it out, giving it a firmer, younger look.

Helena Rubinstein, after studying every great beauty back to the days of Cleopatra, imported volcanic mud from Ischia into her salons in Paris, London, and Rome in the early 1960s, there to use it for masks for the body as well as the face. The mud was a definite circulation zipper-up; it refreshed tired skin and left it rosy and relaxed.

Now there are almost as many masks available as there are moisturizers, and many moisturize beautifully themselves. Their main job, however, is still to *cleanse* better than any other product, sloughing off dead cells from the surface, firming and tightening temporarily.

A dry or dry-to-normal skin should use a mask in the *early* A.M.—and in the bath or shower is a neat idea. That's the time Liza Minnelli puts on a mask, choosing a protein-based one to moisturize and/or cleanse, to sweep away all the impurities that gather on the skin during the night. It's a good start for makeup—and for the day.

An oily skin would be better off using a mud or fruit mask *at night*, either before going out or before going to bed, to take away not only the excess sebum produced, but the pollutant buildup that an oily skin (more than a dry one) invariably attracts during the day.

At home, use masks.

At the salon, try facials that include face massage as well as deep cleansing, steaming (using herbs to get behind any deep-rooted grubbiness), lavish moisturizing packs for dry skin, astringent treatments for the oily one.

Facials

I don't believe in do-it-yourself facial massage unless learned meticulously from a professional.

Elizabeth Arden, who personally inspected the hands of every operator wishing to work in her salons often said, "Do-it-yourself" massage on the face can 'sag and bag.' " She was right. Traumatizing the skin with the wrong set of movements is aging.

The best professional facial massage works this way:

1. Massage of the front and nape of the neck to relax the client, to stimulate local circulation, to work on skin, muscle, nerve endings.

2. Stroking movements start from below the chin up to the forehead, never dragging or pushing, only soothing and relaxing the cutaneous nerves, loosening up underlying muscles, using a protein cream for a dry skin and vegetable oil for a greasy one.

3. Next the more active or *petrissage* part of the massage—knead-

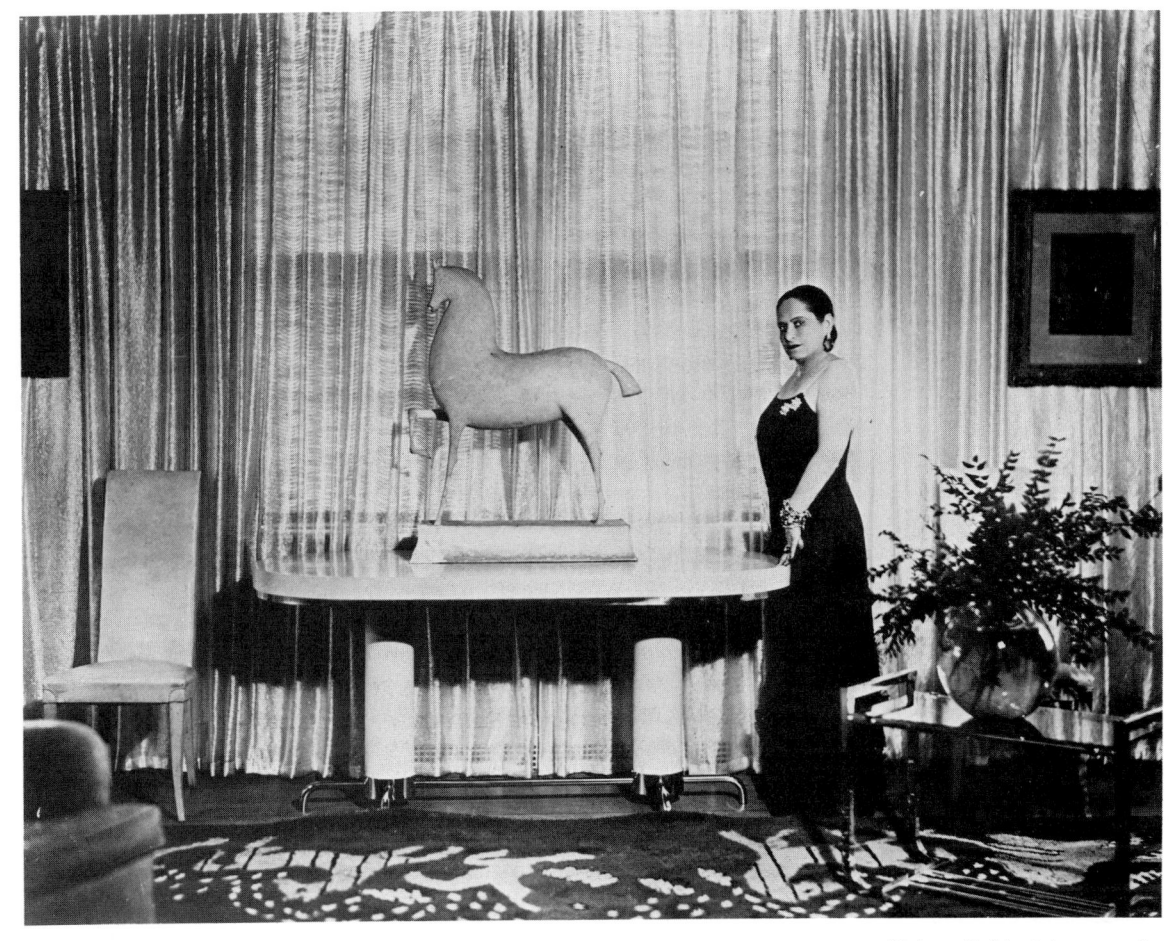

Helena Rubinstein, one of the greatest innovators the cosmetic world has ever known.

ing. With the hand cupped in the shape of a spoon, the masseur takes up just the *right amount of tissue,* enough to be effective, never *too much* to give strain. She starts on the lower right cheek under the ear, moves to the left cheek, covering all peripheral zones of the face, keeping up the same rhythm throughout until the forehead is reached. Here a technique is employed to relax the frontal muscles using a thumb and middle finger.

4. The massage ends with *tapotement,* a light and rapid tapping movement designed to tone up the skin completely, leaving it firmer, revived, rosy, the underlying ambition to reeducate the sebaceous glands, whether too active or too lazy.

A facial from an experienced pair of hands and a mask from your own (remember to read the label) are quick and easy routes to better looks.

Learn from the Models

When I add a new habit to my beauty regime, more often than not I've "ingested" it subconsciously from one of the models I've worked with—from Lauren Hutton, for instance, one of the highest-paid models in the world; in fact and in figures she earns upward of $250,000 a year. Lauren uses herb treatments away from the studio—herbal steaming to deep cleanse her pores, herbal rinses on her hair, particularly rosemary to give it natural lights. From star Cher I learned to use a bar of transparent soap to perk up my eyebrows—she brushes the bar up and over the hairs, so they not only glisten but stay put where she wants them. Cover girl Karen Graham is one who would never dream of putting base all over her face, only in certain areas where she feels she needs it to hide a flaw or to produce a special effect. Now, I do the same.

A good model knows her face as well as a cartographer knows his maps. Increasingly, models arrive at the studio with good skin, not like "the old days" when a retoucher—the man who takes flaws out of pictures before they're in print—was constantly called in to touch out spots and marks on the faces of the famous . . . too often signs of too much makeup, not enough cleansing, not enough sleep, too much of the wrong food, too much champagne.

Here are tips I heard from *Vogue*'s top models that work and are quick:

"When I take a tub, I make it hot enough to last about an hour and a half, then soak and soak, sipping a glass of iced water to induce lots of perspiration to clean out my pores. I like a little baby oil in the water, too, to keep my skin silky. For morale's sake I sometimes substitute ice-cold Dom Perignon for the iced water."

"I find yogurt makes a great facial mask—so does egg yolk and evaporated milk."

"I eat lots of avocados for the sake of my skin—because they're full of vitamin A and E—for the sake of my shape, too. If I'm bulging with a few extra pounds, I eat nothing but avocados for a couple of days to fine down."

"If I cry—rough treatment from the photographer or my boyfriend—my eyes get puffy, so I put thin slices of cold potato around them for an hour or so and they get rid of the puffiness completely."

"I don't often kick over the traces foodwise, but if I feel queasy the morning after the night before, I mix honey, hot water, and apple-cider vinegar for a digestive tonic before breakfast. It cleanses me completely—and makes my skin glow. I always have a bottle of mineral water on my dressing table and drink plenty of it all day long to flush out bad things from my system—and my skin."

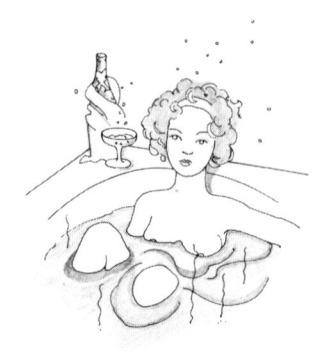

"I eat lots of fruit and vegetables in the summer, the green ones that contain A, the beautiful-skin vitamin. I like rubbing my body with apricot oil, corn oil after bathing. It not only leaves my skin *feeling* like a baby's, but looking like it, too."

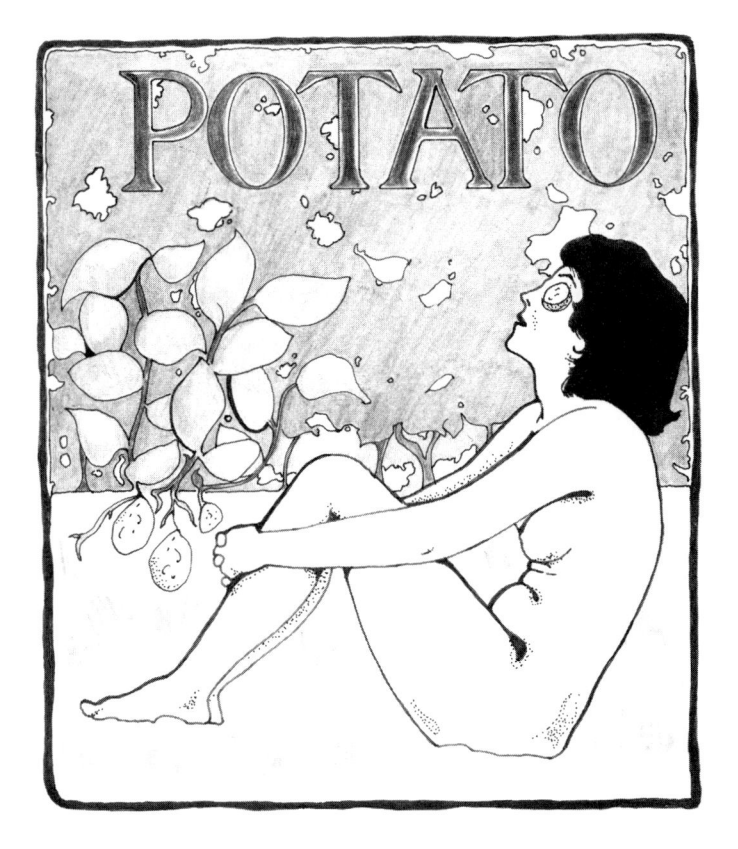

Beauty Secret from Russia

The models learn by trial and error; the beauticians can't afford to—they study and constantly meet at seminars to exchange news and views. Lecturing in Russia at the Institute of Dermatology, beauty authority Aida Grey was really surprised by the good-looking skin of the Russian women and appalled at the same time to learn the Russians like their women to weigh in at 150 pounds—minimum.

The secret of that skin? Aida finally pinpointed it to the enormous amount of cabbage in the Russian diet: "There are piles of cabbages at every street corner, and at every dinner party I was served cabbage soup. In fact, cabbage is part of every meal, including breakfast on cold days." When isn't it cold? No wonder the ladies weigh so much. But why cabbage for good skin? Because of its *hyaluronic-acid content,* the same natural acid that *binds* moisture in our skin, and lying in all connective tissues, acts as a shock absorber.

Since her Russian visit Aida has provided cabbage pills in her salons across the country and urges everyone to eat cabbage in either salad, soup, or soufflé form at least once a week!

Check Your Calendar—It's Time to Change Gear for Summer

Summer is potentially the best time for skin—if you know how to take advantage of the great outdoors. Skin acts younger in the summer—like a lot of people I know.

Take care of skin properly, and it can help you face the worst days of winter that lie ahead.

Take the expression "heating up" as used for making love; it derives from what happens when your skin "heats up," the way it seems to do in summer. Adrenalin flows through your veins; you feel more alive. Everything flows faster, including your surface blood level, its speed increasing with each rise in temperature. What is charmingly described as "cellular garbage" is collected and carried away faster, while the expression "in the pink" literally expresses what all this means: your skin *is* pinker, rosier, and prettier—but *not* because of a glut of sunbathing. (Beware!)

With this increased flow of oils and sweat, your skin needs more cleansing, frequent showers, deodorants, fresheners after every cleanse like a delicious cool frappé after every meal, and light, fresh fragrances.

Sun—Foe or Friend?

The sun *can* be a friend. It all depends on you, because it can also be the most dangerous enemy your skin will ever encounter.

Sun actually makes skin *stronger* when its rays are at its strongest. Exposed to that amount of ultraviolet, skin doesn't change color in the way bread changes to toast under the grill. Tanning results from a process *inside* the skin, when the lower skin cells are provoked into producing extra melanin, extra pigment. This is nature's ingenious way of putting up a defense against possible injury from burns, in the same way that skin protects itself when hurt, thickening into a callous or scab. Without this extra melanin, skin exposed to the full free rays of the sun would shrivel right up.

When a little extra melanin combines with skin's own protein to produce a strong healthy shield, *not* burned, not even really tanned, more slightly flushed (with the extra pigment in force), this helps skin to be more resilient and gives it a glorious glow. This amount of sun is fine—about ten minutes each side maximum; then you are also receiving benefits from the sun's infrared rays—the ones you feel on your body as heat—nourishing certain organs, offering a plus factor in reduced tension and fatigue.

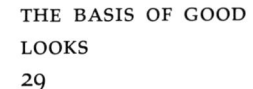

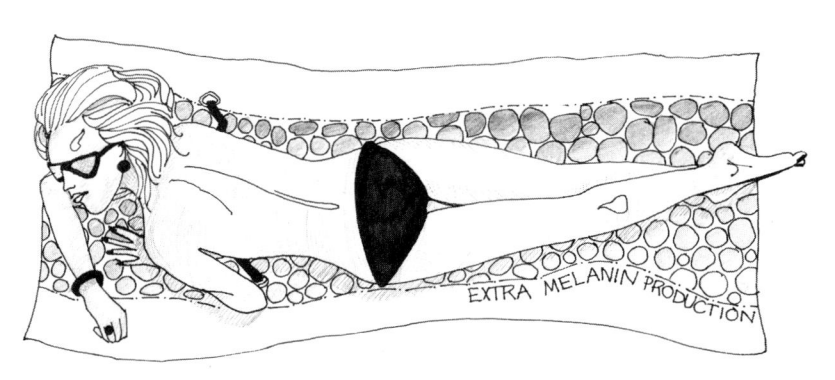

Unfortunately rarely does enough discipline go along with the sun oil. Too much sun—and too much can be arrived at very speedily—is what most people get, however many times they've read or have been told that too much sun spoils skin eventually *irretrievably*, the extra melanin no longer providing only a healthy strong shield but an ugly piece of skin that looks like leather.

Why do women want to be brown? Men don't particularly care. Very often the more tanned the man, the more he wants to keep *his* woman white—however often his eyes move off to some svelte, mahogany figure glistening with sun oil.

It's a conundrum that baffles dermatologists who spend their lives propagating the benefits of shade for they know—and by now I guess *we all know*—that the sun browns, burns, and, alas, *ages* skin faster than bankruptcy if its rays are allowed free play. The reason is simple. Too much sun dries up the corneal layer.

More sinister, it's been proved there's a higher incidence of carcinoma (skin cancer) among those who are constantly exposed to sunlight, notably those who because of their professions have to live outdoors in a sunny climate.

Once upon a time the paler the skin, the greater the distinction. Up to about the middle of the 1920's, the leisurely affluent lived life indoors, rather than out, and lack of tan meant there was money in the family. Only the working classes changed skin tone with the seasons. They couldn't help it; they worked outside.

Social nuances have changed. To some people there's even something priggish about the sight of a lily-white girl guarding her complexion beneath a parasol or covering every inch of herself up on the beach—her very whiteness jars, for today it's a year-round bronze that's wanted.

THE BASIS OF GOOD LOOKS

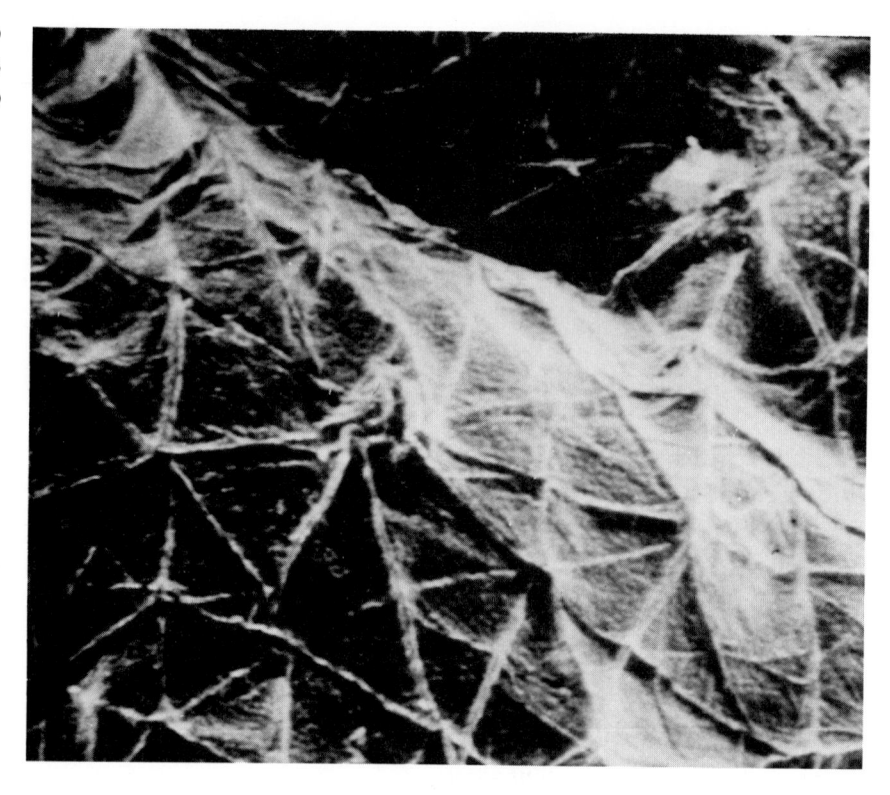

Skin doesn't change color under the sun in the way bread changes to toast under the grill . . . here, surface topography of sunburned skin as seen through a scanning microscope.

So we don't cultivate tans for health's sake or for prestige, so why?

It has to be better looks, a way to differentiate and upgrade winter's gloomy touch—a way to accentuate natural coloring, to change into tropical colors, and look—we hope—dazzling.

The main problem is that most of us want a tan today, not tomorrow or the day after, yet it can't be rushed. Genetically speaking, some tan faster than others, while there's a whole skin type who can't pigment at all—primarily those of Celtic descent, Irish, Scots, Welsh—who freckle and burn all the way to one big peel no matter what they do. They have "holes" in their natural sun screen and need the maximum protection from a sun block to stay looking pretty.

All suntan preparations are sun screens, but they differ in the amount of ultraviolet they let through. Your genetic makeup sets the speed at which you tan, and if you try to hurry it up, you end up *retarding* any increase in color by developing a burn that blisters off the color you already have.

Summer isn't the only time to beware. There's an old mountain myth that says you can't get burned in the snow. Each ski season people painfully learn it isn't true. As Dr. Frederick Urbach, Faculty Member of Temple University's Medical School, Philadelphia, explains "the ultraviolet radiation emitted from the sun that causes sunburn is highly reflected from only two things—sand and snow. Snow is the best reflector, almost 100 percent reflective. When you are outdoors on snow and ice, you get double the dose, once from above, once from below. Sand reflects only about 50 percent, but that's enough to give the skin plenty of trouble, too."

The Worst Thing You Can Do to Your Skin

To go after a tan holding a reflector, sitting on a catamaran skimming across the water, is like putting your skin in the fire, yet more women than I can pack onto the beach in Acapulco do just that every year. Water doesn't *reflect* ultraviolet—that's an old fallacy—but it does *transmit* virtually all of it. When you are out on the ocean with no buildings or mountains interfering with the sky, you have rays radiating on you from all directions—far more than if you were on a lake with trees or in a pool with your house or somebody else's throwing up some shadows and shade.

Because water lets the rays go through, you have to count every minute you're *underwater,* swimming or scuba diving, as time spent in the sun. You should wear a sun screen when you go in the water, when you come out, and when you stay out, for perspiration wears a lot of sun screen away. On a cloudy day you're still not safe. Clouds are made of water vapor, so on a totally cloudy day about 50 percent radiation is getting through. On a hazy day you could be getting nearly 100 percent.

We all know people who say, "I don't *need* any sun oil. I *never* burn. I can take *all* the sun it wants to give me." It may not be this year or next that the results of soaking it all up show, but if they could see their skin in a crystal ball ten to twenty years hence, they might think again. The skin just can't take that kind of third degree year in, year out, without slowly reneging on its identity and turning into a kind of weather-beaten old leather—and *old* is the operative word. Don't do it!

If you're taking any medication, check with your doctor it isn't the kind that can make skin extra sensitive to sunburn, but medication or not, sunbathe only with *proper protection,* and *always* in moderation—however much sun you *think* you can get away with.

Black Skin—Slow to Age . . .
The Black Girl Is Wise to Her Skin

Too much sun ages white skin fast, while the melanin content of Black skin acts like a filter whenever sun rays are strong, letting less of the damaging ultraviolet through. A Black girl rarely sunbathes to excess anyway, for she generally knows how to look after her skin only too well.

When it comes to skin care, from an early age Black women traditionally use many natural substances on their skins. It starts in the cradle, when a mother tenderly applies baby oil, petroleum jelly, and cocoa butter to her baby's skin to make it as supple as possible. All these things the dermatologists would love us *all* to use *every day* as shields against the elements that rob our skin so outrageously of its most precious possession—moisture.

Does Black Skin Age at a Slower Rate than White?

We've only got to think of some ageless beauties to know it's a possibility. Lena Horne's skin is still as smooth as somebody's half her age. Why is it so?

Color counts. The darker the skin, the slower the aging process for a variety of genetic, environmental, and skin-care reasons. Here we go again: the earlier you start to care, the better your skin will be.

Some people think Black skin ages at a slower rate than white because it's more oily, but this is controversial. Black skin is not more oily, some doctors say. The Black models I know say it is. Doctors answer back with, "It appears more oily because light reflects on it . . . and dark-skinned people have more sweat glands."

A spell of cold weather and one can agree with the doctors, for dry skin shows up in the *ashen look* that dark skin often then has.

Basically because the Black woman knows her skin so well and believes in skin care as a natural part of life—inheriting a routine from her mother as *her* mother did from hers—she often appears to have an ageless look.

Whatever the color, ALL skin needs the same amount of cleansing, protection, and stimulation of circulation to offset what the years can do.

Check Your Calendar . . . It's Time to Change Gear for Winter

The reason so many house plants do poorly in winter is because of the lack of humidity. The human skin does poorly in winter, too, unless by chance it's lucky enough to live in a *humidified* atmosphere.

Skin loses less moisture to summer air than to winter's because summer air is obviously more humid. Once you step away from your air conditioner, whatever trouble has been wrought can be rectified outside. For their skins' sake many models live in unheated apart-

FACING PAGE
Black skin—slow to age?

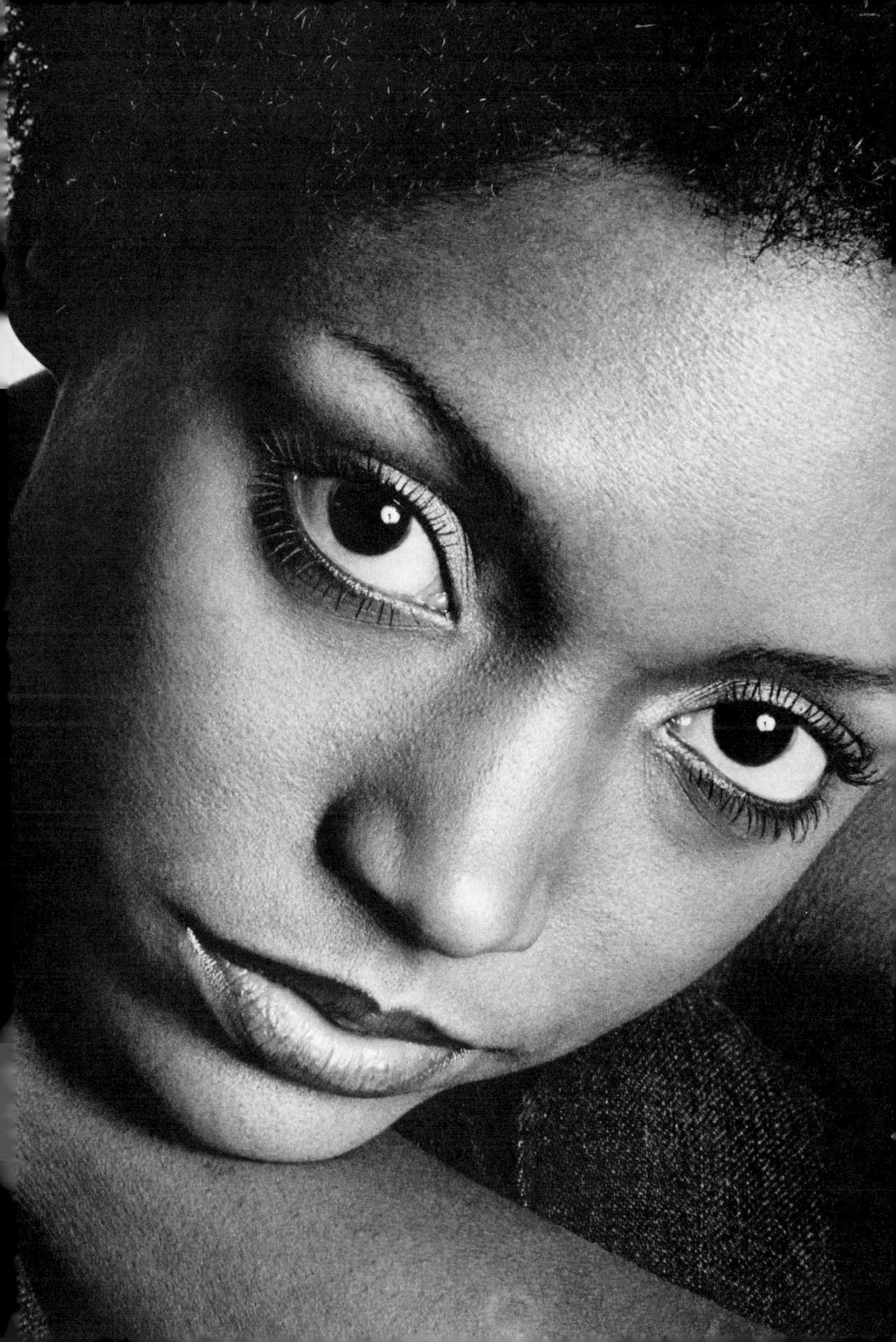

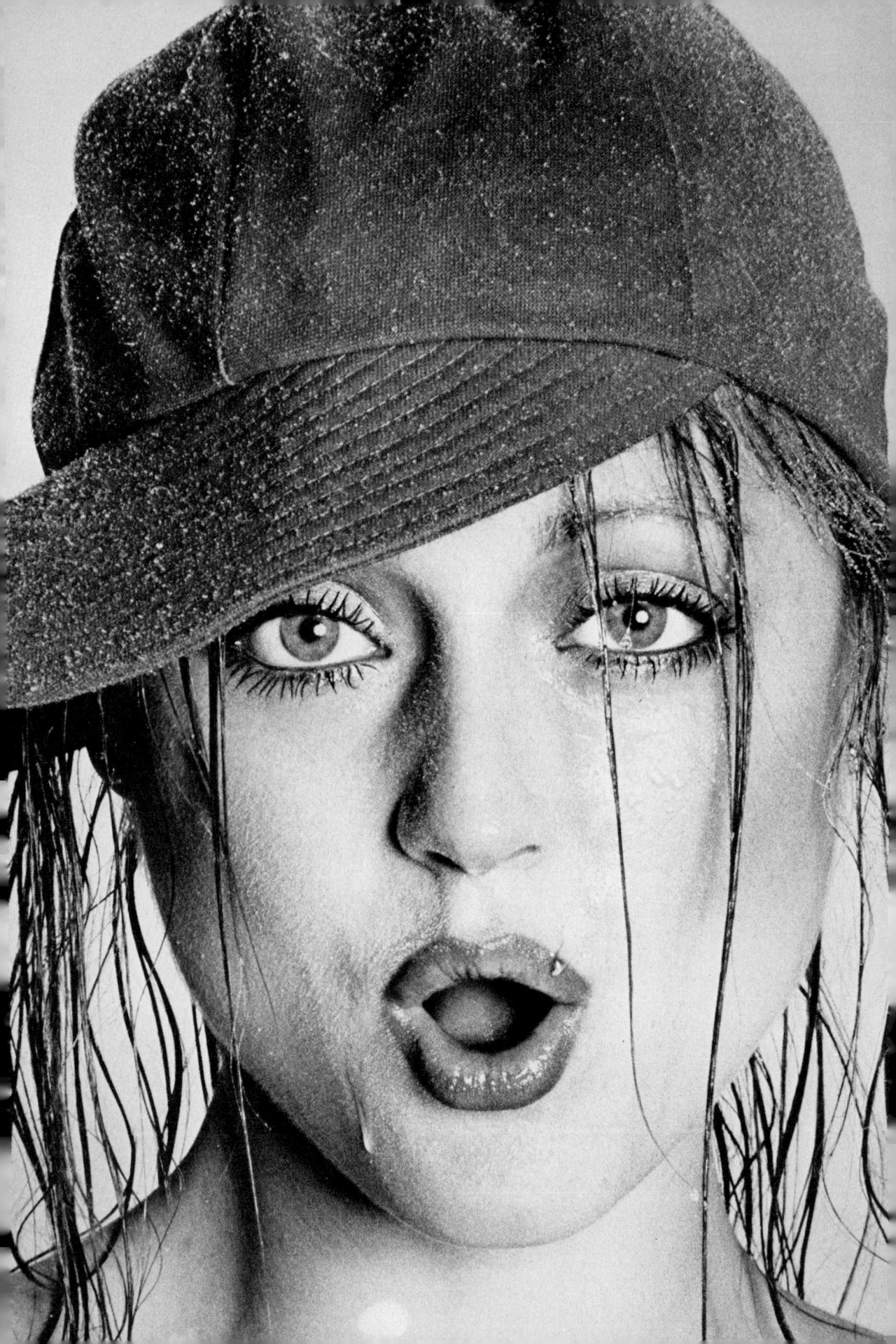

ments, using only water heaters when the weather really gets Arctic. In summer they only turn the air-conditioning on to cool the place down when they're going out, switching it firmly off on their return.

Winter skin is different from summer skin—it's thinner, and thus far more vulnerable and sensitive. As winter slowly moves on to spring, skin's thickness increases according to how much warmth is in the air—then it's at its thickest and most evenly spread when summer finally comes round.

Thin skin needs more help than many women realize, for thin skin can't hold much moisture, dries *fast* on a cold windy street or in a steam-heated room, and can easily begin to look weather-beaten, *old*.

The extreme result of dehydration is when skin is chapped, cracked anywhere it has a chance to be—at lip corners, around nostrils, even at the corners at the eyes.

Left unchecked, cracks and chapped skin can develop into serious problems, but any woman worth her powder puff *knows* they have to be cured fast with double doses of moisturizer, and applications of special creams fortified to increase skin's capacity to hold more moisture than its thickness usually permits.

As products are more and more refined, the oils used for the lotions and potions are light on the skin, yet have such an affinity for it that they "hug" it, insuring a new available "water supply."

Basic common sense in winter is to take fewer baths, avoiding hot water and soap whenever possible, for that combination removes whatever moisture is at the surface along with the dirt.

Bathe at night and, if you must, use a shower in the A.M., a short shower without soap. Bath oil is a *must*, soap or no soap, and this is one time when you can be as narcissistic as you like, *slathering* rich emollients all over your arms, legs, breast, face, while you're soaking.

Don't overclean your face, stripping skin of any natural oils it would rather hold on to. It's better to cleanse with a cream or lotion for safety, leaving it on a few minutes to catch as much debris as it can. Where skin is thin and vulnerable all year round, at eye, throat, and hand level, use even more moisturizer, more creamy luscious stuff.

If you wash your own hair and blow it dry, wrap your skin up in moisturizer before you start work. Hot moving air is an extra attack skin doesn't need.

However much cream you put on your skin at night, only just so much can be absorbed, so after a generous slathering, tissue off what's left on the surface. Nobody needs to go to bed with a creamy mess on her face.

Eat high-energy food for the sake of your skin, winter and summer, and concentrate on everything containing vitamin A and B2—cheese, liver, eggs, leafy vegetables, fruits.

Doctors say people rarely stay out in the cold—skiing, tobogganing, skating—to the frostbite stage, but a pre-frostbite condition can occur without your realizing it. Patches of skin turn white, are then

FACING PAGE
Baby, it's cold outside.

surrounded by a bright-red area, and the patches feel like first- or second-degree burns. When your skin starts to hurt, it's time to get out of the cold—*fast*.

If you wrap your skin up and swaddle it in emollients, just as you wrap up your body in a fur coat, you stand a better chance of defeating Old Man Frost. For those who think to defeat him by migrating with the birds to Barbados and the sun or the ski slopes and Aspen, there's again that other hazard to watch out for—the *s-u-n* and more *s-u-n*. Protect is the word—in the cold and in the sun.

Will Skin Ever Be Recycled as GOOD as New?

If you've been a good girl and stayed away from sunbathing all your life, if you've kept your temper low, and your nutritional intake high, the chances are you don't need to read this section—but it's fascinating just the same.

Rejuvenation isn't a word that slips off people's tongues so easily any more. When Dr. Niehans was alive and well, busily "rejuvenating" in Switzerland, rumors circulated all over the world about how good and valid his treatments really were—injecting the rich (the very, very rich, so they were invariably famous, too) with embryos from unborn baby lambs, taking fatigue away from the weary, replacing old lamps with new, one might say, as far as vitality and a youthful vigor were concerned. Dr. Niehans's work goes on today, as controversial as ever—carried out by his disciples in Marbella, Spain, in Switzerland, and to a lesser extent in London. Here in the United States the omnipresent watchdogs of the Food and Drug Administration preclude anything untried and untested by our medical authorities—so the treatment is not available.

In Europe many women regularly subscribe to a royal jelly treatment, anointing the skin with the same nourishment that enables a grub to turn into a queen bee with a life span of five years, while the worker bee lives only a couple of months. Again, because of the FDA policy, no royal jelly is available across the counter here, although it's bootlegged in by quite a number of women anxious to try anything to retrieve lost looks.

The miracle of the moisturizer—alleviating to a certain extent the dryness that contributes so much to aging looks—is over forty years old. It's time for a new miracle, but where is it?

Biochemists, dermatologists, enzymologists, have been trying for decades to circumvent the sluggish stratum deep in our skin responsible for new cell output, to isolate the protein present in human cells responsible for skin regeneration and every metabolic process in our bodies. Enzymes, once described by Britain's Professor Jevons of Manchester University as "life's basic device," are the same complex proteins we depend on for a radiant complexion.

Various compounds have been mentioned as having a bearing on the subject, and procaine, generic term for Novocain, is one for which the most regenerative claims have been made. The Romanian doctor, Dr. Ana Aslan, prescribes a buffered version—Gerovital H3—at her Bucharest Geriatric Institute, made famous long ago by patients like General de Gaulle and Nikita Khrushchev. It's said that procaine, while forestalling the formation of the MAO enzymes (generally found in aging people, and said to be responsible for the depression that goes along with age), also encourages the body to produce certain hormones, spurring on a more youthful attitude to life and sex.

Because of the *quality* of the case histories—rather than the quantity of "rich and famous"—Ana Aslan's work is now being carefully studied by many scientists in this country. With typical protective reticence, the FDA will only allow that Gerovital H3 is being investigated "through the normal channels regarding its effect on depression." For bootleggers of the product, even this small admission gives rise to hope that one day Gerovital may be available here—on or off prescription.

Scientists are too canny to commit themselves on the subject of the controversial vitamin E. As one spokesman summed it up, "Science will show that if vitamin E does anything at all regarding aging it will only play a small part." Vitamin E *is* the most mysterious vitamin of all, but if a scientist—that most noncommittal of human beings—admits to it playing any part, however small, it *may* be a key to counteracting the aging problem.

Years ago the word *colloidal* was used as a prefix to European skin-care mask-type products in an endeavor to prove they were the result of scientific processes. Today chemists look to the mask area—optimistic that this is where research will pay off and a new "miracle" might occur—while more and more products based on collagen, the protein present in our skin and responsible for its elasticity, are receiving serious attention, too.

It could be that one day we will have pharmaceutical cosmetics or pharmaceuticals for cosmetic purposes only. In this way skin care would obviously be more specific and individual.

As Charles Revson, one of the greatest innovators the cosmetic world has ever known, once said to me, "For *your* skin I have treatments, products that will retard age, take away poor skin tone, eradicate your wrinkles—but for the woman next to you, the products may not have the same sweeping effects. To create sensational products that will produce dramatic results for *everyone*—that is my aim and one day it will happen."

Many spectacular scientific advances have been made for other purposes today *that incidentally have been found to have cosmetic overtones.* It may be that these overtones will provide the keys to future cosmetic progress. Until then, we'll keep on hoping *and* must keep on cleansing, toning, and nourishing.

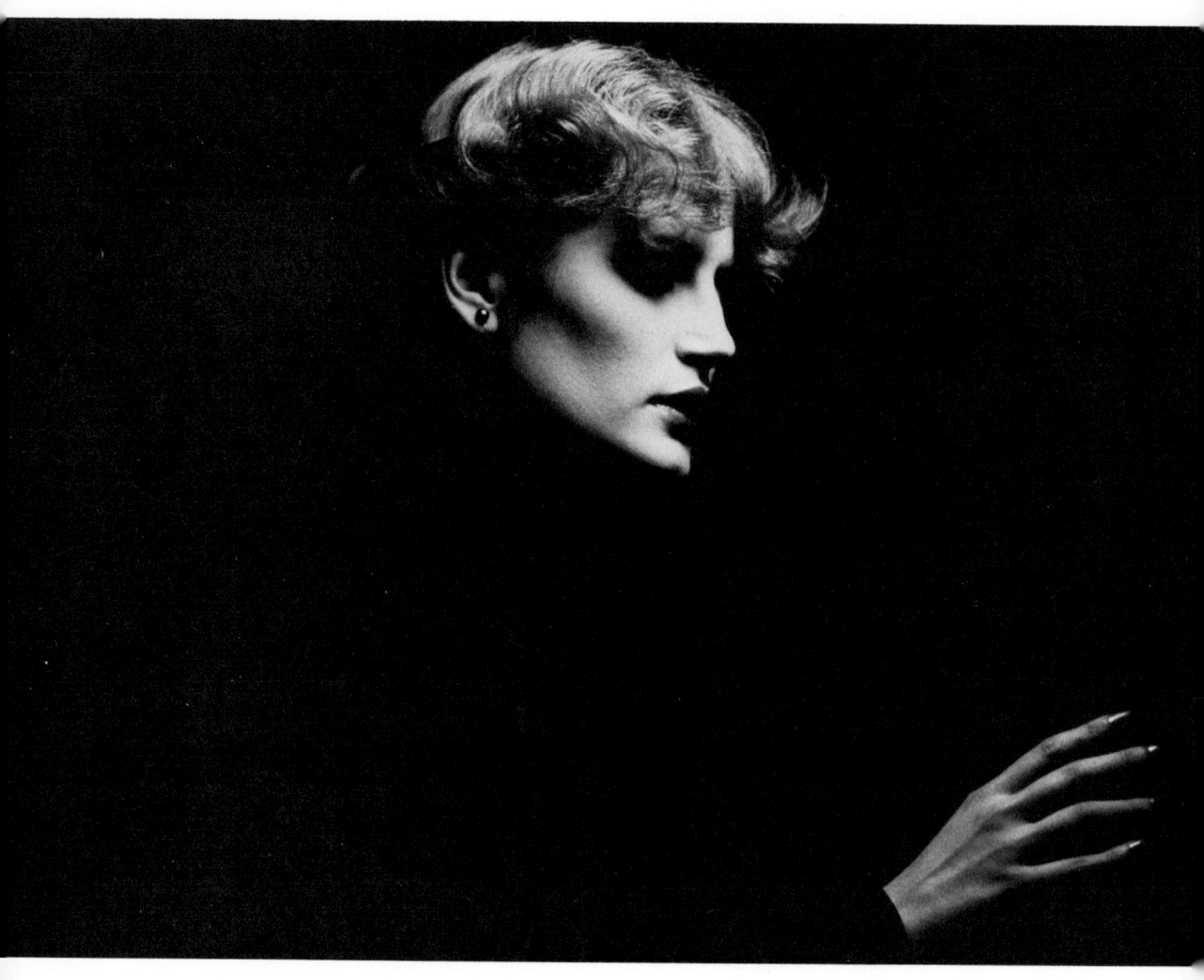

Hands can give the beauty game away.

Hands (and Neck) Get the Worst Deal—Give Them Some Help

Hands, like necks, give away age. Why? Skin coverage is thinner there than anywhere else on the body, and there are few oil glands, so skin dries and "creases" faster while there's little flesh beneath to support moisture. In short, hands show *every sign of wear and tear,* and they get a lot. Necks don't work so hard, even though they have the heavy job of fighting gravity to hold our heads up high. But necks can easily be hidden under collars or scarfs, whereas a sleeve can only go so far. Unfortunately hands, wrinkled or not, have to stay in view.

Can anything be done? Plenty. First, there's that underrated product, hand cream, regularly turning up in Christmas stockings, only to get put away in the bathroom cabinet, and then to be forgotten. It's a pity, for most hand lotions—usually about 80 percent water, 20 percent moisturizing oils—at least help skin cells to *retain* any moisture around and form a barrier against the elements outside, the weather that does so much harm to unprotected skin.

Some hand lotions are sticky and so even more forgettable, but recent developments have introduced polymers that don't stick, allowing the moisture to sink into the thin skin and stay there down deep.

Delicious oils from the avocado or aloe vera plant give hands great protection, while some creams claim their ingredients can penetrate *six cells down*, which sounds useful. Six cells or one, the regular use of hand cream really does preclude that ugly sight—chapped, wrinkled hands.

If you're too busy to remember hand cream, you can catch up in the bath. Keep the richest cream you've got on the side and smother your hands in it. Steep hands in the warm water, hopefully laced with a rich bath oil, too. Run hands through the oily water several times, in and out, in and out, until they're well saturated. You'll be amazed how much oil they soak up because they need all they can get, particularly in winter.

The best hand-care products feed oxygen into the pores, have antibacterial properties, and set out to whiten skin as well as soothe it. *Look for the label* which spells out that *polyunsaturates, vitamins,* and *lubricants* are inside the bottle or jar. Those ingredients mean business. Massage the lotion down each finger as if smoothing on suede gloves—again skin will soak it up. For any brown marks use a depigmenting cream; there are plenty around, and they're getting better all the time.

One Line of Defense for the Hands, Another for the Nails

Nails are in the front line with bright colors.

To start, leave nails naked for a day, then paint them with white iodine and leave it on overnight to encourage growth, discourage flaking, chipping.

In their basic state nails should be pearllike in texture, slightly pink in color like an oyster shell. But beautiful nails don't grow on hands without help.

The matrix is at the bottom of nature's deal, located at the nail base, showing only its top, which we call a moon. Whatever natural sheen and surface you have on top depends on whatever diet is part of your life. The better the natural gloss, the more nutrition you're giving your body . . . arriving to help the matrix and then the nail itself via a myriad of tiny blood vessels.

If you feel you're eating right, yet your nails still let you down, genetic factors could be to blame, for the genes do play their part.

Remember to moisturize nails; they can suffer from desert dryness. Use a cuticle cream, protein-packed, emollient enough to reduce the dryness that makes even those with saintly dispositions start to ruin their resolutions, picking and pulling at their manicures. Use a cuticle jelly to make cuticles soft, easy to push back, leaving nails trim and elegant.

Do have a weekly manicure to help you keep any resolves you make about your nails.

Do file nales square in one direction only—never back and forth—a sawing motion causes snags.

Don't cut cuticles. Push them back with a wooden stick.

Do avoid water at least for a few hours after a manicure.

Do use gloves for cleaning jobs (except when you clean your face).

Do dial with the end of a pencil; using a finger can ruin nails.

Do use the cushions of your fingers to pick things up.

Don't wear a frosted enamel all the time—it's too drying.

Don't overuse nail hardeners, strengtheners, or nail-polish removers. Touch-ups are preferable to redos.

Don't remove polish midweek. If you think the color looks murky, add another coat. If you want to switch color, add it on top. Better to build up enamel than keep using remover on your nails.

The Best Do-It-Yourself Manicure

Scrape nail surface after removing old enamel; this eliminates roughness.

Clean cuticles, and coax them back with an orange stick impregnated with cuticle remover.

File straight across tip toward nail center, using either an emery board or metal file covered in diamond dust (preferred by many manicurists because although the dust gives the metal a smooth surface, it's still abrasive enough to take away snags and split edges).

On weak nails use a strengthener, applied only to nail tips. This works by penetrating and fusing the nail, helping prevent breakages and splitting, plus encouraging length.

Find a hardener that's also a colored enamel; otherwise, use two coats of polish, plus one of sealer, to see the manicure through the week.

Toenails need care, too. Get a pedicure at least once a month or follow the same procedure as you do for your manicure. Both hands and feet should have a pick-me-up at the end of a day—a massage in and out of each toe and along each finger with a fragrant lotion. It can't hurt.

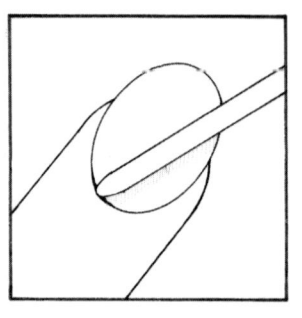

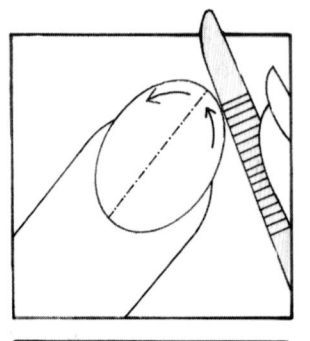

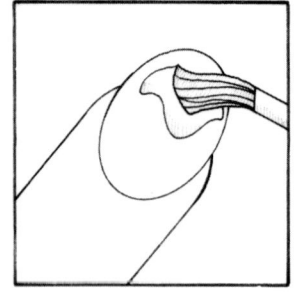

Everybody's Skin Should . . .

Be thoroughly cleansed at least twice a day.
Be diagnosed by a dermatologist once a year.
Follow a prescribed regime of treatment.
Learn how to compensate for dry, oily, or hydrated skin.
Avoid excessive exposure to the sun *always*.
Use a sun screen, if not a sun block, when the sun is at its height.

Everybody Should . . .

Watch for any allergic reaction to a product.
Avoid heavy smoking—it's bad for the skin.
Drink up to eight glasses of water a day.
Have frequent masks according to skin type.
Have frequent facials according to skin type.
Stimulate circulation by lying head-down on a slant board.
Jog, walk, run, exercise for skin's sake.
Remember *neglect is aging*.

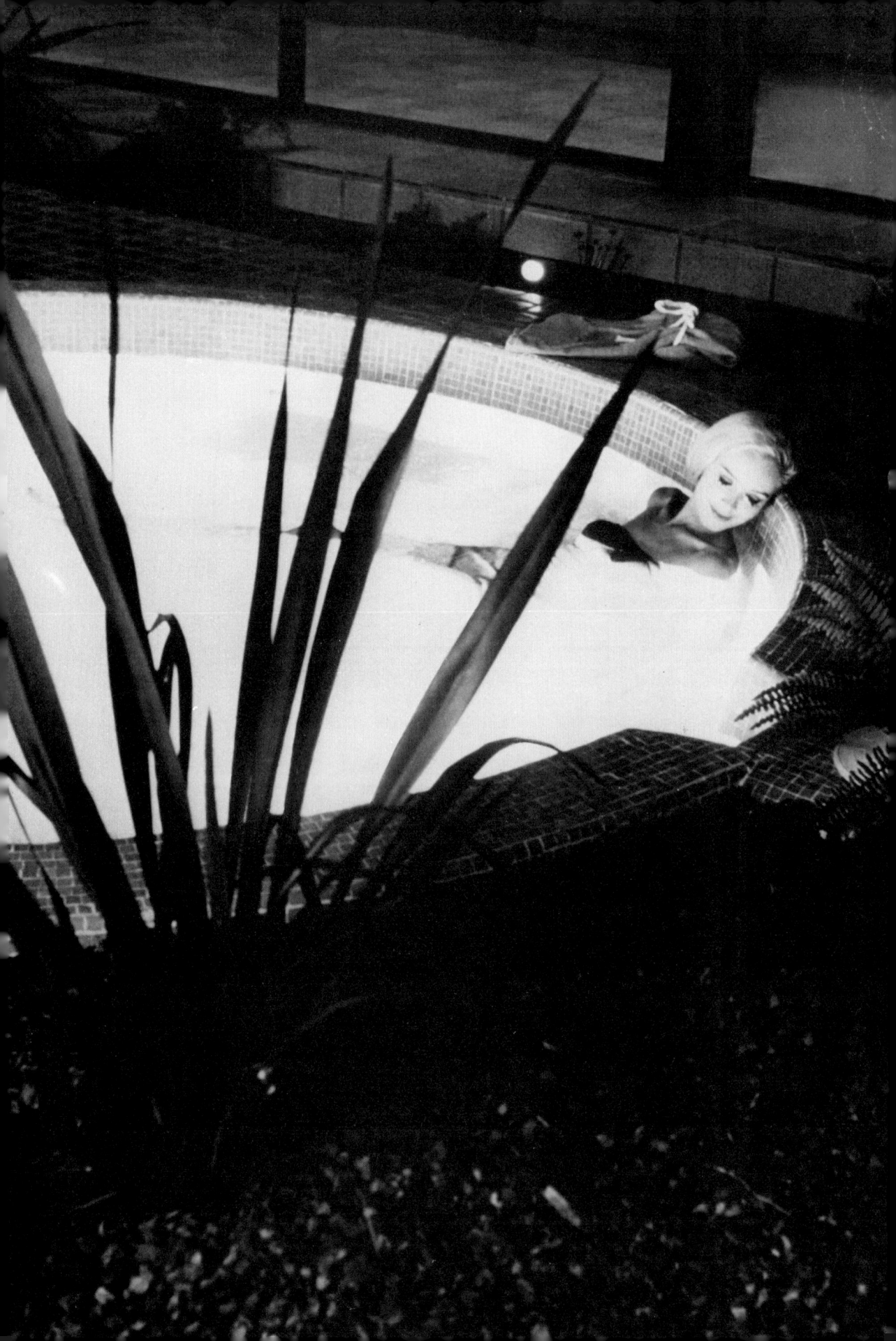

2

Dressing the Skin

From the Deodorant to the Bath
and
What Each Can Do for You

It's no longer merely a question of whether your best friend will ever tell you. Every skin worth its epidermis should be dressed A.M. and P.M. these days not only with treatments and makeup for the face, but with lotions and potions for the body—the choice grows daily. There's no longer anything remotely narcissistic about bathtime beauty rites—oiling, foaming, nourishing, powdering, whooshing fragrance literally all over from top to toe. Today *cleanliness just isn't enough*.

Before I dwell on the powers and pleasures of the bath, which ladies from Poppaea, empress of Rome, to Elizabeth Taylor, once empress of Hollywood, have enjoyed, the power of the deodorant and antiperspirant must be recorded.

FACING PAGE
The bath—perfect place for beauty treatments.

Deodorant power has grown over the past few years, since research established more exactly the cause of body odor, the iniquitous BO or sweat. "Not to be mentioned in refined conversation," says the Oxford Dictionary.

Why do we sweat and why does it smell? It seems an unfair process but it isn't. In fact, it's all part of a well-run plot, as practical as the rest of the body's mechanisms.

We sweat mainly to keep cool, and it isn't the sweat or perspiration that smells, but what it meets up with on the way out—bacteria, present on everyone's body.

There are two kinds of sweat because we have two kinds of sweat glands—eccrine and apocrine. The output of neither smells on its own; perspiration is, in fact, almost odorless.

You wouldn't put a deodorant or antiperspirant all over your body where the eccrine glands are distributed—about sixty-five hundred to the square inch—with a concentration on the forehead, palms, and soles—for their secretion is about 99 percent pure water plus a few salts. Exuded from a clean, healthy young man or woman, this secretion actually has a slightly salty smell—apparently an aphrodisiac to some.

The eccrine glands mostly handle the job of keeping us cool, plus eliminating waste, working around the clock regulating the body's temperature at or near its normal level, using the evaporation of water from the skin's surface as a cooling system.

You *would* apply a deodorant or antiperspirant to those areas where the other type of sweat gland—the apocrine—secretes not only water but some protein and waste substances, providing a better environment for bacteria to thrive on. Larger than the eccrine, the apocrine glands are restricted mainly to the underarms, the anogenital region, and the nipples. Their growth, closely associated with hair follicles, is stimulated by the same hormones that cause hair growth under the arms and around the genital areas. That is why body odor is rarely a problem in children and old people where hormone and therefore hair supply are less.

Stress and Sweat

Recent research has proved that body odor occurs more often during times of emotional stress—sweating from heat alone doesn't cause the same sort of smell and so the same sort of problem. That's because it's during times of stress—fear, excitement, tensions—that most apocrine sweat is secreted, although it also handles some normal air-conditioning for the body. Merging with the eccrine sweat secretion, this is all added inducement for bacteria and so odor.

Diet can affect body odor, too, generally not noticed by humans but apparent to keen-scented animals like dogs, who can distinguish vegetarian natives from meat-eating Westerners, and lions, who can spot a man a mile away when the wind is in the right direction.

In Western countries, where emotional problems are frequently countered with an annual consumption of billions of tranquilizers, the *stress factor* plays a significant part in producing excessive apocrine sweat.

While some products are efficacious enough to control bacterial action and so odor for the majority, the minority who suffer from excessive perspiration problems are still waiting for a major breakthrough. Research goes on, but medical opinion is divided as to whether it's a problem that can really only be solved by nerve-blocking drugs under medical supervision.

Viva la Difference!

Many don't realize there's considerable difference between a deodorant and an antiperspirant. A deodorant is formulated to mask or diminish odors, plus inhibiting to a small extent bacterial growth, without affecting the flow of perspiration. An antiperspirant, composed of chemicals, actually *reduces* the perspiration reaching skin's surface by partially closing pores and inhibiting the sweat glands. The pores are not completely blocked—they couldn't and shouldn't ever be, for if they were a prickly-heat situation would quickly result. The curious thing is that the physiological processes involved are still something of a medical mystery.

The advantage of using an antiperspirant is that by checking perspiration, bacteria growth is also retarded—it has less to grow in, feed on. Almost all antiperspirants contain one or several aluminum salts, which means sensitive skins can experience a slight irritation if used every day. Alternating between a deodorant, which has a gentler action, and an antiperspirant is the wisest choice for this type of skin. The one simple act often overlooked in choosing this sort of product is TO READ THE LABEL.

A friend of mine with a heavy perspiration problem (nerves are the culprit here, too) said there was nothing on the market to help her condition. When I asked her what she used and when she used it, I learned she had never read the instructions, which clearly said she should put the antiperspirant on *before* going to bed. An early A.M. shower or bath doesn't dislodge its ameliorating effects. She carried out that instruction and has had no problems since.

Another fact often overlooked is the question of shaving or getting rid of underarm hair, for hair is just another place where bacteria love to thrive, turning the combination of apocrine, eccrine secretions, and bacteria even faster into odor.

We need to sweat for our body's sake and for comfort, too. To reduce perspiration to the minimum required for our "air-conditioning" is the goal, and the choice of a product has to be based entirely on personal requirements—so, once again, don't forget to read the label.

Whatever the commercials imply, however, no product can become a substitute for cleanliness. Bathing comes first and last, with deodorants or antiperspirants fitting neatly in the middle.

Beauty In—and Out of—the Bath

Before the modern advances of science, and therefore the advent of the deodorant (Mum in 1888, Odo-Ro-No in 1914), bathing was the answer. The Hebrews believed in it; the Romans even more so, evidenced today by the remains of their many elaborate bathing establishments all over Europe.

The great cover-up of body odor with fragrant oils and essences used instead of cleanliness (phew!) began in the fourteenth century and lasted till the beginning of the eighteenth—all because church dogma then equated nudity with lewdness, so that any public bath had to be a place of debauchery.

As the *Guide Michelin* points out, in the thirteenth century there were twenty-six public baths in Paris. Under Louis XIV there were only two—and he himself boasted he never took a bath. The one bathtub left in the palace was thought to be so superfluous it was moved to the garden as a fountain, while Marie Antoinette bathed in a white flannel nightshirt, brainwashed from birth into believing that bathing naked was a cardinal sin. Earlier, Queen Elizabeth I of England, forever emphasizing her individuality, left behind the big news that she bathed once a month "whether it was required or not." Of course, her best friend never told *her*.

For the last one hundred and fifty years the importance of regular bathing has become increasingly obvious. The only controversy left lies between establishing which has the more merit—the bath or the shower. Americans generally regard the British as a less clean race because of their antishower, bath-mad attitude, but whether you bathe or shower, the end result is the same if you use soap. You get wet and clean—for soap makes water work more efficiently, the kind you find in a jar working best of all, being the mildest, approximating to a cleansing cream that needs water to activate it.

Water, Water Everywhere—but Where's the Softest Kind?

The best kind of water to bathe or shower in is the soft kind. It allows a rich lather with less soap, and rinses off that soap more easily, too.

With hard water—which unfortunately exists in a good proportion of the United States—a thin film is likely to remain on the skin after washing, causing irritation and drying, especially on the face. The remaining film has the potential to entrap small amounts of bacteria and dirt, hazardous to any skin that's sensitive or already a victim of acne or breakouts.

Shampooing hair in hard water is a hard task, too, leaving a film on the hair that dulls it however much elbow grease went into the work. Anyone living in a hard-water area (see below) has to rinse harder than a soft-water dweller—unless you invest in a water softener, a much more practical buy than many people think; you can always buy the small sink-size if the large size really eats up too much space and money. For beauty's sake, it's worthwhile having at least one area in the house with soft water.

Very hard water (10.5 + grains per gallon) is found in most of Montana, much of Idaho, small patches of Washington, the northwest corner of Kansas, the southeast corner of Texas, most of Kentucky, all of Tennessee.

Hard water (7–10.5 grains per gallon) is found in Arizona, New Mexico, half of Texas, all of North and South Dakota, Nebraska, Minnesota, Iowa, half of Wisconsin and Illinois, Indiana, Ohio, western Pennsylvania, West Virginia, parts of Georgia, and most of Florida.

Moderately hard water (3.5–7 grains per gallon) is found in California, Nevada, Utah, Wyoming, Colorado, parts of Texas, Kansas, Wisconsin, Missouri, Oklahoma, Arkansas, most of Louisiana, parts of Georgia and Florida, Michigan, and the far eastern corner of North Carolina.

The remaining states—from New York and Maine in the East to most of Washington and Oregon in the West—have the best water in the country, as soft as you can get with 1 to 3.5 grains per gallon.

Temperature plays a big part in determining how good the water in your bath or shower is for you. Extremes of either hot or cold are bad. *Too hot* shocks the system, dries and ages the skin. *Too cold* can cause blood vessels to constrict and reduce the blood supply to the skin—dangerous especially in the case of older people or anyone with a weak heart.

The best temperature for relaxation is warm (from 85° to around 90°). The best atmosphere (discovered during the energy crisis and kept as a good habit in many people's lives) is candlelight, or at least low lighting, with a background of whatever music happens to send you, from Cole Porter to Verdi.

Apart from the restorative powers of the bath, relaxing and refreshing after a long hard day at the backgammon board, skin is at its most receptive *underwater* when wide-awake pores can receive, without resistance, all manner of benefits, banishing parch at least till you step out into the great outdoors again.

Bath Accompaniments

The well-dressed bath these days is never without . . .

A loofah: the dry, rough-textured gourd that swells and softens when wet, yet sloughs off dead skin with accuracy leaving the body tingling. A natural loofah is about fifteen inches long—long enough to get to hard-to-reach spots on your back. Underwater massage with a loofah makes do-it-yourself leg shaping easier—providing you move every day, day in–day out, with steady firm strokes *up* toward the heart, water pressure helping the movements.

A friction strap: usually made of hemp and blended with horsehair can be at the bathside for the same reason as the loofah—sloughing skin, helping do-it-yourself massage.

A body brush: the best are made of stiff, natural bristles, useful for brushing up circulation—particularly on shoulders and back, while a natural-bristle hand brush can be put to work nicely on legs, arms, abdomen.

Pumice stone: this piece of ultraporous volcanic lava fits into the palm to work away at small rough spots on ankles, elbows, heels.

Soap and water go together as far as the body is concerned, but some soaps are better for some bodies. Oily skin will benefit from a glycerine soap, which does its cleansing job without adding any extra oil; cucumber soap is good for oily skin, too.

Any superfatted soap (rich with lanolin, cold cream, cocoa butter, or coconut oil) lubricates dry skin, which needs every bath aid it can get in the way of oils, foams, milks. Submerging dry skin in a fragrant oil bath is a fast easy way to soothe it thoroughly.

Supersensitive skin has more and more to choose from in the way of fragrance-free soaps—the mild Castile or transparent kind, plus soaps with added vitamins.

Poor skin, prone to breakouts, needs medicated soap plumb full of antibacterial agents, which do their bit toward controlling infection, clearing up problem areas.

Normal skin—perfectly balanced between dry and oily—has the whole world of soapsuds to choose from, can indulge any fragrant whim and enjoy a bath like no one else. Soap for the face is something else again, for soap with a high degree of alkalinity removes acid in the same way detergents do. The natural guardian of the skin, called the acid mantle, can be broken down in time by the use of such a soap, leaving skin wide open to any irritation going. If you *must* use soap on the face, use the mildest one you can find—often transparent.

Gels, milks, foams, and oils—produced from things as diverse as the avocado pear to the juniper plant—attach minuscule globules to receptive skin, to get "polished" in afterward by the towel, soothing any dry patches that may appear naturally on skin's structure or that have been caused by the onslaught of the elements. All these products leave a light allover aura—which can be intensified later by wearing a perfume from the same fragrance family. They differ only in slight ways. Gels will clean you as you soak; they're gentle on the skin and don't leave a ring around the tub. Oils contribute more lubrication than gels, while milks, rich in fats and oils, contribute still more. Bath salts and crystals can soften water, plus adding color to soothe the weary spirit.

Pampering and soaking isn't only for the sake of the skin. It's great for the mind, too. Some women, like sculptor Louise Nevelson, dress designer Pauline Trigère, and actress Arlene Dahl, use the bath as a think tank—the place to go when they have a particularly knotty problem to solve. Others, like Cristina Ford, consider the bath as part of a workout regime, staying in fragrant hot water for only a few minutes to perspire, then getting out to work on their bodies hard with loofah or friction glove, finishing off by making their bodies glossy with baby oil. Cristina Ford says, "My bathroom is the room I take the greatest care of. It's always well stocked with salts, oils, sponges, brushes, but I don't like heavily scented bath products. They would clash with my favorite perfume, and in any case, there's nothing like the odor of clean skin following a bath."

Sonia Rykiel, the Parisian designer, treats the bath exactly the same way—out of the water in five minutes to her exercise period—whereas nightclub owner Régine spends most of her bathtime standing up, rubbing herself all over with a friction mitt, sitting down only for a few minutes for a massage from her "nanny" of twenty years.

The Japanese attitude to the bath—dirty if it's used to wash in—is accepted by writer and historian Lady Antonia Fraser. She spends twenty minutes relaxing in a clean tub of fragrant water—after washing herself thoroughly via the shower. "This is the time I like to discuss the day with my six children."

Some people resort to the bath to counter a horrible day as others rush to an analyst's couch. There are a number of tried-and-tested homemade pick-me-up baths—from the euphoric cucumber one, where slices are scattered on the water and two pieces placed on the eyelids (cooling and calming), to the oil of rosemary and wheat-germ bath. Old-fashioned remedies soothe sunburned skin—like adding baking soda or oatmeal to the water (tied in cheesecloth, so you don't clog the drain). This sort of bath helps the feeling of burning heat to escape from the body. One tablespoonful of mustard to each gallon of water eases tired aching feet, but mustard or half a pound of Borax won't do anything like as much for the psyche as say a lily-of-the-valley milk bath.

An hour spent in the bath can be good for looks—not for books. I've never seen the joy of trying to read either the paper or paperback in the bath, when soggy edges only fray nerves, don't soothe them.

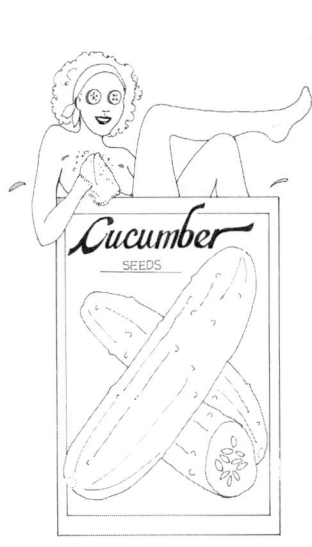

Set up supplies on a bath tray or stool next to the tub. Include a facial mask, pumice stone, razor, tweezers, nail file, cuticle oil, bath oil, small brush, magnifying mirror, deep cleanser and plenty of cotton. Then dampen your fingers and apply cleansing cream all over face, neck, shoulders, sliding back under the water so that a little steam opens up pores. Clean off thoroughly with the cotton, then apply the mask. Relax for several minutes, working on your nails with file and cuticle cream, working the cream in deeply around each finger. Brush your brows up, so you can see the natural line clearly, then tidy them up with tweezers. Pumice all rough spots away and apply bath oil directly to skin, turning what was rough into silky smoothness. Finally lather yourself all over with the most sweet-smelling soap, shave off any superfluous hair, empty the tub, then shower off every vestige of soap with a cool direct spray. Out of the tub, rub your body all over with bath lotion, before wrapping yourself in a huge turkish towel, patting yourself dry. It's a soothing experience—especially just before bed.

Bath Habits to Get Into

A.M. Make up before getting into and quickly out of a tepid bath. The warmth softens lines, keeps makeup looking fresh. Add a last touch of translucent powder before leaving the house to help makeup last still longer.

A.M. Try an algae or seaweed bath, a sulphur or mineral one, to untense muscles; each one can give an allover pick-me-up feeling to skin and liven morale. Stretch in the bath and try to do early morning exercises there. You have to expend more energy to do exercises in water, and moving muscles against its force causes you to make smooth unjerky motions. Press your feet against the end of the tub, brace your arms on the sides, and slowly raise and lower your hips as many times as you can. Or brace your head on a soft bath pillow, hold sides of tub, and raise legs, bending the left knee slowly, then straighten. Repeat with the right. Sitting, raise one leg, grasp calf and pull leg slowly toward you—five times each leg. Flex and then relax muscles underwater. Contract buttocks for a count of five, then in turn abdomen, bosom, neck, shoulders; relax and slide shoulders under water for a few minutes before repeating the movements.

P.M. Just before bed, lounge in a warm foaming milk bath; drink your warm milk there, or hot buttered rum. Relax for ten minutes, then quickly dry and into cool, clean sheets. Lights out.

P.M. Give yourself a double double face cleanse in the bath, using first cleansing cream, then a skin tonic, then a light peel-off mask—ending with another pat of astringent or freshening, clean-up lotion.

Love Me, Love My Shower

For the antibath, love-my-shower brigade, instant energy seems to shoot out of the nozzle along with that fine jet of water. Certainly a shower can and should liven up the skin, and no area need be neglected—backs of ears, nape of neck, under each foot, in between each toe. Temperature changes can be useful to help the freshen-up idea, too. If you start with warm water, washing with a soap-filled mitt, switch to tepid midstream, and finish with cool to rinse off *thoroughly.* If you direct the jet to individual parts, switching from hot to cold and back to hot again, it zips up circulation in every area. If you have backache, you can alleviate it sometimes with the shower treatment. Sit on the floor of the bath, resting your head on your knees and let the warm to hot water pour down over back, shoulders, and back of neck—three minutes of this relaxes all muscle tension.

Whether you love the relaxation of a bath, the energizing quality of a shower, or sensibly combine both—bath first, shower second—after-the-bath therapy is another time to dress up your skin.

Moisture can be replenished with lazy strokes of body lotion, helping keep the skin as supple as it was meant to be. Smooth it on when you're damp and pores are still relaxed.

Maxi-coat yourself with an antipeel bath-oil spray, leaving skin as silky as broadtail and twice as pretty.

Splash yourself all over with a cologne version of your favorite fragrance to help it last all day if you remember to add one touch more of the Big Strength as you leave for the day or night.

Massage face, neck, shoulders, bosom, with creams that have special jobs to do, emulsions that help skin cells absorb 20 percent of their water content, "plumping" out layers, diminishing bad color, sallowness, dullness, often caused by lack of moisture (see Chapter 1, page 14).

Some emulsions are called *isotonic,* which means they are correctly balanced to the skin's own oil and moisture content (pH), so do that plumping easily, making all the difference between facing the day looking your best or not so good. All these body accouterments, lotions, bath-oil sprays, splashes—not forgetting the good old standby of yesterday and today, talcum powder—are now so refined that their *effect* alone is noticed, leaving only an aura behind via their perfume.

Rounding up the bath business, here is a neat guide:

For a wake-up bath. Test with a thermometer and aim for a temperature between 70° and 80°; bathe briskly, don't linger, don't forget the bath oil. Dry fast, powder well.

For a warm-up bath. After you've been in the snow and hail, take it at above normal body temperature—about 102°—comforting, but don't stay in long. Soap, rinse, jump out, and dry vigorously with big nubbly towel.

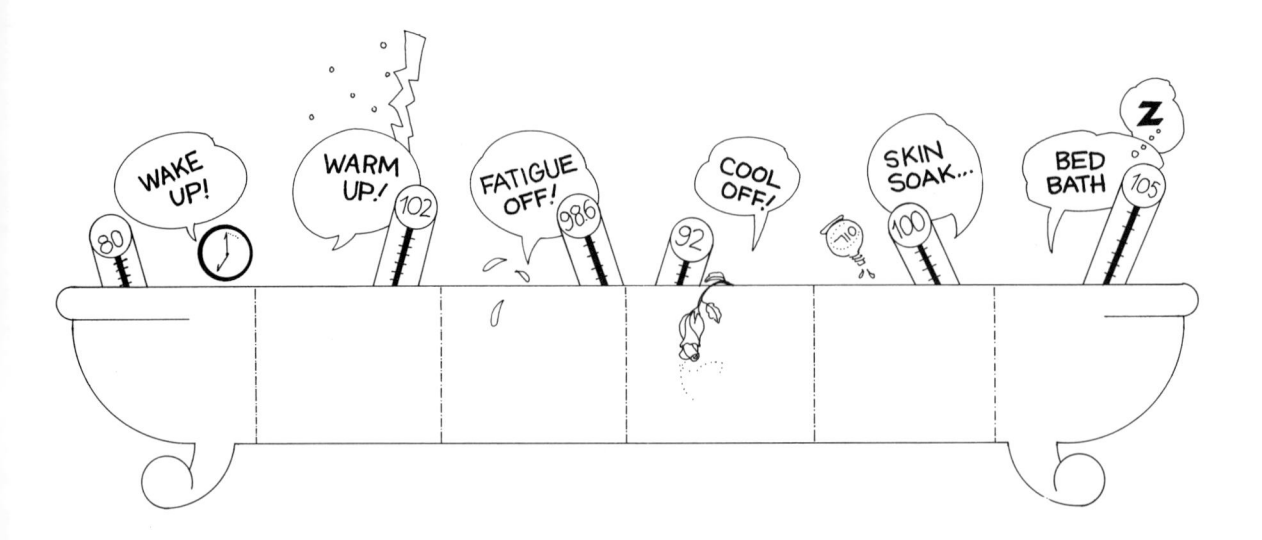

For a fatigue-relieving bath. Keep temperature at normal body heat between 98° and 99°, and soak in the hot soapy water for at least fifteen minutes, finishing with a cool rinse. Blot dry, use body lotion all over, particularly at tense spots, shoulders, nape of neck, wrists, ankles, calves, feet.

For a cool-off bath. When it's over 100° outside and humid, a cool bath will cool you down for longer than a *cold* one. Take it at about 92°, soak for twenty to thirty minutes with your fragrant bath essence along, the more floral the better. Blot skin dry, then lavishly powder, so clothes will slip on without sticking. This should cool you down for at least four to six hours. Repeat as often as you like; it isn't enervating.

For skin relief. If you're burned, chapped, or simply parched, take a warm 95°–100° bath, laced well with bath oil. Start the tub at body temperature, then let warmer water trickle in as you soak—the length of the soak is important—the longer the better. Don't use soap, don't rinse, gently blot your skin dry, leaving a slight film of oil on top for protection—no bath powder.

For a bedtime bath. Always a good move for insomniacs—particularly if it's the day for sparkling clean linen—turn the bed down before you turn the tap on to 98° to 105°. Soap yourself before you relax for about ten minutes, then rinse in warm water, gently blot and powder well before rushing between those sheets. Lights out immediately. *No late, late show, please!*

Water is good, it benefits all things, said the Chinese philosopher Lao-Tzu way back in the sixth century—and he was right. Nothing affects the body more profoundly. It's the fluid of life itself—70 percent of our body weight is water. More than half of most of the food we eat is water, and best of all, *water* in all its many forms can be a great beauty tonic.

Spas—Where to Go and What Happens When You Get There

Not so long ago the word *spa* meant miracle water place in Indian language, mineral spring to the well traveled, and a place to rest and, hopefully, rejuvenate to most of us.

Today a spa has more the connotation of a resort—one where there's an emphasis on health, leading to perfect shape and condition via a medley of treatments, often the *least* being a mineral spring on the property.

The true spas, like those of Wiesbaden, Baden-Baden, Vichy, and Aix-les-Bains, still offer programs under medical supervision based on drinking the waters (all-day-long drinking from the fountains is actively encouraged), bathing in the water and—sometimes—using the steam or water itself in specific treatments. A recent medical study provided the following statistics of people taking "cures" via the waters in Europe:

Russia	6,000,000
Germany	1,000,000
France	400,000
Italy	1,500,000
Czechoslovakia	700,000

In the United States, however, the spa has mostly lost its "mineral spring" label, while the habit of "taking the waters"—at Stafford Springs, Connecticut (America's first spa), Poland Springs, Maine, or at the springs in Saratoga—died long ago.

Today anyone who goes to a spa in the United States is probably not thinking of the daily quart of restorative water he or she will have to drink but of sauna baths, mud packs (for the body as well as the face), and beauty pampering in general, either at a rule-bound, totally nonpermissive health and beauty establishment, like the Golden Door in California, or a permissive do-it-if-you-like beauty pleasure park, like La Costa a few miles away.

A century ago people dutifully drank and bathed in the mineral waters of this country, but it was still more of a social occasion than a therapeutic one. Visiting Hot Springs in Virginia at the Homestead (more famous today for its haute cuisine than its special H_2O plus) was known to be a husband-chasing occupation. There was even a Billing, Wooing, and Cooing Society set up there in the 1830s to lay down some ground rules.

It was a pleasant life. After rising at 8 A.M., an obligatory drink of the mineral water started the day. Then came a lavish breakfast with no calorie counting. Midmorning champagne and watermelon were served, followed an hour later by a big luncheon and more mineral water. A siesta was necessary before afternoon tea, followed by a concert or a garden party. Then in the evening more mineral water was followed by supper, more champagne, and a ball or cotillion. This round of pleasure still existed up until World War II, and the Duchess of Windsor remembers it well. It seems ironic that, although the meals were as lavish as banquets and with champagne served as often as mineral water, most of the figures were as trim as her own. Or did fashion conceal more than we can imagine?

Today, just as the European spa is gaining in popularity *because* of the stringent rules and the emphasis on medical help, the American spa in the true sense of the word has declined. To stay in business, the old spas like the one at Saratoga have had to introduce other lures—horse racing and an arts center, built close to the bathhouse where the mineral springs still bubble out of the ground.

If you yearn for the natural life and to drink of earth's goodness, there are still sixty springs or "real spas" to be found in the United States—offering a variety of rules or no rules, luxury or Spartan living, beautiful surroundings or built in the middle of nowhere. In Alaska there's a spring at Bell Island, as rugged and as wild as you could possibly want, with moose and bear on the doorstep—plus gallons of thermal water that keeps the open air pool at a constant 84°. In midsummer, because of its location, there's eighteen hours of daylight for swimming.

At the other end of the pendulum is the Palm Springs spa, built around the old hot springs of the Agua Caliente Indians. "Built around" does not mean with rough-and-tumble wigwams. Here is a lavishly appointed hotel with Olympic-size pool, whirlpools, steam rooms, salt packs, saunas, and every kind of water treatment devised to make you feel better on your feet . . . plus king-size beds for when you're off them, Bloody Marys, sunsets, and orchestras.

People who go to Steamboat Springs, Colorado, to ski—a relatively new "in" place—may not think the last part of its name implies anything to drink—but there are over one hundred springs in the area with a combined flow of two thousand gallons of water a minute. Once you've taken off your skis, you can drink a glass, go for a swim in an indoor or outdoor pool, or take a soak at the bathhouse. The water's always warm, but if you're there for skiing, the weather won't be—wait till May.

Making use of a natural spring, first discovered in the mid-sixteenth century, is the Safety Harbor Spa, situated between Tampa and Clearwater, Florida, where, if you sign on, you are supposed to follow a program tailor-made for shape and condition. After a medical checkup, you get your marching orders, and drinking the water is always part of them. But there's more to it than sipping or guzzling, depending on whether you like the taste. Yoga is part of the program, a special diet for sure, and plenty of sport—two eighteen-hole golf courses are on the property, tennis, and chess after six.

No springs but plenty of slogging hard work if you want to work for the sake of your looks takes place at another medically supervised beauty and health establishment at Palm-Aire, near Pompano Beach, Florida. Called the Spa at Palm-Aire, it epitomizes what the word *spa* means in the United States today—offering every kind of aid to make a body beautiful *except* the natural elixir of spring water. At Palm-Aire, discipline is remedial, coaxing along all clients with a low-calorie diet or a put-on-weight program for the lucky few who never seem to be able to put on an ounce. It also has an enormous array of equipment plus plenty of experienced—and attractive—instructors.

Arriving at Palm-Aire may be bewildering—because the spa is but one of a number of elegant-looking buildings scattered over seven hundred acres. You can buy a condominium in the sun at Palm-Aire, spend a vacation at a luxury hotel, also on the property, where the emphasis is on haute cuisine and haute couture, or—the antithesis of all that—make the journey for the benefits offered by the spa. If you sign on for the spa program, you're expected to follow it, but rules are by no means stringent—unlike Maine Chance in Arizona, founded by Elizabeth Arden, and the Greenhouse, outside Dallas, which *really* looks like a terrarium, all human "plants" being firmly nurtured according to house rules and no deviation allowed.

Permissive or Nonpermissive—Take Your Choice

One of the first things you have to decide on the day that you—or your husband—decide you and/or he ought to go to a spa to reduce, increase, or just maintain, is exactly how strict you want that spa to be.

If you know you get better results on a long rein, Palm-Aire and similar permissive spas are for you. If you know you need an instructor breathing down your aching back, then it's best to put yourself fairly and squarely into the hands of people long experienced in delivering a tough get-fit program, which includes low-calorie foods, well-programmed exercise and activity, and medical supervision.

At Maine Chance, the Greenhouse, and the Golden Door, for example, no alcohol is a way of life—and anyone caught smuggling in an airline pack of daiquiris is sent to her room, or sent home without refund if she's unrepentant.

At all reputable places, a medical checkup comes before any attack on daily habits. With health well documented, a weekly program can then be planned, hopefully well balanced between rest and activity, willpower and cosseting.

Imagine you're at Palm-Aire with your husband—another bonus, because most spas like to concentrate on one sex at a time, so that the majority divide their year into male and female weeks or don't allow the boys at all. You will wake up in the spa hotel—a few orange trees away is the "other" hotel, where all the self-indulging ones will be wondering what to do with their day, but not so at the spa, spic and span with white paint, pale citrus-green and yellow furnishings. On the breakfast tray will be the daily program, taking up most of the room on the tray, for there won't be much in the way of breakfast—an orange, a piece of wholemeal toast, and a cup of weak tea in all probability. As on the lunch and dinner menus, each item will have its calorie value clearly marked, so there's no way you can eat more than a maximum seven hundred calories a day—unless you're one of those ambiguous people who like to cheat between rigorous workouts with secret nibbles on strawberry cheesecake.

The program usually starts at the civilized hour of 9:30 A.M., so arm in arm—I've learned over the years self-control in diet makes one very affectionate—you will stroll with your other half to the Spa headquarters where, in a sumptuous lobby lined with modern paintings and sculpture, you will go through the "Her" door while he goes through "His." Once on your side of the fence, life takes on another meaning. It's Wizard-of-Oz land. Piped music is of the low, soothing never-never-land variety; your fellow workers in various stages of undress are suprisingly all smiling, going with purposeful steps to whatever part of the agenda awaits them. Whirlpools whirl; bar bells twirl and blue pools, indoors and out, look improbably blue.

Directed to your own locker, you will find pinned to it a replica of your breakfast tray program, which quite likely will read like this: 9:30 A.M., jazz exercises; 11 A.M., whirlpool bath; 11:30 A.M., yoga lesson (generally the teacher demands a headstand the first day); 12 noon, massage; 1 P.M., lunch—hot or cold. If you choose hot, you will be able to join your husband back in the spa dining room; a cold choice can be eaten around the pool in the ladies' section—and it can be a delicious mix of citrus fruits, kiwi, lichee, mango, fresh raw vegetables, and iced fresh Florida juices. There are tropical gardens and pools in the female workshop, just as there are in the men's, where it's encouraged to sunbathe in the nude—and even on a cloudy day, it looks as if the sun's shining through the glass roof. Sunbathing—just like everything else—is timed so that the sun becomes a friend, not an enemy.

Watching over all this is someone described by many Palm-Aire regulars as "the iron hand in the velvet glove"—Lisa Dobloug, a striking Norwegian, who first learned about spas from another great one in California—the Golden Door. She graduated at the Greenhouse, then went on to become director at Palm-Aire. Lisa works meticulously with dieticians to produce good-tasting food that's also easy on shape, plus supervising every facet of the programs available.

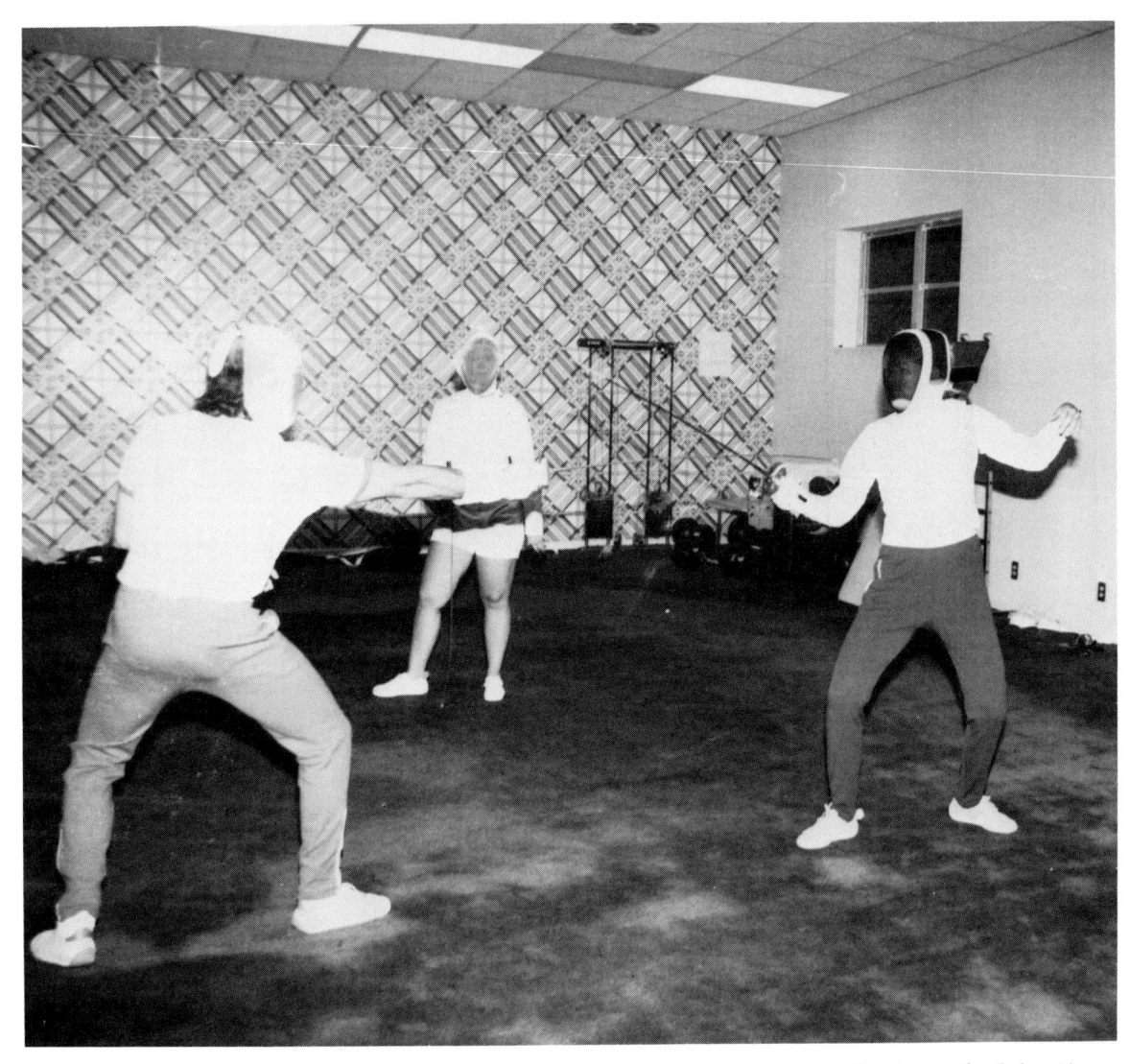

Fencing at the Palm-Aire Spa—good for your figure, good for developing quick reflexes.

At 3:30 perhaps, there's another exercise class—this time in the water—followed at 4:30 by a herbal wrap, where you're swathed like a baby in swaddling clothes that are hot, herbal, and scented, and where you perspire your toxins away. A facial might end your hard day's work, so that you're fresh, glowing, and ready to meet your date—also fresh from his labors—outside in the no-man's-land lobby, before relaxing in one of the many lounges before a devastating vegetable-juice cocktail and dinner.

La Costa, three thousand miles away, near San Diego, California, must be the largest spa on earth, if you count every one of its seven thousand acres as participating in the keep-fit endeavor, but it follows closely the Palm-Aire permissive principle: "If you want to leave looking better, slimmer, and so feeling healthier, it's entirely up to you."

No shot gun to get you up, and here the spa dining room is part of the resort dining room, so it's no wonder temptation rears its fat, flabby head and people are liable to find themselves saying, "Well, just one and no more this week," as they down a neat Bloody Mary.

Everything is king-size at La Costa except the spa's portions of food. Beds are huge; the golf course has twenty-seven holes—making the nineteenth playable for a change; there's a private beach on the Pacific, where I found facilities to be surprisingly tatty in comparison to everything inland; and both "His" and "Her" spas have their own enormous gyms, swimming pools, whirlpools, Swedish saunas, Finnish rock steam baths, Oriental massages, classes in karate, judo, yoga, and dance, with a beauty salon for the girls (where Mrs. Burt Bacharach regularly gets her hair done) and a barber shop for the boys.

In keeping with its size, choice of accommodations is huge. You can stay in a spa apartment, the main hotel, rent your own cottage, hacienda, or villa—and the size (and price) goes up each time. Personally I found La Costa too permissive to achieve any serious results, but it's great for having fun without paying for it in *excess pounds* along with excess baggage.

Another Southern California oasis, Murrieta Hot Springs, as the name suggests, really does have mineral springs emerging from an underground realm at 170° plus tule mud baths—which means a kind of muddy root bath on which you lie, the mud, smoothed all over you, heated by the same hot springs. A minimum stay of four days, three nights, is required before you can enroll in the spa—although you can stay at the hotel and enjoy a regular sort of holiday. It reminds me of when I was a child and my parents solemnly weighed both themselves and me at the beginning and end of each vacation. Any gain in weight meant the holiday had really been a success—times *have* changed.

For over three decades the emphasis has been on food at Rancho La Puerta, just over the California border at Tecate, Mexico, and under the same management as the Golden Door in Escondido, California.

Rancho La Puerta was originally created by Edmond Szekely, an early environmentalist, who was sent by the French government to study and report on various regions of the earth and their relationship to human health. Finding himself in Southern California at the outbreak of World War II unable to return to France, he observed that San Diego County had the most healthful climate in the world, because of its soil, average temperature, mountain, desert, and sea atmosphere. He decided to stay and to create a spa there—Rancho La Puerta—offering a vegetarian health cure with diet based solely on natural foods grown in soil without fertilizers or sprays.

Professor Szekely's choice of a site was based on yet another reason. He observed that the area is in exactly the same latitude as Canaan, the ancient Promised Land, the land of plenty. To make a land of plenty at Rancho La Puerta three decades ago, Professor Szekely planted vineyards over acres and acres. In those days visitors to the "spa" might easily find themselves put first on a grape-juice cure—nonstop grape juice and only grape juice for fourteen days.

Today the meals are still vegetarian, and all the food is grown on the property. Grapes—and grape juice—remain abundant, for the vineyards still prosper, but Mrs. Szekely Mazzanti, the professor's former wife, is now in charge, and the menu also includes the Rancho's own crusty dark bread, a blend of several whole grains, made daily in an outdoor stone oven, plus organic honey from local hives.

Over thirty classes, treatments, and activities are available, but if you opt for the sedentary life, cacti watching is allowed, even encouraged if it's thought you need peace and quiet more than anything else.

Rules and Regulations

You may have got the message that Mrs. Mazzanti, whether married to Professor Szekely or not, still believes a healthy mind is as important as a healthy body and that one can't be achieved without the other. To that end, at the Golden Door, also under her watchful eye, the reasons for wanting to come are studied as thoroughly as blood pressure, metabolism, and all physical readings.

The Golden Door is *not* permissive. Once in, *you join in:* and that means an early call—7 A.M.—for an *up* the mountainside walk, back for breakfast in bed, then a day that is neatly divided into forty-minutes sections of activity until 6 P.M., when mind-stretching occupations are on hand. Meals are in the nectar category, for here also all produce is grown on the spot, most of it being picked fresh for every menu.

I love Maine Chance for all its rules and regulations, its tut-tutting if somebody sighs for a brandy sour on the rocks or a double martini with a twist of lemon. Elizabeth Arden was a shrewd lady, finding some of the best operators in the business. To this day, there are still some of her original choices working at Maine Chance, massaging, soothing, caressing, delivering a feeling of *joie de vivre* to the most double martini-ed jaded body. Miss Arden always chose girls with "fat finger pads," stating that without them, nobody could possibly make a good masseur, facialist, or makeup expert. "Fingers talk, explore, know what a face or a body is all about," she used to say.

At Maine Chance you realize she was absolutely right. I've had the best massage there, the best facial, too. Fingers talk—so do their owners.

One member of the staff, as she put me with great care into a wax

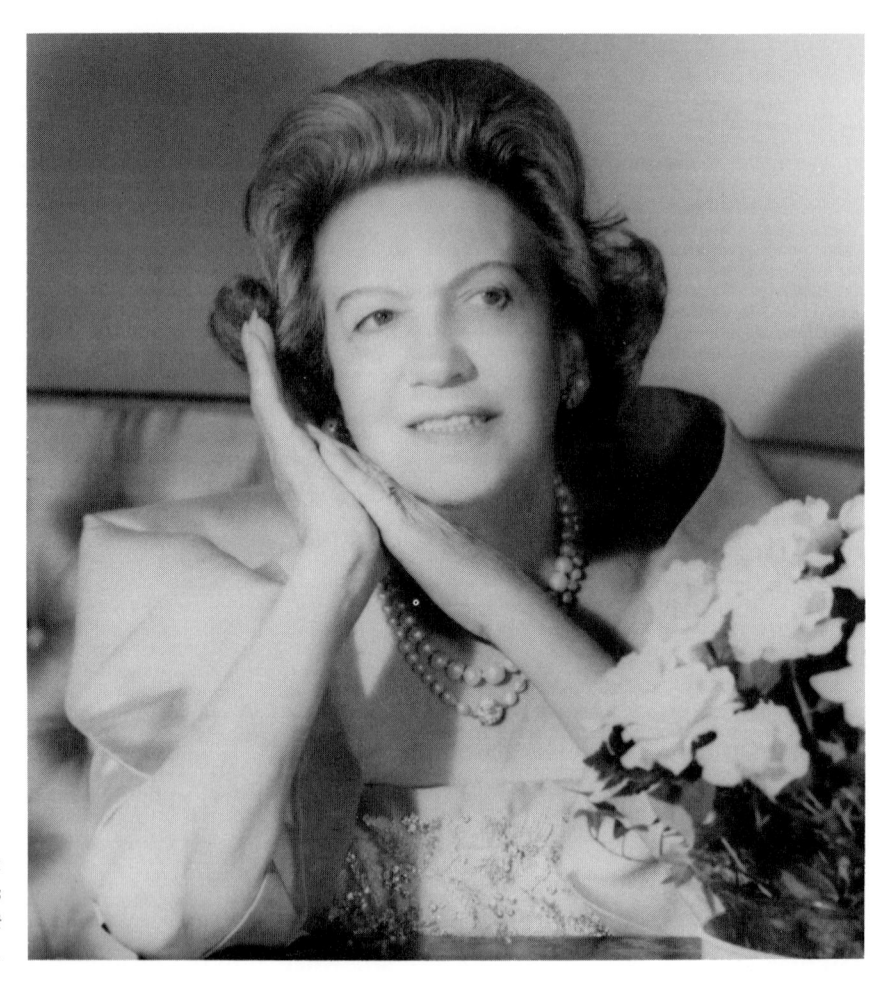

Elizabeth Arden, no mean masseur herself, always chose spa operators with fat finger pads . . .

bath, told me she had studied medicine as a young girl at the University Hospital in Berlin, where zone therapy was taught (see page 201)—as part of the benefits of socialized medicine. Still with a faint trace of German accent, she told me she was taught how to massage the foot to treat another part of the body, to activate the palms of the hands to affect the spine, and to massage the trapezius muscles surrounding the spine to help neck and shoulder tension disappear. Another part of her training involved knowledge of lymph drainage to rid the body of cellulite—moving the fluid deposits along the lymph canals, still an important treatment of cellulite in Germany now, although not well know here. Having escaped from Hitler's Germany before the Second World War, this particular operator was interviewed by Miss Arden here in the United States: "She examined my fingers, exclaimed over the fatness of them, and I had the job."

Apart from the experience and efficacy of the Maine Chance

beauty experts, the chef is worth a line or two, if not a few bouquets. From Chile, of French origin, Josef Bello enjoys the challenge of Maine Chance, really enjoying the look of disbelief on the clients' faces as they eat his mousse of grape with yogurt, lemon, and honey dressing, or his hamburger with special onion and shallot stuffing, or his papaya plate (the papaya is flown in to Maine Chance twice a week from Hawaii)—disbelief because they are eating so few calories, yet it tastes as good as coq au vin followed by crepes suzette.

At the Greenhouse, a staff of eighty-eight looks after eighty-six women, which is another way of saying it isn't one of the most commercial enterprises in the world. Instead the Greenhouse is a magical place for more than one princess, if you count Grace of Monaco. Lady Bird Johnson wouldn't dream of giving up her annual visit, and everyone is quite happy—although they have no choice—to wear the compulsory uniform of pale-blue leotard and yellow terry robe during the day, changing to a little Givenchy—noncompulsory—for their nonalcoholic pick-me-up at 6 P.M. Texas zing gets into the atmosphere, although it's rarefied and controlled, all under glass. You don't have to venture outside at all to go to the sauna or to the beauty salon or even to the exercise track—run by one of the greyhounds in the business, Toni Beck. The food, surprisingly, is sometimes laced with wine or cognac, but they say the extra calories are cooked away, leaving only that delicious and—to most of the Greenhouse regulars—familiar flavor.

This sort of spa is obviously expensive, and the rooms reflect it, equipped with the sort of comfort you might have or hope to have at home—private phone, sunken tub in bathroom, deep, deep rugs, lighting with dimmer switches, color TV, masses of closets. When you are spending money, it makes sense if you go where you will get what you came for. Otherwise you might just as well have a splurge at your favorite restaurant.

Beauty at Sea

Some time ago, before the *France* was taken out of service, the French Line approached me and asked me to help them with a cruise—"something to do with beauty." I suggested they turn the *France* into a floating spa on the basis that as it then was considered the greatest ship in the world, it couldn't help but become the greatest floating spa.

I ran a beauty clinic on board, and a patient queue of ladies would gather outside my door with every kind of beauty question. My favorite visitor was plump, fair, and pretty and she told me in great depression she'd once been a member of Esther Williams Water Ballet but had "let herself go." Her husband had put her on board with strict instructions she was to return looking "her old self" or else!

Disliking him immediately, I worked with the rest of the experts on board not to return any "old self" but a much more confident, pretty, and poised "new self." She went on a diet—not easy on the France, although in keeping with the spa trend there were calorie-counted menus, too. She went through exercise classes with Eileen Ford of the Ford Agency; she had her hair toned down to a paler blonde with color wizard James Viera running the color courses; she had makeup lessons every day from Lancôme. There has to be a moral to the story. The last day at sea, prettier and more poised, she met a dashing ship's officer and confided in me that she was seriously thinking of never returning home at all. . . . I'm sure she did return, but it just goes to show—floating or otherwise, a spa can do wonders for a girl's morale.

Baths You Won't Find at Home

Apart from eating and drinking differently at the spa of your choice, you can also bathe differently—deliberately—for health's sake. Here is a brief rundown on the baths you can expect to find and what each does for you.

Mud baths—the mud of volcanic origin—draw out toxins in the skin to clear up a spotty back, for instance, and help to ward off arthritis but DON'T cure it. Helena Rubinstein used to import vast quantities of mud from Ischia to use in her salons in the top European cities and in her New York salon, too.

Oxygen baths are great pepper-uppers for both psyche and circulation. Pure oxygen is pumped into a whirlpool bath, so a good mix of oxygen and water swirl around you, the oxygen-suffusing skin donating a revitalizing effect. These baths can be found in many Swiss spas—at the Grand Hotel Beau Rivage at Interlaken, for instance.

Paraffin wax baths were introduced to the United States by that disciple of beauty, Elizabeth Arden. The wax bath is likened by one of the operators at Maine Chance to "causing a storm in the river, causing it to overflow its banks." This is a neat way of saying that the wax bath causes a flood of perspiration, sweeping away as much impurity from bloodstream and skin as possible. You lie for half an hour encased up to the neck in melted wax to which various oils have been added. While the wax isn't uncomfortably hot, the process is a demanding one, stimulating the heart, which is one reason no one can have a wax bath without a medical OK first. The skin afterward looks and feels as near to silk as it ever will.

Vitamin baths mean many vitamins plus minerals are added to a whirlpool bath by a separate pipe; you find these baths where there's no natural mineral spring on the property. Otherwise, where there is a natural spring, as at Hot Springs, Virginia, you bathe in water gushing out of the ground, loaded with good minerals, iron, potassium, lithium.

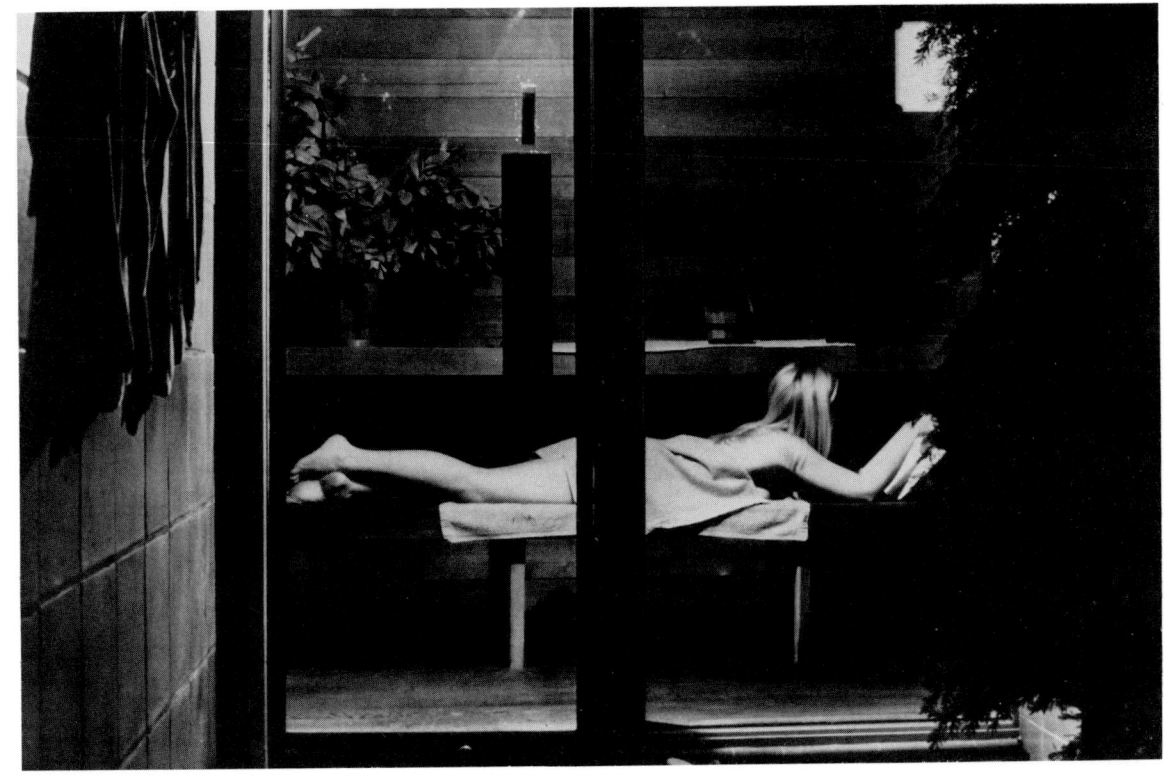

The sauna bath—great place to while away the time—and the excess pounds.

    Sand baths are rare, but they do exist in the East, where they are taken as part of a special beauty regime. On the island of Kyushu at Ibusuki, Japan, the sands beside Kagoshima Bay are heated by an underground stream. At low tide, health seekers are buried up to the neck in the hot sand by attendants, only to be dug up again when the tide turns. No, the results are *not* the same on the beach at Waikiki—or Westhampton for that matter.

    Sauna baths, originating in Finland, are now almost commonplace—but in Finland there is usually an ice-cold pure stream or lake outside the sauna for constant dipping between dry heat sessions, all wonderfully good for circulation, *providing* you're in A-OK condition as far as your heart and blood pressure go. You're advised *not* to take a sauna or steam bath if you have diabetes or while you are under the influence of alcohol or taking drugs such as anticoagulants, antihistamines, hypnotics, vasoconstrictors, vasodilators, narcotics, or tranquilizers.

    You can also bathe in camomile in Scandinavia, seaweed in France and England, peat moss in Germany—all to soothe, purify, and heal.

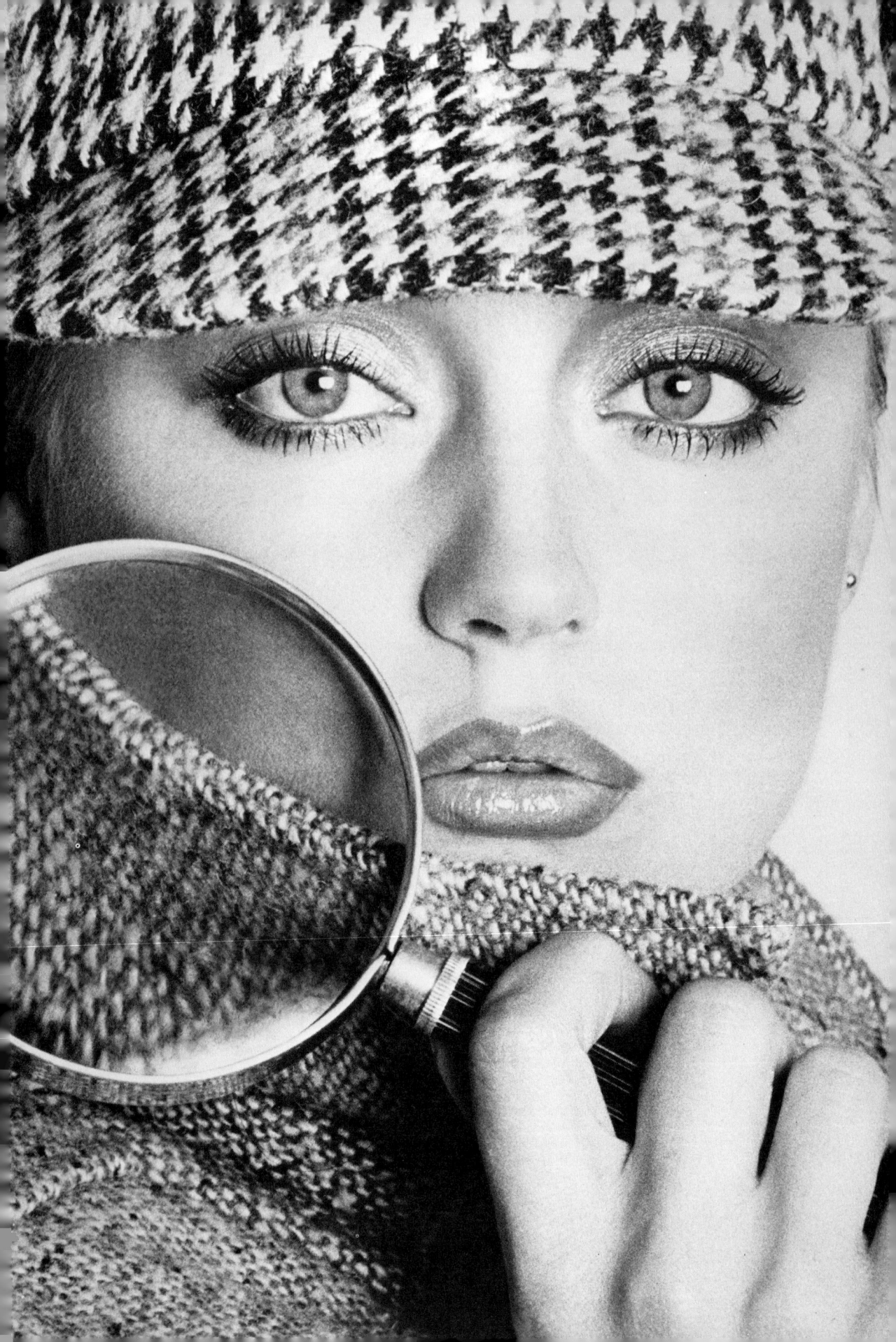

3

Your Makeup
Tyranny or Therapy?

Way Bandy is one of the top face designers, makeup artists, visagistes in the country today. There are many ways to describe his contemporary profession, and he'll answer to all of them, providing he can get on with his work, which, in fact, is transforming many of the familiar faces you know from anonymities into luminous beauties ready for the camera.

Way, who doesn't mind admitting to a face tuck or two before he reached thirty-five, said to me a few years back, "Makeup should be *psychiatry for the face,* not tyranny, but therapy. I wish women didn't feel they *had to* follow this or that trend . . . and then get depressed out of their skulls when they find they can't wear the current look."

FACING PAGE
Do check your makeup with a magnifying glass when you switch locales and lights.

YOUR MAKEUP

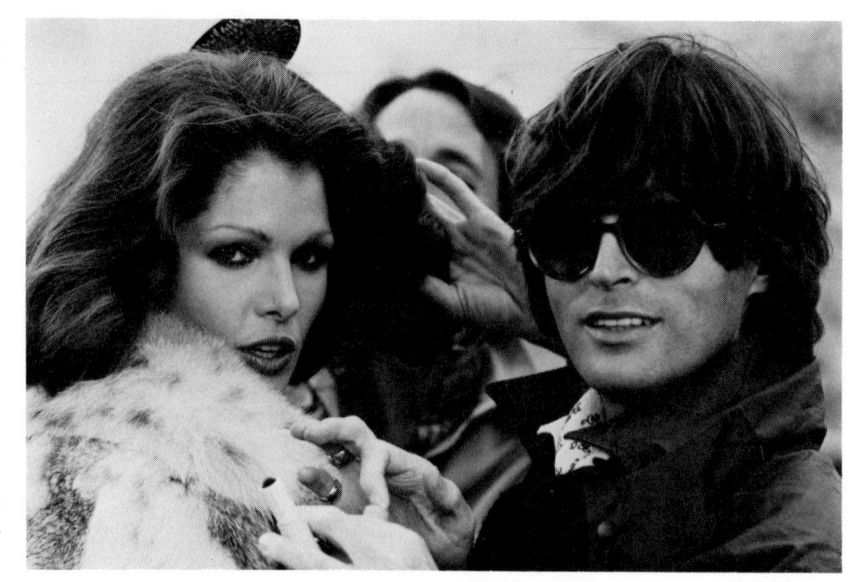

Top face-maker Way Bandy with one of his favorite faces, Lois Chiles.

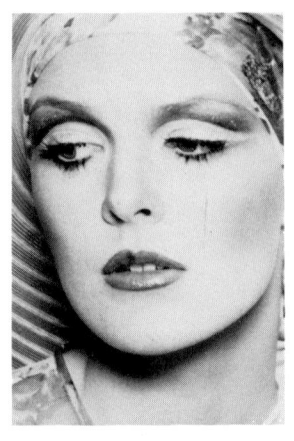

"No top model ever wears base all over her face," says Way Bandy, "only where she feels she needs it."

He was exaggerating the picture, but once upon a time, not all that long ago, we *were* copycats, trying to emulate Marilyn Monroe's pout, Rita Hayworth's high gypsy cheekbones, even Doris Day's dimples.

It wasn't fashionable to be ourselves, so we didn't give ourselves a chance.

Today, more health-conscious, serious, and above all, *busy*, we don't want our looks to be rubber-stamped. We're learning how to look like more beautiful versions of ourselves with the help of makeup.

Way, who works daily with professional models for TV commercials, *Vogue* fashion and beauty pages, and for the bigger-than-lifesize billboards you see on routes all over the country (except in Virginia!), knows the art of makeup backward and forward and agrees there's been a definite change of heart.

Along with the demise of the Louis Quinze salon, the little black dress for after six, and the foot-high hairstyle has come a fervent desire to look "natural"—but as pretty as possible at the same time.

How Much Does Your Face Cost You?

In 1972 I wrote an editorial for *Harper's Bazaar* that caused comment. Called "The Two Billion Dollar Face," it related to the American woman who then spent that much annually on a package deal of makeup ($930 million), treatment ($535 million) and fragrance ($620 million). Since then the treatment graph has shot up, and today's face must cost several million dollars more. There's one positive result. *We look younger today* than we did a decade ago because we buy the right products and know how to use them to bring the right look about. This encourages the development of more along the same lines—products that improve our skin as they color it, products that produce a "natural" beauty or as near to beauty as we can manage.

The products we left on the shelf were eventually shelved forever. We didn't buy them because they were too heavy, too perfumed, too "artificial."

We all know you can't make a good painting on a poor canvas. Skin has to be right first before makeup can do its best job, so we buy more treatment products to take care of that basic requirement.

As Way Bandy believes in the emergence of the natural look, so do other notable makeup experts like Count Pablo Zappi Manzoni (discovered in a Via Veneto salon in Rome by Elizabeth Arden herself). As Pablo puts it, "In makeup one should try to follow nature as much as possible. A woman should look clean, soft, subtle by day, more dramatic by night, but never as if she's wearing on her face everything in her makeup case, even if she is."

"The natural look" requires talent and time; perhaps more talent (or practice), but less time than the old-fashioned "made-up" face.

The idea is to look as nature would have made you had she been more of a designing woman, not by changing features—something Pablo particularly disapproves of: "The important thing is to play up one's advantages, play down the unattractive or average. I see elegance in imperfection. A flaw can be of value, a mark of distinction."

To that end he works to emphasize the character he sees in a face, even if that character is illustrated best by a big nose or wide-apart eyes. He works to make the face *memorable,* because he makes it handsome or lovely—and a big nose doesn't seem to stick out because it works so well with the rest of the face.

Although Pablo works a great deal with plastic surgeons, helping patients with post-plastic-surgery makeup ("their makeup almost always has to be changed"), he is one of the first to try to dissuade a client from surgery if he feels nothing would be gained by it, showing her instead how a new makeup might be the answer.

Hair First

Before *Vogue*'s contemporary Beauty Annual in 1973, makeup editorials frequently urged the reader to study the shape of her face and put color on it accordingly—rouge or color gel high on the cheekbone for a round face, lower down on a long, thin face, and so on. When I started to work on the annual with Pablo and a talented hairstylist called François (then working at the celebrated Kenneth Salon), we experimented and found that hair—seen at last in its true light as an incredibly adaptable natural fiber—could also play an important role in governing where makeup should go on the face. All because a hairstyle itself often gives the face a new shape.

It was a new thought and a great idea. To that end, Pablo plotted his makeup *after* François had with brush and comb given a new shape to our model's face with each style he created.

With bangs he made her face appear smaller, shorter, wider. With another style he elongated her face shape.

All this affected Pablo's makeup ideas until we came to the simple conclusion: *Hairstyle comes first. Makeup contouring should always be plotted afterward for the best results.*

Easy Tips

Here are some easy basic tips everyone can follow to accomplish in the shortest possible time the free and easy pretty look we all want:

Base Coat

No top model ever wears base *all* over her face—only where she feels she needs it, perhaps for skin tone to be more matte, covering up poor (sallow) color, tiny lines, or blemishes. Nothing looks more fake than a one-colored skin, for skin wasn't born that way.

- The better the skin, the thinner the base can be. Choose a gel or translucent liquid that gives glow but minimum cover and lets your makeup's best asset—a naturally good skin—show through. Gels are tightening, too, good for firming up makeup, particularly good when skin is lightly tanned. A translucent liquid product is often a powder suspended in liquid, so it must be shaken before application, and is good for an older skin because it doesn't emphasize fine lines.
- A tinted lotion or emulsified makeup base is fine for dry or normal skins (dry sides, more oily center panel). Oils in the formula give a dewy look. Frequently this type of product is moisturized, too, for extra skin help.
- To test you're not using too dry or too oily a base for your skin, drop a little into a glass of water. If it disperses and looks like café au lait, it's oil-in-water, *water-based,* and therefore right for oily skins. If it stays put in a little puddle, it is water-in-oil, *oil-based,* and the right one for dry skins.
- Dry skin should always wear a moisturizer beneath makeup to help it glide on and stay on longer. All bases are best applied with a damp sponge. That way residue is removed even while the base is being applied—all to ensure a smooth, even surface.
- If you have something to hide—a blemish, broken capillaries—or irregular features to balance, a cream or cake makeup does the job, again best applied with a damp sponge to give the smoothest finish.

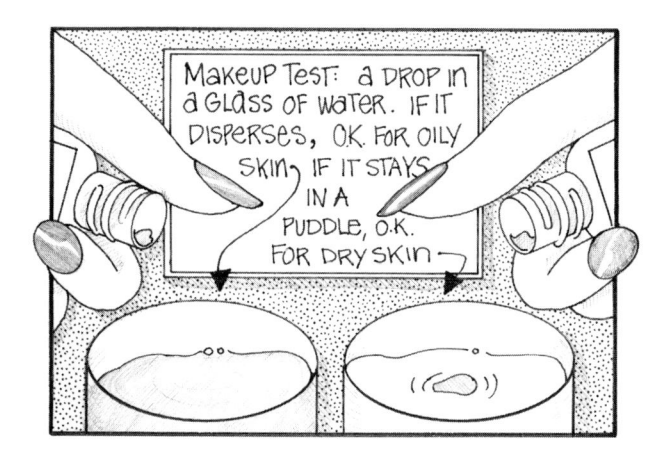

□ A cover-up product is labeled that way to show it's heavier—made with heavier waxes. Read the label when looking for a medicated product—all the ingredients will be listed and have been chosen and blended to help a problem skin, antibacterial power calming down breakouts and blemishes while at the same time coloring.

□ For allergic women there's more choice in makeup now more and more cosmetics are deliberately made fragrance-free (perfume is often the allergy culprit). This specialized type of makeup is low in common allergens. In fact, today most makeup has as few allergens as possible for obvious reasons.

□ If you have dark circles or lines under the eyes, *do* touch them out with a conceal-type stick, then put base on top.

□ *Don't* apply base to an area where there's fuzz; it only accentuates it.

□ *Don't* create a demarcation line between face and neck—makeup and bare skin.

□ *Do* stop short with your base about an inch above the jawbone, then blend down from there. By the time you reach your neck, the base should have dwindled down to match natural skin color.

□ *Do* practice using two shades of the same base, one darker than the other, if you feel your face is too long, too wide, too round. Actress Vanessa Redgrave, for instance, has a longish face, so uses a darker shade of foundation across her forehead just below her hairline for a depth of a fraction of an inch. She also uses the same darker shade on the tip of her chin. On the rest of her face she uses a lighter shade, but the dark touches tend to reduce the look of *"length."* In the same way, actress and Las Vegas star Ann-Margret slims down her wide face by blending a darker shade of base along both sides of her jawline diagonally out toward her earlobes. She traces an imaginary straight line from the pupil of her eye to her lower jaw—and this is the point of her jaw where she starts the darker color.

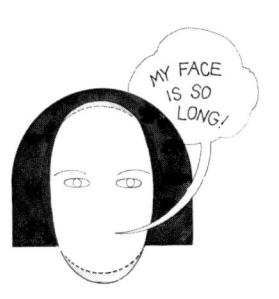

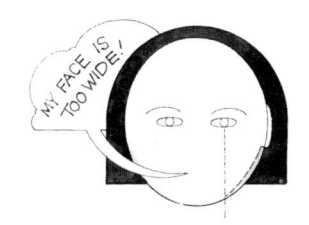

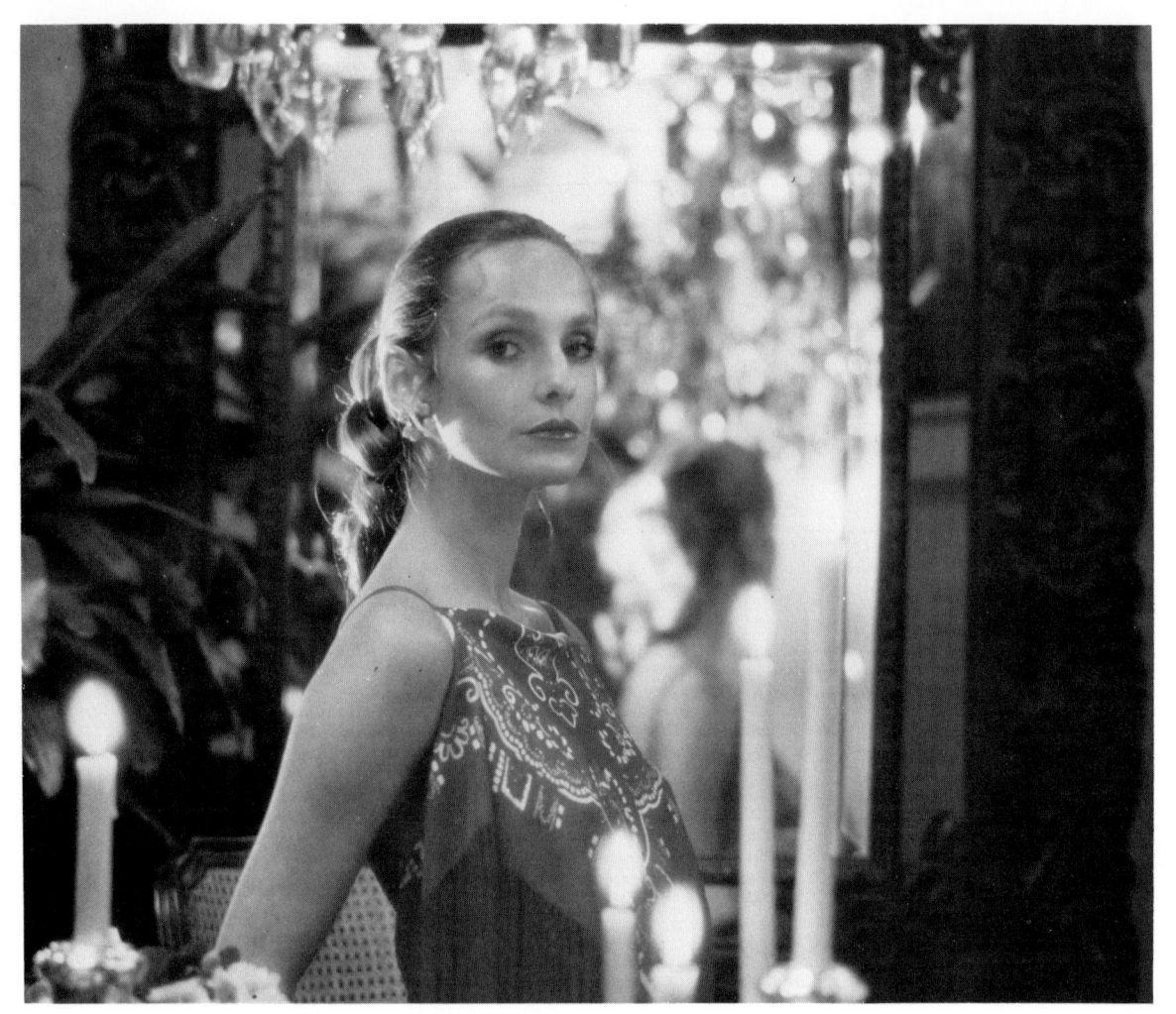

Light is the catalyst, and electric light can make or break your makeup. After dark, a new set of color rules . . .

▢ *Don't* wear the same base year in, year out. Skin changes from season to season as I've already explained (32–36).

▢ *Don't* wear the same base day and night either. Light is the catalyst, making or breaking makeup's effect. Just as electricity affects the way your makeup is going to look, so does geography. Latitude and the position of the sun are as heavily involved in the final result in the mirror as are fluorescent or candlelight.

▢ *Do* check with a magnifying mirror when you switch locales and lights. Take a frank look at yourself in the most telling place of all—above the clouds in a plane, where truth is there for the seeing.

If you remember the higher the latitude, the stronger and more revealing the light, you will know how to even up the score. In New York, for instance, (latitude 41) the light is more flattering than in Stockholm (latitude 59) where skins have almost a natural searchlight on them, tending to "blue" everything, making colors more intense or spectacular depending on makeup skill.

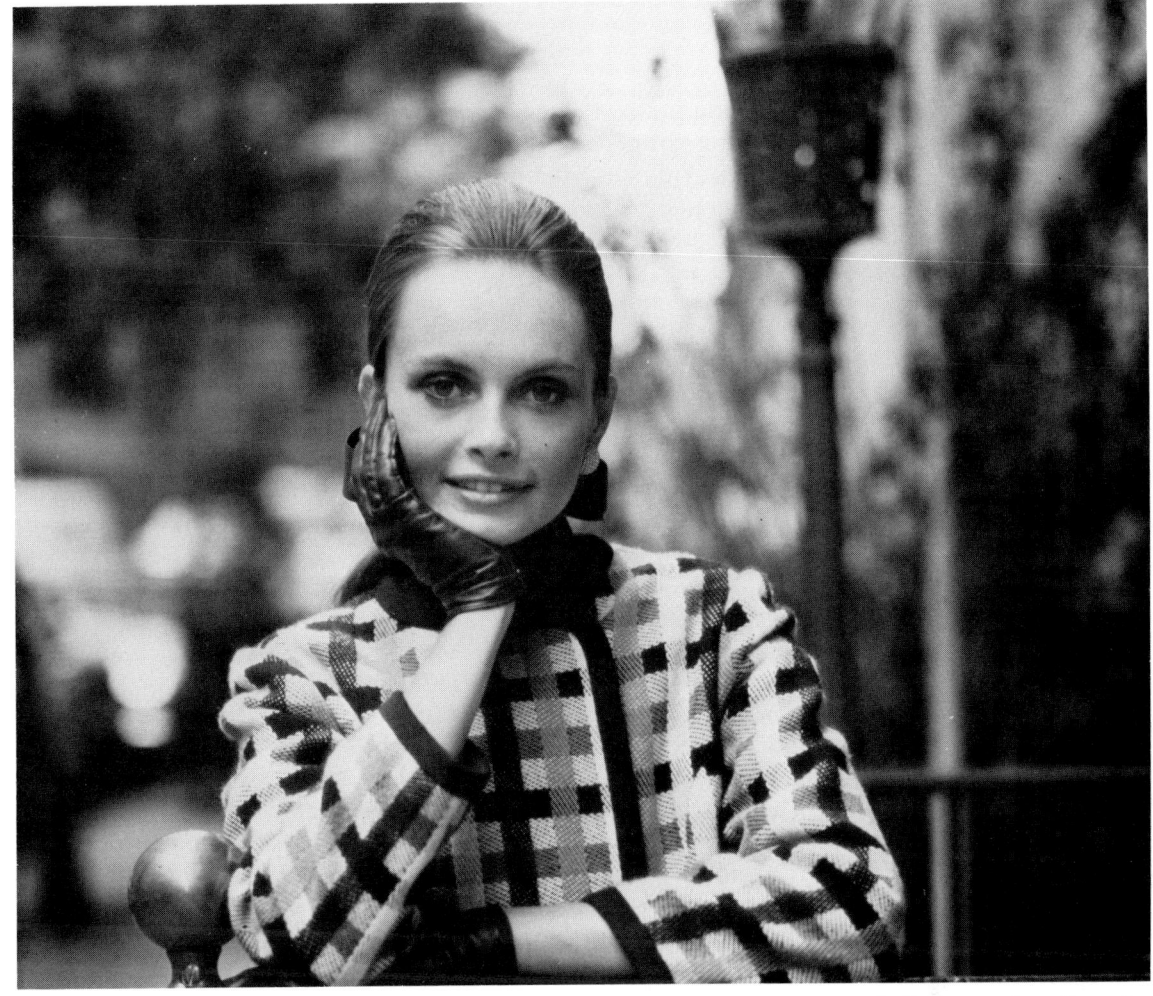

Smile to see where the natural "apples" of your cheeks are, then apply color dead center to get the most natural effect.

In low latitudes nearer the equator (Miami, 26°, Barbados, 13°), the light cast is warm, adding yellow to orange to gold tones to makeup and hair color. This counts more than that skin-damaging tan toward making you feel you look so well there.

After dark, the best lighting to aim for is incandescent, equating with low-latitude light, giving you glow, plus hiding circles and other facts of life. At the other end of the wattage is fluorescent lighting, which equates with the light found in high latitudes, hard and revealing.

When choosing makeup base for evening, avoid anything with a yellow tone (this includes nail enamel) because artificial light can have a yellowing effect. Foundation should have pink undertones to warm up color.

Remember that *pink warms, blue harshens, yellow turns sallow.* A degree or two lighter or darker can make all the difference to getting the maximum mileage out of makeup.

The good news is that today's makeup is *actually good for the skin*. Far from enlarging pores or creating disturbances, a good base now protects the skin, sets up an invisible barrier against pollution and its inherent dangers. If you use the right foundation, you are doing your skin a good turn, a healthy turn.

SPECIAL TIP: Raquel Welch uses a bronze gel-like base on cheekbones, cheeks, and chin only—all to give a spotlight effect to her own all over natural tan.

Contour Color: Rouge, Cheek Gel, Blusher

Whatever it's called, contour color is an increasingly vital piece of makeup equipment, appearing in as many guises as it has names—in a stick, a jar, a sponge, a pencil.

Contour color basically highlights "good bones," or "creates" them for the face born without. Whenever there's a suspicion good face shape exists, a contour color emphasizes it. Above all, it adds just the right blush of health when used correctly.

Models use a contour product for many things today—even as eye shadow—but for most of us it's enough to know how to use it for its original purpose.

There's a difference between a glosser and a blusher—the former adds luster, gloss to the face without adding too much additional color; the latter gives generous color and can warm up the entire face.

Contour color is as important to a face as eye makeup. It can fight the downward force of gravity and even "lift" a face with its illusionary powers. Pablo sometimes applies a touch of pink/brown at the hairline, plus a little under the brows for the same reason.

If you know you're heavy-handed and liable to smudge color, use powder blushes (the same goes for eye shadows), easier to blend than the gel or liquid variety. Most can be put on damp with a little sponge when you want to intensify color.

To add warmth to your base, brush contour color over the high points of the face—cheekbones, chin, tip of nose, and forehead. For definite shading, use under chin, on the forehead, in cheek hollows, and along the jawline.

If you only feel happy with cheek color, *never* suck in your cheeks to see where to apply it. Remember the key word is *natural*. Smile broadly to see where the natural "apples" of your cheeks are, then apply color dead center to get the most natural effect.

Don't bring color too far up the sides of the face toward the eyes— too near beside or below, cheek color can take sparkle away from the eyes. Too near the nose, it can make a nose appear larger.

Remember matte and glow produce different effects, a matte look coming from a blusher or a powder product, a glow from a glosser or gel. Anything light—glow—*emphasizes* by leaving a larger impression, while a matte, flat shade will absorb light to diminish size. If the matte shade is dark, it also *conceals*. Some makeup artists use both blusher and glosser on the face, the blusher lower down on the cheeks, the glosser immediately above on the cheekbones, the contrast reflecting face shape even more dramatically.

At night cheek color is vital. There should be plenty of it. To avoid calling attention to any facial lines or under-eye circles, a warm chestnut-red cream rouge can be blended lower than usual on the cheek and more to the side. Color on the fattest part of the cheek is not becoming at night.

If you're blonde or fair-skinned, try a bright-pink gel gloss (applied with damp sponge) over base (which should match skin tone as closely as possible), then after a brief touch of translucent powder to set makeup, use the same pink in a powder blusher product on cheeks, under brows, lightly down nosebridge, and on the throat down to the hollow.

If you're brunette with warm coloring, try a bronze cheek gel during the day, a gold one at night.

Gold works perfectly for a true *redhead*, too, day or night, using a gel to add shiny color.

Never rub in contour color, always pat it on first, then gently brush to blend. Practice your blending; then you can begin to mix two or three colors together, blending one into the other for extra shading and vibrancy . . . just as the visagistes do.

The merest touch of rouge at eye corners just *below* the brows gives eyes more emphasis, whereas if you wear glasses, a touch of blusher *above* the brows can help give eyes more life and sparkle.

The contour color that lasts longest, stays looking freshest is the cream variety. The brush-on blusher works wonders as a finishing touch, but for staying power (even underwater), cream rouge leads the field.

SPECIAL TIP: Model and beauty Betsy Theodoracopulos uses coral cheek gel on cheek, forehead, and earlobes to spread the warmth of her personality. Top model Lauren Hutton draws stripes with a bronze contour stick under her cheekbones, then blends them straight down onto her cheeks with other little stripes of orange and pink. A quick dot of bronze blended on her chin also gives a healthy look.

Eye Makeup: Woman's First Choice for Desert-Island Living

Once a woman would have chosen to take her lipstick in answer to that old desert-island question. Today if she had only one choice, it would be her eye shadow or, if a model, her "contour color"—to be worn on her eyes just as much as on her "contours."

Eye makeup is a personal matter—but experimentation is the key.

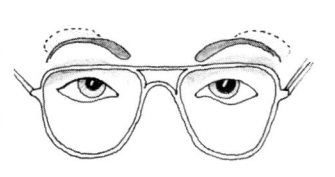

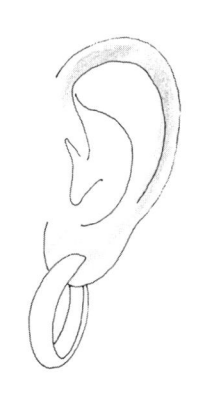

YOUR MAKEUP 74

The amount of color and where to put it varies from face to face, so copying Barbara Walters or Catherine Deneuve may seem a lovely idea, but you won't know until you've tried it on yourself.

Easy Tips

As matte and glow produce different effects, matte making smaller, glow making larger, a woman may choose a *frosted* green (glow) shadow to match her green to hazel eyes and because it's a frosted (glow) color, it will emphasize her already large eyelids. If she chose a *matte* green, it would still leave a large lid but would not look so prominent. Then the green chosen would make one notice her lovely *green eyes* rather than her green *eye makeup*. Eye makeup can be matched to eye color, but it isn't a crime if you don't. There are so many shades to try, and to reiterate: experimentation is all important. You don't know what you're missing until you've tried it.

Remember the matte and glow rule. Add to it: *dark colors conceal; light colors highlight.*

Work it out for yourself—if you haven't much "lid," use a light color to emphasize what little you have. If your eyes tend to protrude, use dark colors, but highlight with a spot of *white* under the eyebrow to bring brow bone into prominence.

□ *Eye shadow* (whoever thought of the word goes to the top of the class) comes in cream, liquid, or powder form, and all give best results when applied with a brush.

□ A *cream shadow* gives a moist soft look but is apt to smear and smudge unless you have a practiced hand.

□ *Powder* is long-lasting and easier to apply.

□ *Liquid shadow* is lighter but still long-lasting if put on with care.

When it comes to liquid or cake eye liners (not used so much since the introduction of the fat easy pencil), both need practice. Lines should *never* be the object, rather soft blurs or smudged dots to add a smoky look. Cake liner is easier to use than liquid, and lasts longer if the brush is dipped in hot rather than cold water.

Mascara is vital and for best results should be painted on each lash separately, working from the root up, using only the wand tip. For bottom lashes it's best to work *down* with tip used vertically.

If you're timid about eye makeup, start slowly—and try only the most subtle effects—patting on color with the index finger, gently stretching eyelid skin away from the nose to color only over the eyeball. Always stroke shadow *up* toward the crease or brow, and avoid moving beyond eye shape until you're experienced.

To prevent shadow "creasing" on the lid, delicately pat eyelid skin with toner first, to make sure there's no natural oil lurking there. Use a powder shadow rather than a cream and set it by dusting over lightly with translucent powder.

FACING PAGE
Today, the eyes have it.

Try to use liner only in lash line to create an effect of lushness and

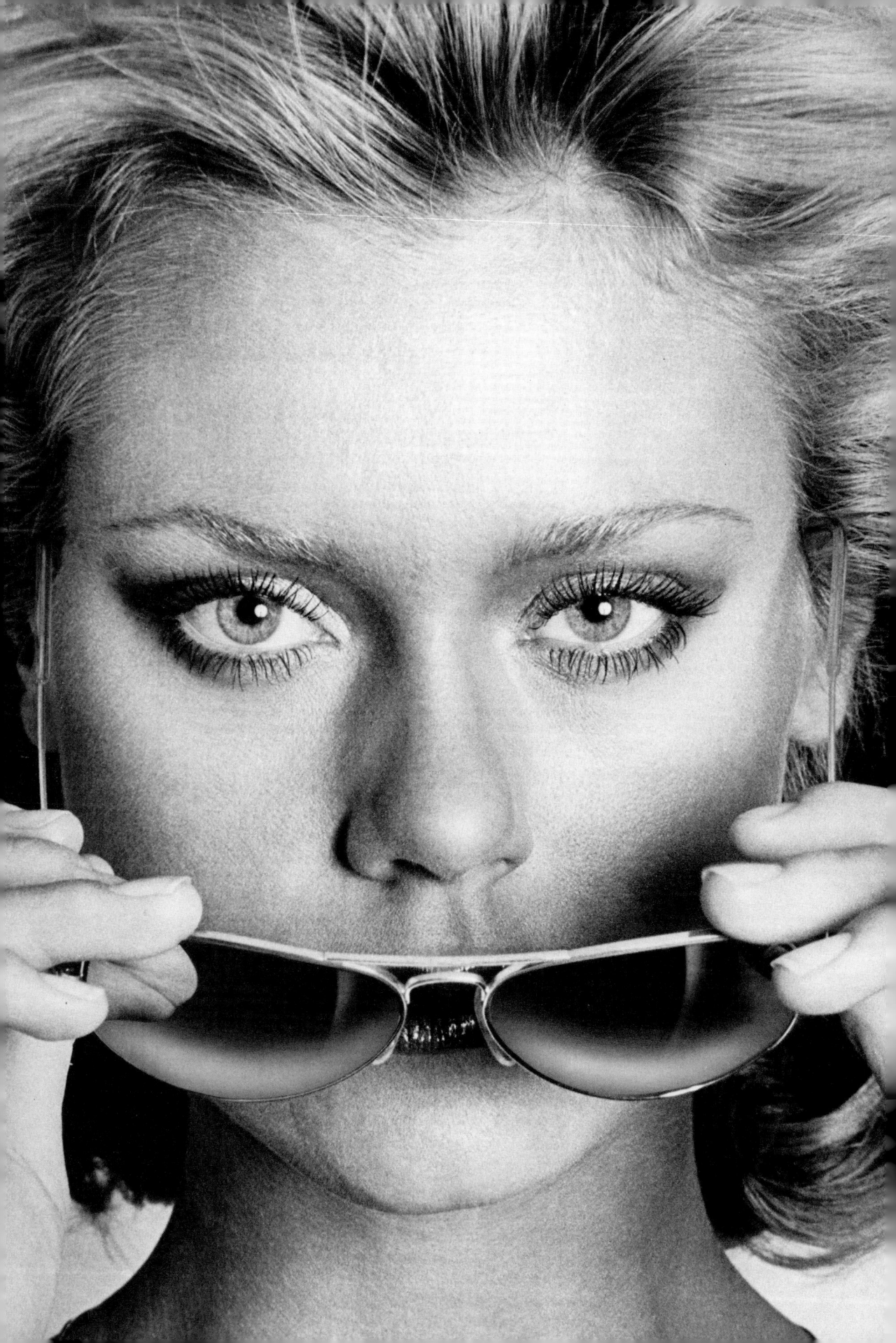

thickness. Use a color deeper than your natural eye color, yet still in direct relation to it. Hold the brush parallel, and for softness always break or blur the line you make, stopping at eye corners.

□ *For small eyes,* use a bright shadow on upper lid only, close to lashes, drawing a fine line along upper lashes, finishing before the inner corner, extended very slightly at outer corner. On the outer upper lashes use a lash-lengthening mascara or a small swatch of false lashes.

□ *For very round eyes,* apply shadow only *above* the crease toward the brows. Use liner above top lashes, thickening line at outer corners, sweeping it slightly upward—use mascara more heavily on outer lashes.

□ *For eyes too close together,* blend eye shadow so that it is *deeper,* darker at the *outer sides of the lids* to give an impression of width. Using a light base beneath brows also gives an illusion of width, plus a thicker line drawn above upper lashes starting about a third of the way along to the outer corners. Eyebrows could be slightly thinner toward the nose to make more "space," too.

□ *Where eyes protrude,* dark shadow should be applied right up to the brows.

□ *Where eyes are deep set,* a light shadow should be used above crease all the way to the brows, a darker shadow on lids.

If you hate false lashes (which most models rely on for "instant plus"), curl your own with a lash curler, available at any drugstore, remembering to apply lots of mascara once they're curled.

If you want to try false lashes, use a trick from another makeup maestro—Nicholas Guercio. He instructs his customers this way:

"Hold lashes in an outstretched hand and think of them as a plane coming into land. Bring hand in slowly, steadily at eye level to 'land' lashes in place. It's extraordinary, but this movement makes putting lashes on easier than if you crouch over a mirror, using little movements.

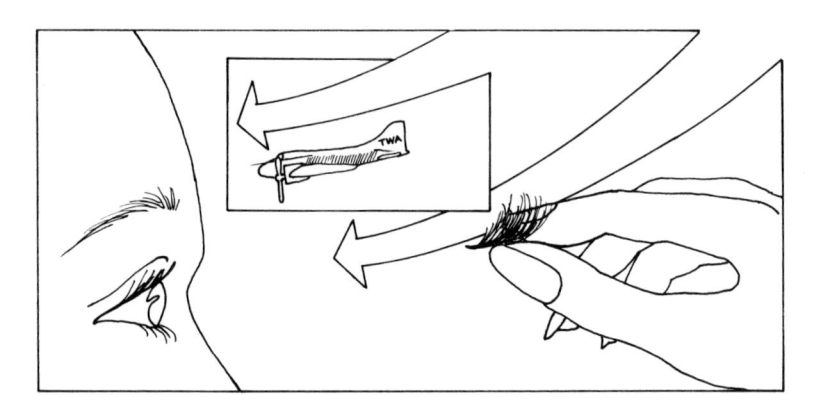

"Of course, first you must apply adhesive to the lashes—and some lashes may need trimming as they tend to be made extra long to suit all eye shapes. Adhesive should be applied with a toothpick *sparingly*. You should aim to 'land' your lashes on the center of the natural lash line, gently pressing them into an arc shape and into place with fingertips."

Individual lashes *can* be put on at home, but except in the case of professional models, look better when an expert is in control.

Special Eye Tricks from Vogue

An easy way to ensure eye makeup comes out looking pretty and soft starts with a dotted line of soft brown pencil drawn along the bottom lashes, lightly smudged in with fingertips until almost invisible. You'll be surprised to see how this immediately makes eyes appear fuller, prettier. Continue by lining the upper lid from corner to corner, this time keeping to the top lash line with the same pencil, being careful not to extend the line beyond eye shape. Stop at the last lash to make the eye look wide-open.

If your hand is shaky, start the line at the inner corner of the eye to the center, then from the outer corner in to meet it—then softly blur all together.

Shadow should start at the eye's inner corner, keeping close to the top lashes, and not carried above the crease or fanned out toward the brow. Cover the lid with a taupe color—it suits most colorings—or something you *know* suits you, then blend a little white in under the brows—all this to open up the eyes and make them look "smiling."

You can never use too much mascara, and dark brown is prettier than black for day, except for the really black-haired senoritas. The cake variety gives a very lush look, providing you let each coat dry, building up lashes to look thick and beautiful.

If you prefer to use eye liner instead of pencil, start by pulling your eyelid taut at the outer corner and work from the inner one, keeping close to lash root. Use small strokes, and make sure before you begin that your brush has no loose ends, has a fine, small but not sharp point. *The right equipment is all important.*

At night, retrace your steps, using *eye makeup that is stronger, more dominant.* Use a colored, iridescent shadow in place of the taupe, either blending color up toward the outer corner of the brow in a diagonal shape, or add a slightly lighter color at the crease to move toward the brow.

One trick is to use dark-brown cake eye liner diluted with water, to create a light-brown "wash"; brushed all over between crease and brow, it gives a more delicate effect than that achieved with pencil or powder. A touch of gold beneath the brow looks gala; then finish with lashings of black mascara—better for all colorings at night, even the lightest blondes.

The New Importance of the Brow

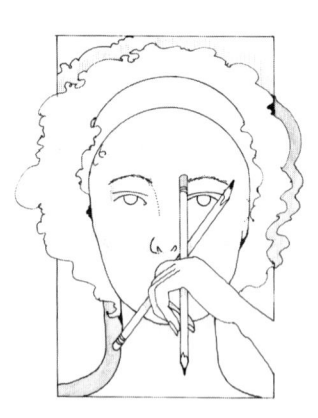

A clean light brow is essential if eye makeup is to get off to a great start—and the most "natural"-looking brow is the answer, with no straggly ends. The brow shape you were born with may not, however, be the best "natural" shape for you. Eyebrows count a lot where eye makeup is concerned—so check yours out with an expert if you can, or if not, try the pencil trick to determine whether you have the perfect shape for your face. Look in the mirror and hold a pencil vertically in front of your face, so that one end touches your nostril—the other end (if held straight) is where your brow *should* begin. To check where your brow should end hold pencil out at 45° from the nostril to your brow. The other end of the pencil points to where your brow should end.

To check brow curve, look dead straight into the mirror—the highest point of your brow should be directly above the pupil of your eye.

Don't draw harsh lines on your brows. Use short, close-together strokes with a soft brown or grey pencil.

Don't tweeze eyebrows from above.

Don't cut them with scissors or tweeze the wrong way—follow the way each hair grows.

SPECIAL TIP: Sandra Linter, one of the few top *female* makeup artists, first learned her craft selling makeup at Bloomingdale's. Now she is an integral part of many *Vogue* photo sessions, making up many of the models you see on the fashion and beauty pages. Sandra is an innovator, believes brunettes should wear dark plums and aubergine shadows for day, bronzes and deep golds at night, while blondes should go for auburn or rose tones on the eyes. She says redheads can get away with "the whole metallurgic bit from copper to bronze to gold"—not yet to tin. Redheads with pale lashes need plenty of mascara and liner; they can wear yellow shadows, particularly the frosted variety, although most other colorings shouldn't try it.

The Best Natural Finish—Powder

Powder is with us again—better than ever—often encapsulated, where all sorts of moisturized benefits are "encapsuled" within each tiny grain, breaking invisibly on the skin as powder is applied, adding a dewiness instead of a "powdered" look to makeup.

Because pigmented powders tend to change color when in contact with some skin oils (oh, the horrors of that faint orange moustache as touch-up follows touch-up at the theatre in the dark!), a better touch-up choice is the transparent kind, unchanged by skin's oils, giving instant luminosity. Powder should always be one or two tones lighter than your base.

A powder puff is still the best applicator, helping powder cling without smudging. It should be used lavishly at the end of all coloring, then brushed off with a fine sable brush, enabling makeup to stay intact all day, so that even if perspiration and skin oil shine through, they don't spoil anything.

To touch up too often—even with translucent powder—takes away makeup's fresh edge. Far better to blot with a tissue, or if possible, give the face a quick spray with atomized water to freshen up literally. Skin is always thirsty, especially in the city.

Powder has the added advantage of reflecting light, so that tiny lines become less visible, which means at night it really comes into its own. It doesn't matter if skin type is dry. Powder today is generally moisturized.

Pressed powder is a neat portable idea, but when a base is incorporated with the powder, it should be left at home on the dressing table as, obviously, it's not good for touch-ups—an accumulation of base and powder looks stale and certainly doesn't help the health of the skin. Pressed powders without base are meant to be taken along on the trip for touch-ups when you need them.

To go gala all the way, a pearlized or gilded powder gives a superb luminous effect, especially when blusher is pearlized, too. And to correct too much ruddiness in the complexion, choose powder that's pale green—it works like a charm.

When you really want your makeup to last around the clock—on that still-too-long flight to Australia, for instance—*press* in your powder (the encapsulated kind is perfect) with a slight twisting movement rather than just casually brushing it on. This *presses* home the fact it's meant to stay and stay—unless you're a crybaby. The chemical composition of tears is a sure annihilator of any makeup, pressed in or otherwise.

How to Make Your Lips Seductive

Lipstick is still a very important accessory, and likely to stay that way. We need lipstick, for the mouth is a very seductive part of the face and extra color there proves it.

Whether you like a creamy, opaque, translucent, or pearlized lipstick, working with a brush is key. The most *lasting* form of lip color is first with an opaque stick, followed by pearlized color or gloss.

If you like pale lip colors, cover the mouth with one shade, but add a gloss or darker shade in the *middle of the mouth only*. It's sexy.

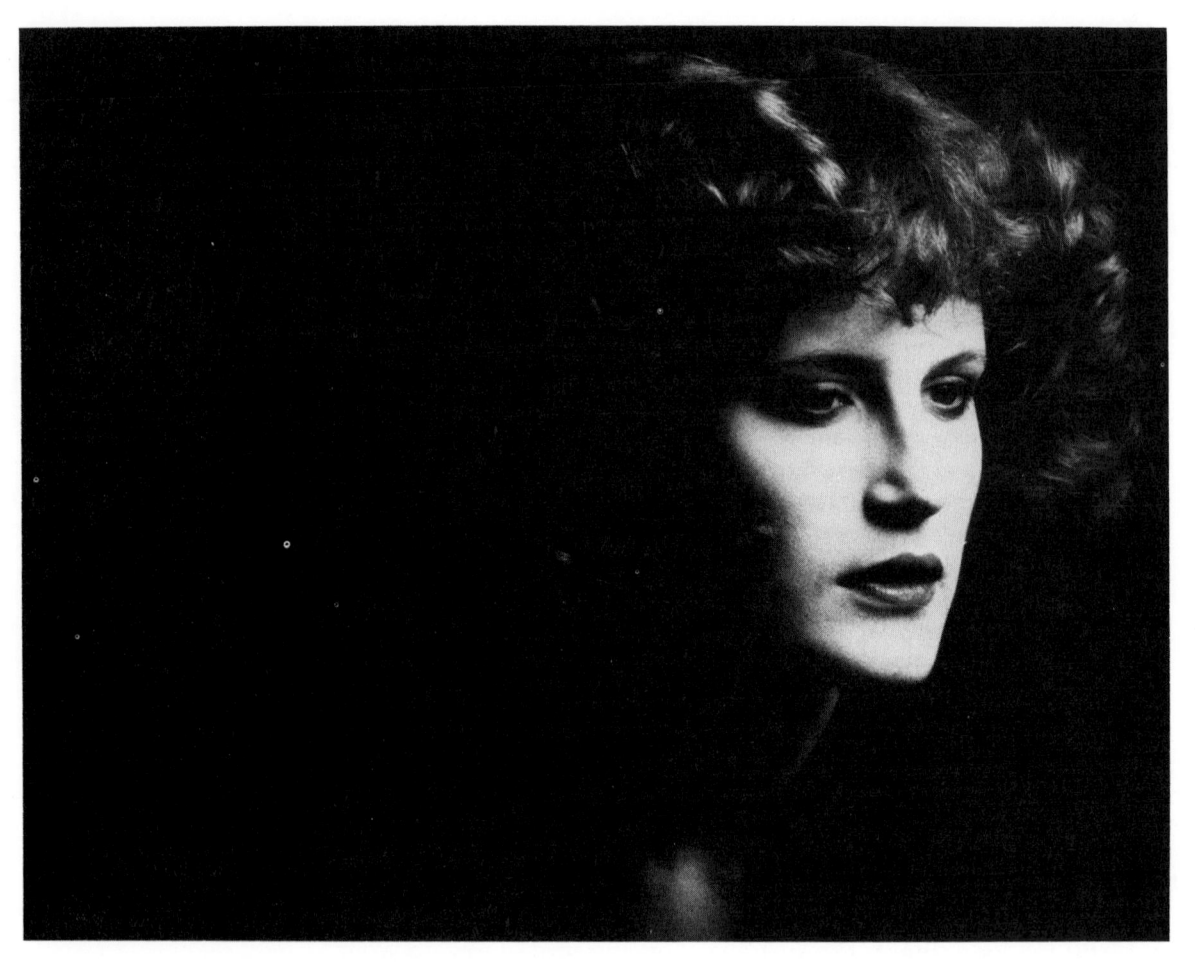

A lip brush is the key to making better lip shape.

If you like dark colors, line lips with a dark shade, using a brighter one to fill in and gloss the middle of the mouth. That's sexy, too.

For a bright *vivid* mouth, fill lips with the *brightest* color, then coat with gloss to soften.

Sometimes you might add lipstick color *over* gloss instead of the other way around—starting from the center to the inside edge of upper and lower lips, just as if you were sucking a red Popsicle. Start with a little, then add as much color as you like to intensify. If handled correctly, the color blends, so no hard edges are noticeable.

A lip liner is useful, and when it's a pencil, it's child's play to outline, preventing smudging or seepage of color into fine lines that can be around the mouth. If you're an apprentice with a lip brush, pencils are easier to handle and practice with—until you graduate to a brush.

The reason a brush is so key is simple. It can follow mouth contour easily and exactly or, if that isn't all it should be, invent a new mouth contour without any strange blurred lines or smudges.

Making Mouths Pretty

For a soft pretty mouth, coat lips with lip balm (winter and summer, too), let set, then wipe off—flaky unwanted skin goes, too. Next, outline the mouth with a pale lip color (Ideally you need a brush for this so that the "highlight" appears around the rim to make mouth fuller, richer). The final appealing touch—a bright, transparent color in the middle of the mouth, plus another coat of shimmering gloss on top.

Easy Tips

□ *If your face is small,* don't exaggerate your mouth. Remember to keep the highest points of the upper lip (the "cupid's bow") within the area defined by the outer edges of the nostrils. Make sure lower lip is not fuller than upper lip at the corners—the mouth should have fullness in the middle.

□ *If your face is large,* outline mouth on the outer rim of the natural mouth with bright color—only gloss inside.

□ *If your face is long,* keep width in the mouth from corner to corner rather than any fullness from top to bottom. Avoid any indent or "bow" on the top lip.

□ *If jawline is heavy,* paint mouth wide with more color in the middle than at the sides.

□ *If lips are too thin,* round upper lip and make middle indentation shallow. Extend upper lip slightly out beyond natural corners, then bring lower lip up and out to meet corners of the new upper outline.

□ *If lips are too thick,* outline mouth *inside* natural shape. Use a darker shade on top lip, lighter on the bottom.

□ *Mouth too sad?* Accentuate "bow" and slightly extend color up and out on lower lip. Use a bright shade with a touch of gloss dead center in the upper lip.

SPECIAL TIP: Mary Tyler Moore sprays mouth color with atomized mineral water to keep color looking "dewy" through the day.

Colors for the Black Skin

Makeup has to be special, for Black skin is special. For instance, there are thirty-five variations of basic shadings in makeup colors for Black skin, only twelve for white.

Bases and powders formulated for white skin are no good for Black, because of the fillers that can turn dark skins grey, while other filler substances like umber can turn Black skin unnaturally red or yellow.

The solution was a long time coming, but finally a whole range of cosmetics for Black women arrived—created by Black women who knew exactly what was needed. Glamorous actress Barbara Walden was one of the first to launch a line, and it's said that six-foot Black model Naomi Sims, one of the most exotic-looking women in the world, will bring out a specialized line, too.

Because Black women have a *natural* bronze tone, they don't really *need* much foundation, but they do need to give their skin a lot of care—particularly in winter, when they often wear an overcoat of moisturizer to help prevent their skin from turning grey from the cold, while in summer a sun block is necessary to prevent uneven dark patches developing.

To even up Black skin tone—the main problem—a deep bronze gel is often the best answer, plus a tan powder brushed over the middle of the face, between brows, around the nose and mouth—to take right away any grey notes, while a bright-red cream rouge blended around the cheeks above the brows and on the forehead add the sort of "big glow" the Black girl can get away with.

Her eye makeup has to be bold, imaginative to live up to her exotic skin color. She can wear the most vivid turquoise, emerald, and grass-green liners, gold-flecked bronze and beige shadows under the brows *and* lightly under the eyes—all to reflect the vivid pupils that most Black women have.

Lips look better out of the conventional bright reds and into the transparent chestnuts or coppers, softened with pink gloss, outlined in auburn or glossed over with the Black woman's favorite (the dermatologists' favorite, too), petroleum jelly, followed by a touch of bronze gel on top. It sounds sticky, but it can look devastating.

Beverly Johnson is a top model with light Black skin who outlooks most models away from the camera because she is so outstandingly beautiful. (Many models, top and otherwise, as I may have inferred, aren't beautiful at all in real life—the camera "creates" beauty through the magic of its lens.)

Because many Black women have dry skin—not, as is erroneously thought, oily (see page 32)—Beverly is a nonstop moisturizer, carefully and lavishly applying a plant-based moisturizer from the bosom up to her forehead before a touch of makeup goes on.

A regular trick she uses is to apply a stark-white highlighter on eyelids, under eye area, on nose bridge, and just above upper lip—all to "lift" areas she feels need it. Beverly brushes on a soft-brown shadow to widen her brows and eye shape, drawing a line half in brown, half in white on the *inside* of her lower lids.

She likes to use lipstick for paint jobs other than her lips. On her eyes particularly she likes to apply a plum lipstick all over the lids, then on the forehead, cheeks, and chin, blending color here outward on both sides to decrease her chin width.

"Using a powder on top of a cream stops color fading" is Beverly's belief. After working for ten hours a day for weeks on end in the world's major studios, she should know. . . . *Another regular trick:* she always whisks transparent powder *all over her face* except her eyelids to give a together look.

SPECIAL TIP: After Beverly Johnson's mascara has dried, she curls her lashes with a drugstore curler, then adds a touch of *black honey lip gloss* to the ends of the lashes to deliver a beautiful glossy look.

This is the way Beverly likes to make up, which she has to do six days out of seven, and often several times a day for each photography session. Some of her tips will apply to you, some not, for the question of "how to make up" is not one that can have a simple, rubber-stamped answer.

Apart from the fact that new ideas, new colors, new methods of application, happen everyday, all of us have to discover how best to *adapt* these new ideas for ourselves. But makeup can improve everyone—it's a lot to do with practice.

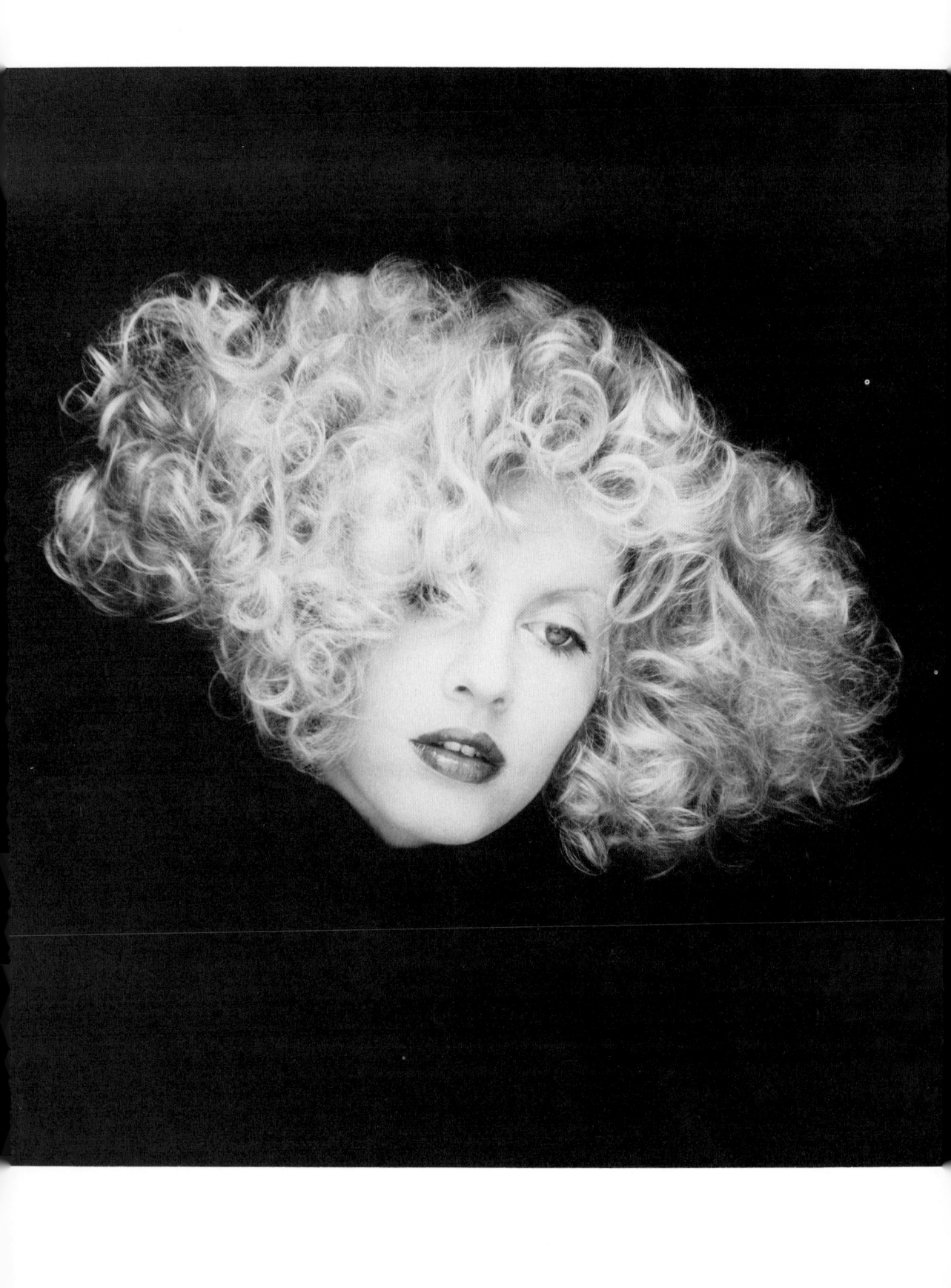

4

Hair

Our Best Asset with a Little Care

Our hair can be our most reliable asset, *if* we give it the loving care it deserves. It doesn't "break out" as skin does when our plans go awry. It doesn't sag the way the body does when age catches up with our muscles. As Kenneth, one of the noblest practitioners of hair care, style, and color, says, "Hair's tensile strength is incredible. You wouldn't wear a skirt or dress every day for three or four years and expect it to be in good shape; yet hair, whipped by the wind, polluted by the atmosphere, dried by the sun, is expected to look great after only one shampoo and set and stay that way."

Hairdressers with a conscience believe women still make too many demands on their hair without giving it proper care, and that is why it *seems* to let them down.

FACING PAGE
Healthy hair—the first requisite for any style today.

"You shouldn't demand from your hair more than it can do," says New York stylist François, another name up in lights as far as model girls and editors are concerned. François is a stylist who can transform anyone's looks for the better—but he refuses to deliver any hairstyle *on demand*—if he doesn't think hair can stand it—however illustrious the client.

This attitude is gaining ground for the most valid reason in the world—hair health, ironically the most attractive selling concept in the hair business today.

Hair health is sweeping the beauty world as the New Look swept into fashion back in 1948. Condition comes before style, cut, and color; in fact, hair's *condition* is now *the* basis for the style—uncontrived, untortured, free, unfettered.

How did it happen? Because the bouffant, backcombed jobs of the 1960s had to topple as soon as the new, easy, carefree clothes came in, accompanied by the more natural look in makeup.

The *fiber* is what counts, as more and more women realize—from Cher, who wears hers thick and straight to the small of her back; to the Queen of England, who hasn't changed her simple style in nearly thirty years; to her sister, Princess Margaret, who cuts and grows, cuts and grows, according to fashion, but who now wouldn't dream of going without her monthly hair-condition check-up and treatment.

How to Look after Your Crop

It isn't called a crop for nothing. Hair *is* a crop as dependent upon the food you eat for its structure and well-being as is sugarcane upon the rain and sun. Sugarcane has to worry about the soil in which it's planted. You have to worry about the state of your follicles—a hundred thousand of them, slightly more for blondes, slightly less for redheads—from which every hair on your head emanates. Poor follicles and your crop will be poor, showing in a variety of miserable ways.

How your hair looks right this minute also depends on the sort of hair your great-grandmamma had, for inheritance plays a big part.

Today more and more dermatologists ascribe women's hair condition to the way women think, pointing out links to emotion, extra responsibilities, stress—all factors, they say, in how much shine and bounce your hair has or hasn't.

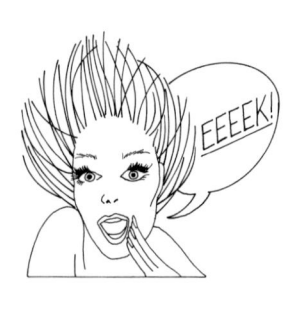

All of us, male or female, start out at birth with a full complement of follicles; each follicle has a blood supply and a muscle, and it's this muscle that causes our hair to stand on end and our skin to pucker into gooseflesh whenever we're scared to death—a primitive defense mechanism inherited from our hairy ancestors, who, just like frightened animals, increased their bulk significantly whenever their fur stood on end! Each follicle produces one hair that grows upward from an area called the papilla, where the hair bulb and root are located.

Unlike some mammals, our hair follicles follow a cycle independently of each other. While some hairs are growing, others are falling out, and it's not abnormal to lose up to a hundred hairs a day. Whether your hair grows quickly or not, again depends on your ancestors.

The usual life-span of a hair is in the region of three to four years—and its life is divided into three stages: (1) anagen, the growing stage, about three years long to reach full growth; (2) catagen, the regression period, lasting about two weeks; then (3) telogen, the last stage, when the follicle becomes dormant for about three months before the hair falls out, to be replaced immediately by an anagen—growing stage—growing on the average about half an inch a month.

On the scalp, the growing stage is long and the resting stage is short: 90 percent of the hair is growing, while 10 percent is resting, a situation that fortunately is reversed on the body.

The three-way cycle operates for each of the hundred thousand hair follicles about fifteen to twenty times before it starts to slow down and malfunction, having the same limited capacity to regenerate as any of our other body processes. This is the law of aging, whether we like it or not, differing from individual to individual according to genes and hormones—and depending on *how much care we give ourselves.*

Although the follicles act independently, they're all affected by outside stimuli, so for climatic reasons more hairs are shed in March and April than at any other time, the lowest amount in July, one reason hairdressers "with a conscience"—the name I give the caring ones—deter their clients from having their hair cut at that time.

Hair Fallout

Keeping your hair has become as controversial as keeping your cool. Hair loss can be temporary ("reversible" as the dermatologists put it) or permanent. In the temporary cases, it means the follicle is still alive, so there's hope of a new hair.

A number of reasons are responsible for the warning signal of more hair left behind on the brush than there should be.

The innocent-looking ponytail can produce a temporary spot baldness, providing medical terminology with a new label, "traction alopecia," where the prolonged pulling of hair back into one position causes inflammation on or below the scalp's surface, invisible to the naked eye. If the ponytail is worn constantly, the inflammation eventually hinders normal growth. The injured hair gives up the struggle, breaks off, perhaps to be replaced during the next cycle, perhaps not. If breakage is continual, the hair bulb and papilla on which the hair is

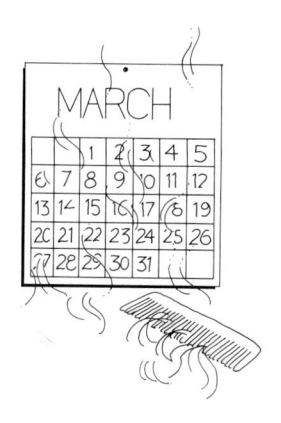

1 YEAR   3 YEARS   5 YEARS

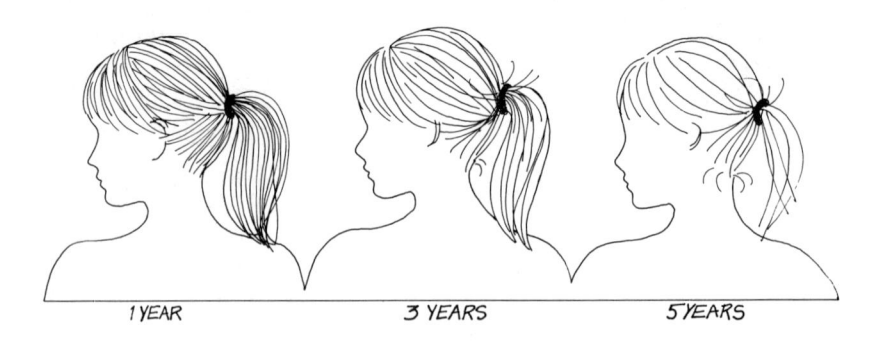

lodged shrinks, dries up, stops manufacture of new hair. Sometimes a new hair breaks through, but it will be thinner in texture, dull and brittle. The reason the ponytail is a potential hazard to hair health is that its success depends on the degree of *tightness* that can be achieved with ribbon, barrette, or worst of all, elastic band. *The strain on the hair can be intolerable.*

After studying twenty-four cases of traction alopecia, Dr. Albert Slepyan, Clinic Professor of Dermatology at the University of Illinois, reported, "Once the ponytail was abandoned in favor of a more relaxed hairdo, there was complete regrowth of scalp hair in every case except two. In these two instances, there was some return of new hair, but after six months the remaining bald spots on the sides and back were taken to be permanent." Scary, to say the least, so beware of too much traction—even when you use heated rollers. Hair curled up too tightly too often is harmful.

Continuous hair-straightening, overvigorous brushing, excessive intake of vitamin A, overbleaching, overperming, over*anything* that isn't a natural way of life for the hair is harmful, too, and means *hair damage*. The irony is that statistics show we really inflict the greatest hair damage on ourselves.

The Pill Is a Pill

The effect of the Pill on hair (and skin, see pages 17–18) is still under investigation. A few years back Dr. Frank Cormia, of Cornell University Medical College in New York, presented a series of papers showing that women who had taken the Pill over a long period of time found their hair had thinned. After further observation, Dr. Cormia divulged, however, that hair loss was greater a month or so after they *stopped* taking it.

He drew a parallel between women on, then off the Pill with those who *after* having a baby experience sudden hair loss, reasoning that just as pregnancy increases *estrogen hormone* production, helping to prevent baldness, similarly the Pill keeps hormone levels high.

When pregnancy is over or the Pill is abandoned, the hair cycle eventually returns to normal, but begins by rapidly producing the telogen and last phase of the hair cycle when hair is shed.

If you take drugs or any medicine, then suffer from hair loss, the two things could be related. If the problem warrants a visit to a dermatologist, even aspirin intake should be recorded—it could have a bearing on the problem.

Women Are Losing More Hair

The amount of hair you lose you may be able to blame on your grandparents—for heredity has a long reach. Your parents may have had thick heads of hair; their parents may not—and it could be *their* unwanted "hair-loss genes" that have been passed on to you.

Age is another factor in hair loss—age and menopause, when women start to produce less female hormone, but go on producing the same amount of male hormone, about two thirds the amount men do. Because the hormonal balance is disturbed, some women find themselves losing hair faster.

Hair loss among women is on the increase—that fact dermatologists have noted over the past decade—ten times as many cases a week being the conservative estimate.

A group of keen doctors have an answer for it. Their research is based on their theory that women are making more male hormone since they assumed male attitudes, responsibilities, and tensions under the banner of women's liberation.

More androgen, says the dermatologist, and the more women will suffer from "the hitherto mainly masculine privilege of baldness."

The normal ratio of hormones in a woman's body is one part androgen (male hormone) to eight parts estrogen (female hormone), the estrogen giving her fine skin and high resistance to hair loss—only 5 percent of women ever go bald.

As Dr. Irwin Lubowe, Clinical Professor of Dermatology at New York Medical College and one of the prime believers in the women's lib theory, explains, "Once that ratio is disturbed, the genetic force takes over. In the case of the woman making excessive androgen, it means the male side of the family tree dominates. If her father or grandfather had a disposition toward baldness, the rate of her hair fallout can surpass the normal rate of regrowth or replacement."

Not every dermatologist goes along with this point of view, but it is agreed that extra *stress* results in an output of androgen which, in turn, affects hair follicles, causing a noticeable change in the hair cycle.

What Can Be Done About Hair Loss?

Dr. Lubowe is optimistic about counteracting the bald facts—eventually for both sexes. Every one of his patients is given a thorough examination, which includes a thyroid test, kidney, calcium, enzyme, and liver studies plus, in the case of female patients, an Estrogen Maturation Index (commonly called E.M.I.), a vaginal smear that tells whether the body is secreting enough estrogen.

A scalp injection aimed at breaking the genetic tie that may develop when a woman produces excess androgen is in the experimental stage. So is an anti-androgen pill to neutralize excessive male hormone output without producing extreme femininity.

The medically approved method of transplantation, pioneered by Dr. Norman Orentreich, is forging ahead, although the situation isn't easy—donor hair is sparse, while baldness is extensive.

Dr. Orentreich's method involves transferring small circular scalp plugs from an area where hair flourishes to an area where it doesn't. Some patients have responded well, others only fair so far, but it can be a viable proposition helped along by injecting small amounts of steroid every month into the transplanted sites.

Research is also going on involving transplants from a healthy scalp to an ailing one, hoping for the day when this kind of treatment can be successfully carried out on any two people with the same color and type of hair.

The Egyptians wrote they had a sure cure for hair loss: "Rub into the scalp a mixture of equal parts of crocodile, lion, hippopotamus, and serpent fat." Unfortunately, there's still no modern product any more effective in *curing* baldness, BUT, according to Dr. Orentreich, the cure may be only years away now, not decades.

Help Your Hair Yourself

What you eat affects the way your hair looks and feels. There's a simple reason: for each hair growing out of the scalp, there's a blood supply feeding the papilla, the blood converted into energy to produce that hair. The success of the output—the difference between a poor and a strong hair—depends on whether your diet is nutritious or not.

According to the most recent research, for the papilla to manufacture perfectly healthy hairs at least one hundred grams of protein should be a daily part of your diet.

Another nutrient for beautiful hair: yeast pills (vitamin B). No-no's: excess sugar, salt, animal fat.

If you have baby-fine, impossible-to-set hair, your hair bulb may not be getting the right sustenance. Add more nutrition to your diet for starters.

Once the hair becomes visible on the scalp's surface, it's an appendage, not fed by anything internally—commonly referred to as "dead"—subjected to the environment, and to the lotions and potions we apply to it.

First requisite: a healthy diet to grow healthy hair.

Second requisite: protection for hair against an environment that can take away all of its healthy qualities through exposure to pollution, salt water, chlorinated water, air-conditioning, steam heat, and too much sun. Now there is a product specifically devised by Helena Rubinstein to *protect* hair from all of the dangers just mentioned.

The important thing is to match your hair products to your hair type and to hair behavior. Choose your shampoo with as much care as you choose your eye makeup and think of a conditioner as part of your hair-care program.

Positively pH

This little symbol means hydrogen potential. It's mentioned more and more in relation to hair-care products these days because pH is the measurement used to determine hair's level of acidity versus alkalinity—and, incidentally, nearly every substance from raindrops to tomatoes.

New hair has a *normal* pH—between 4.0 and 6.0—which means it's mildly acidic, good-looking, and *naturally* shiny, showing the minimum structural damage.

Maintaining the acid mantle—which produces this condition through proper care, the right choice of products, and the right hair handling—is advantageous, because a contracted (acidic) cuticle reflects light (producing the true shine mentioned) and also provides 35 percent of the hair's elastic strength.

Many hair preparations like color treatments, permanents, straighteners, and some shampoos are alkaline, falling into the 7.0 to 10.0 range—some may be even higher.

With continued use of these high pH products, hair itself can rate a higher pH, become more alkaline and more porous. Instead of lying flat and close to the hair shaft, the cuticle scales open and expand to leave the inner structure more vulnerable. The hair swells when any moisture is applied, tends to feel "spongy," and is really prone to damage.

Hair is in serious trouble above 10.0 on the pH scale.

To illustrate the point, I only have to tell you that drain cleaners are able to *dissolve* clogging hair in the pipes completely when their pH level is far *above* this "safe" range.

This would infer that nonalkaline products with a low pH are the ones to buy.

As far as shampoos are concerned, the truth is you *need* some alkaline in order to *cleanse* well, so the ideal shampoo cleanses hair with alkaline compounds, but then adds acid factors to rid hair of dull residue and lower pH to "normal." This is what our mothers and grandmothers used to do when they followed soap shampoos with vinegar or lemon rinses for their acidic value. Read the label on the shampoo before you buy it—pH rating you now know, is important.

Feed Your Hair

As electronic radioactive studies have proved, hair *can* absorb protein and needs protein, too, for its health and strength. Choose shampoos and conditioners with protein or collagen (a good source of protein) built in—and know they're good for your hair.

Do You Know Your Hair Type?

Dry or oily—between the two? Doctors aren't too sure our self-analysis is always (a) correct, (b) helpful. They point out that subjective observations are frequently impossible to substantiate—fine thin hair often showing oiliness faster than coarse thick hair—although both may not accurately be described as "oily."

The condition of the scalp relates directly to the health and *look of the hair,* and although scalp skin is quite similar to the skin on the rest of the body, the glandular secretions are more profuse, allowing sebum from the sebaceous glands to cover both scalp and hair.

A certain amount of natural oils is vital for hair and scalp protection, and the aqueous sebum from the sweat gland is normal and functional.

Oily Hair

Oily hair simply means *too much* oil is secreted and combines with sebum to provide too good a nest for bacteria.

As a result of all this excess oil production, there's the problem of dandruff. When it's more forbiddingly described as seborrheic dermatitis, it means there's inflammation around the oil glands of the papilla or base of the hair, causing itchiness, redness, scaliness, white flakiness. It can be kept under control with products containing tars, zinc, or sulphur, but what happens after a period of time is that a dandruff sufferer can build up resistance to one product, so should switch to another.

Psoriasis is sometimes mistaken for dandruff, but it is a far more serious state of affairs. Then the actual *cells* of the scalp turn over more rapidly than normal, the scalp becoming encrusted and blocked. Psoriasis needs medical help.

How to Cope With Oily Hair

Never brush it, only comb it with a wide-tooth comb.

Never wear a wool or fur beret or hat—this aggravates the condition, gives bacteria more encouragement to breed in a cozy, warm atmosphere.

Ozone is good for oily hair. Dip it in sea water.

Backcomb roots to allow air to penetrate scalp.

Don't shampoo too often. Overwashing promotes greasiness.

Use only lukewarm water. Hot water activates the already overactive sebaceous glands. Only one lathering. Lots of rinses.

Don't be dictated to by your hair, washing it according to how you think it looks. Establish a hair-control program. Wash your hair every three days at the same time if you can.

Choose products formulated to control the amount of sebum released—mild, soapless, herbal-based shampoos.

Avoid any tight curling either with heated rollers or pins.

Avoid effervescent drinks, high carbohydrate intake, cheese, nuts, egg yolk, fats.

Eat more spinach and watercress (iron), egg white, fruit; drink plenty of skimmed milk.

Between shampoos wipe your scalp with cotton soaked in a clear medicated lotion if you feel itchy. An astringent formulated for oily *skin* will do nicely.

Towel dry rather than blow dry if you can, but if not, always use the blow dryer on "low."

Once a week massage your scalp, starting at the back of your head, placing both hands against the scalp and gently rotating skin. Repeat at sides, crown, and forehead, then "walk" fingertips (not nails) over the scalp making small circles with the fingers at each location until you've covered all the ground. A dandruff preparation can be applied as you massage, but hair should then be combed through and shampooed.

Use a nonoil-based conditioner (read the labels!) or a pack of refined clay that coats hair, helps to give it body and become less porous. If hair isn't too fragile, an oily condition can benefit from henna, coating hair to give it body. As it also adds color, henna should only be used three times a year. Otherwise, color buildup can produce too harsh an effect. A vinegar rinse is good for oily hair.

Dry Hair

Dry hair signifies a poor oil supply from the scalp and a lack of moisture in the hair. As hair's norm is only 3 percent moisture to 97 percent protein, it can't afford to lose one drop.

If hair is dry, skin is probably dry, too, or hair can become dry from lack of care. Too many treatments, permanents, tinting, or bleaching jobs, shampoos that overclean and strip hair of its natural oils—all these things can dry hair and spoil it. Too much sun, wind—wind blowing hair particularly in an open car—and overheated air are harmful, too. Dryness means hair will not be easy to manage, is flyaway, supercharged with electricity. It's telling you it needs help.

How to Cope with Dry Hair

Use a shampoo designed to remove soil but not natural oils, incorporating lanolin or other fats. Pure castile soaps have high oil content, so are good for dry types; so is camomile.

Use only the mildest shampoos and a big sponge for washing, gentler than fingers on the hair, better able to flood it with water.

Brush, but only with natural bristles, never nylon and only for a short while each evening, to distribute natural oils evenly throughout the head. Brushing also boosts circulation by "massaging" scalp. Forget about one hundred strokes a night; they are positively bad for thin, fine, or damaged hair.

Match bristle to hair type—soft for soft, stiffer for thick.

Brush by bending over, up and out from nape, again as a circulation booster.

Never brush hair when wet. It stretches, then breaks.

Oil hair the night before a salon visit. Try mink oil—it's good.

Use products after shampoos that calm flyaway ends and add shine and luster, coating hair with a water-soluble barrier thus offering protection from the elements, especially harmful to dry brittle hair.

Use a conditioner regularly after a shampoo. Conditioners help make the hair cuticle (outer layer) smooth, manageable, and neutralize any excess alkaline residue left over from shampoos.

Replacement of moisture balance gives hair shine, adds various humectants, decreases split ends by reducing friction between one hair and its neighbor.

For extra benefit, use conditioners that aim for deeper penetration of the scalp, aided and abetted by heat to dilate cuticle and set off a chemical action.

A head massage with warmed baby oil is helpful.

Saran Wrap is a useful ploy. Wrap it around hair that's saturated with baby oil or conditioner and secure with bobby pins. Grab more heat by covering "the parcel" with a shower cap or thick towel. Stay that way overnight if you can. Rinse thoroughly in the A.M. and dry with moderate heat.

To contain flyaway hair, use a setting lotion that deposits chemical resins on the hair, making it easy to separate strands, then hold hair in position when combed. Some give body by externally coating hair shaft, adding a "plumping" effect.

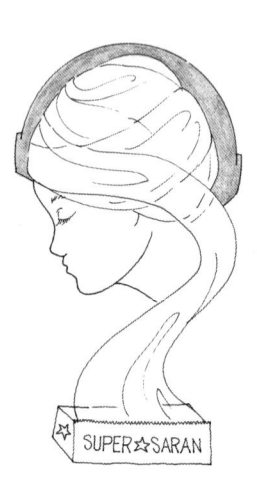

If hair is brittle, it can signify lack of protein. Apply protein externally, choosing an appropriate product, and internally by eating more better-class protein—meat, beef, eggs—green-leafed vegetables, vitamin B in supplement form as well as in natural foods.

Avoid spices, alcohol, too much carbohydrate.

Damaged Hair

When hair is damaged, the parting can give you your first clue, even before poor hair begins to show. The scalp looks grey, dingy, or unnaturally pink from irritation. An expert can *feel* when a scalp is not well. It feels tight from poor circulation, no elasticity, no movement.

Hair that refuses to take color or perms or falls out of shape in an hour may have your diet to thank for it. The wrong, low-nutrition diet means the hair bulb is not receiving the nutrients it needs to produce lovely hair, so it atrophies, causing improper formation of the hair cuticle, weakening hair shaft, leading to easy breakage, or at the very least, hair with no stamina. Even premature grey can be caused by a missing link in the nutritional network—for grey is simply a sign of a poor pigment supply in the cortex.

How to Cope with Damaged Hair

First, whatever program you decide on—under expert supervision at a salon or at home—it has to be followed faithfully. Damaged hair is *sick* hair, and the patient won't recover if treatment is slapdash.

Intensive conditioning has to be the long-term part of the program, but first, hair should probably be trimmed. Damage is most noticeable at the ends, where the oldest hairs are.

Instead of a trim, a much shorter look may be the fastest route to healthy hair renewal. Getting rid of all the old, weak hair, to replace it with a sharp, new look—and new start.

For new hair to be healthy, it's vital to have plenty of blood rushing to the scalp—and an expert massage is one way to achieve this. One pair of healthy-hair–producing hands belongs to expert Don Lee, who believes knotted shoulder and neck muscles—which the majority of city dwellers have—cut off blood flow to the scalp. The capillaries constrict, the oil glands go haywire, and as he says, "the scalp comes down with a virus." If a scalp is smothered under layers of foreign material, it means the hair-growth cycle is interrupted or blocked.

After consultation, Don Lee's method of solving hair problems begins with a stupendous head, neck, and shoulder massage that lasts for about fifteen minutes. Then, depending on the problem—the scalp may need exfoliation—one of six variations of a special formula containing vitamin concentrates and organic substances is massaged into the hair with a miniature bristle brush. Polyunsaturated and water-soluble, all formulas get to the follicles where bacteria can cause a load of trouble. The finale is a fifteen-minute session under an electrically heated cap, enabling the special solution to go as deep as it can. The solution stays on when you leave his clinic to be washed out a few hours later at home with a mild, preferably baby, camomile, or herbal shampoo.

Regular conditioners are necessary to continue the good work, especially to bolster protein that binds the moisture in the hair shaft, reviving damaged hair by smoothing down rough chipped surfaces.

Never rub damaged hair vigorously—or, for that matter, any hair—it snarls it unnecessarily. Instead, blot, pat, and dry on a *low* heat, never on a high one.

Avoid going bareheaded in cold weather—it gives hair the "shivers." Each hair shaft contains water, a speedy conductor of heat or cold, so outdoors on a freezing day, hair can get chilled, chapped;

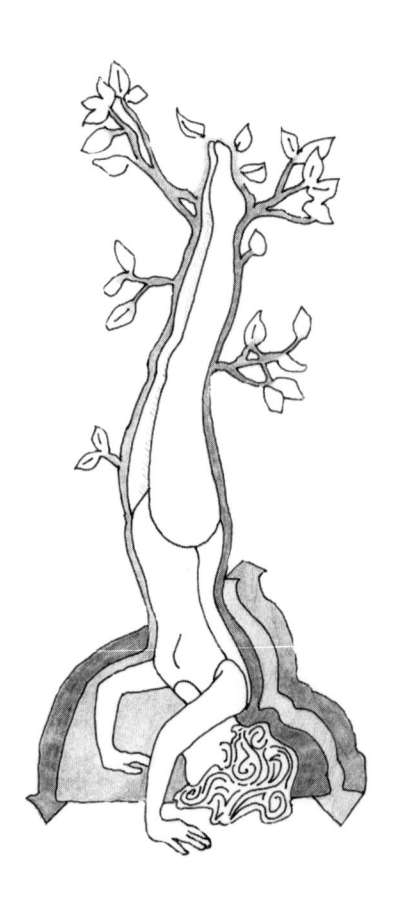

then when you go inside to a heated—often overheated—room, the sudden change can shock hair, and disrupt its moisture balance still further. Wearing a hat or scarf in very cold weather prevents this trauma, and maintains a good supply of blood and nutrients circulating to the scalp by keeping it warm.

Hair should be covered on hot days, too. It may not show sunburn, the way skin does, but hair can be burned, too.

A daily headstand does wonders for circulation, which in turn benefits hair, scalp, and skin, too. Remember, your blood flow is your beauty flow (see pages 22–28).

If hair is *really* hurt and so looks terrible, don't try to cover it up with a new color, a new perm. It will never work and can only cause more harm.

Never color and perm your hair the same week—there should be at least ten days between.

Avoid excessive quantities of vitamins A and D (sun), both capable of causing dry-scalp symptoms, inflamed hair follicles, leading to eventual hair loss.

Change your parting periodically to expose another section of your scalp. Give your hair a chance to hang free at least once every week.

Hair Boosters

The beautiful Baroness von Thyssen (Denise) has blonde hair a yard long that she washes regularly twice a week wherever she is—an arduous three-hour job. She believes her hair might not be so beautiful if she didn't give it a tremendous amount of attention—and she may be right. Extra-long hair is weak hair, because it has obviously been around quite a time. To ensure it always looks and feels its silky best, this young baroness relies on three hair experts, each of whom she visits several times a year: Philip Kingsley in London, Rita at Kenneth in New York, and the one she sees most frequently—Mademoiselle Mad in Paris. In her salon on the Fauborg St. Honoré M'selle Mad concocts all her own brews, treating the heads of many Paris-based beauties like model Marisa Berenson, society types like Susie Dyson, La Baronne de Rothschild, and Madame David Rothschild.

Hair's Secret Weapons

To build up hair strength, Mademoiselle Mad recommends her clients take intravenous or intramuscular shots of *Bépanthène* (panthenol) for twelve days every six months. The Baroness von Thyssen has been taking this advice for ages for the best reason—she finds it improves her hair out of all recognition. Why? *Bépanthène* is said to donate panthothenic acid—B_5—to the body, and B_5 is known as the antistress vitamin.

A lack of panthothenic acid can lead to seborrhea, even hair fallout, breaking nails, and poor digestion, so conversely it would appear an extra dose does give hair—and nails—new strength and growth. Easily available in Europe in ampule or pill form, *Bépanthène* is only available on prescription through your doctor here.

Other vitamins from the vitamin B family, it's said, can affect hair color. In Europe the prematurely grey are advised to take a complex supplement of vitamin B that supplies fifty milligrams of each component, all in an endeavor to restore pigment to the cortex and eradicate grey, the sign that pigment has practically run out. When it *has* run out, hair color is obviously white. You can find vitamin B in natural foods, too, such as oysters, liver, broccoli, crab, mushrooms, and skim milk.

Another secret weapon to guard against hair damage can be found on the top floor of Kenneth's exotic salon on East Fifty-fourth Street, New York. There a small hurricane called Rita uses a high frequency "ray-gun" that fitted out with different attachments "exercises" each hair by sending a burst of ultraviolet light straight through it. She "rakes" the hair and scalp with this special ray-gun, and a tingle goes right through the body. You can actually *feel* your circulation improving, sending fresh blood to the scalp to cleanse and tone it.

Rita has another trick that involves shampoos. She whips each one in a blender to ensure it's lighter than the hair it's going to wash—for she firmly believes too much heavy lather *deadens* hair and so dulls it.

She also always rinses hair *first* before using the whipped-up shampoo, so forcing top dirt out, preventing it from being massaged into the scalp. One shampoo only, so as not to wash out too much of the natural oils, followed by *many* warm water rinses. Water must only be lukewarm, she says, for hot water makes hair swell, while cold makes it limp.

Expert Rules for Hair Care at Home

Whip shampoo diluted with a little water—using an egg beater if you don't have a blender. This ensures hair is not "traumatized" with too much weight from lather.

Rinse hair first only with warm water, then wash with whipped-up shampoo. Rinse again thoroughly.

Blot, pat dry, never rub vigorously.

Dry hair immediately after it's shampooed. If it's allowed to dry too slowly, the slow evaporation causes loss of natural moisture, resulting in a lifeless, dry, brittle look. Excessive heat must also be avoided for the same reason.

    Brush hair only when absolutely dry.
    Never brush dirty hair—it can spread bacteria on the scalp.
    Wash every two to three days if you live in the city, three to five in the country.
    Watch diet. Build hair strength by eating nutritiously—good protein, vitamin C, and the vitamin B family.
    Keep hair pruned like a plant—trim every six weeks.
    Always wash hair gently, rather like washing pantyhose.
    Use only brushes with natural bristle—boar is best.
    Do change style occasionally to give hair a change, a rest.

The Experts Say . . .

    Don't curl hair too tightly with hot rollers, too tightly with *anything*.
    Don't use any broken equipment—it can scratch scalp, break hair.
    Don't use an elastic band for your coiffure. Always use a covered band.
    Don't use a sizzling hot dryer.
    Don't oversunburn, overtease, overspray, overperm, overcolor.
    Don't forget a six-inch strand of hair is about a year old at its end, has been through a minimum of fifty-two shampoos and sets, perhaps two thousand combings.
    Don't ignore split ends, or they will continue up the hair shaft.
    Don't use dry shampoos more than once a month at the most. They should be for emergencies only.
    Don't use just any shampoo if your hair's colored. Look for those that are specially formulated for colored hair.
    Don't wait for hair damage before you use *conditioners*.

How Conditioners Work

    The basic job of the conditioner is to detangle, unsnarl, reduce frizz, make smooth with antistatic ingredients that calm down flyaway hair, add *body* and so life and vitality to hair.
    Some conditioners smooth down the platelets on the cuticle, fill in lost patches of body and seal split ends.
    Fine, limp, color-treated hair and hair abused through too much wear and tear (even overshampooing) should use protein conditioners. The protein coats the hair, is absorbed by it, and each strand actually becomes thicker as well as more springy. Protein, in any case, is a key ingredient in any conditioner for any type of hair. By adding body, it obviously adds *life* to any style, straight or curly, long or short.

Balsam is also frequently used in conditioners today. A fragrant, aromatic and usually resinous substance oozing from a variety of plants, its prime job in products is to add sheen and luster.

The "instant" kind of conditioner relates to the setting kind, helps hair hold shape, curl, plus depositing protein on the shaft to "fill out" hair strands.

Corrective conditioners encourage hair to hold moisture, soften hair that's dry and brittle to make it more supple and resistant to breakage.

The Newest Sex Symbol

When master builder William Levitt, of Levittown fame, extended by fifteen feet his yacht *La Belle Simone*—at that time one of the largest privately owned in the world—it didn't cause any comment.

When La Belle Simone herself, his dashing French wife for whom the yacht was named, cut off fifteen inches from her long, almost waist-length dark hair, it made the papers, caused remarks everywhere she went—and took ten years off her looks.

Alexandre of Paris, possibly the most famous manipulator of a pair of scissors in the world, did the job, and Simone was so delighted she went back the next day to ask for more pruning.

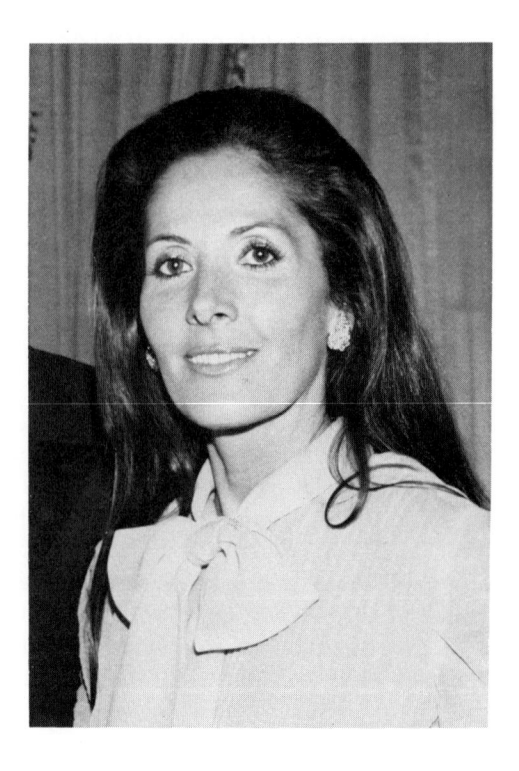

To cut or not to cut—a tricky decision for any woman with long, long hair like Mrs. William Levitt. She cut —and liked the result.

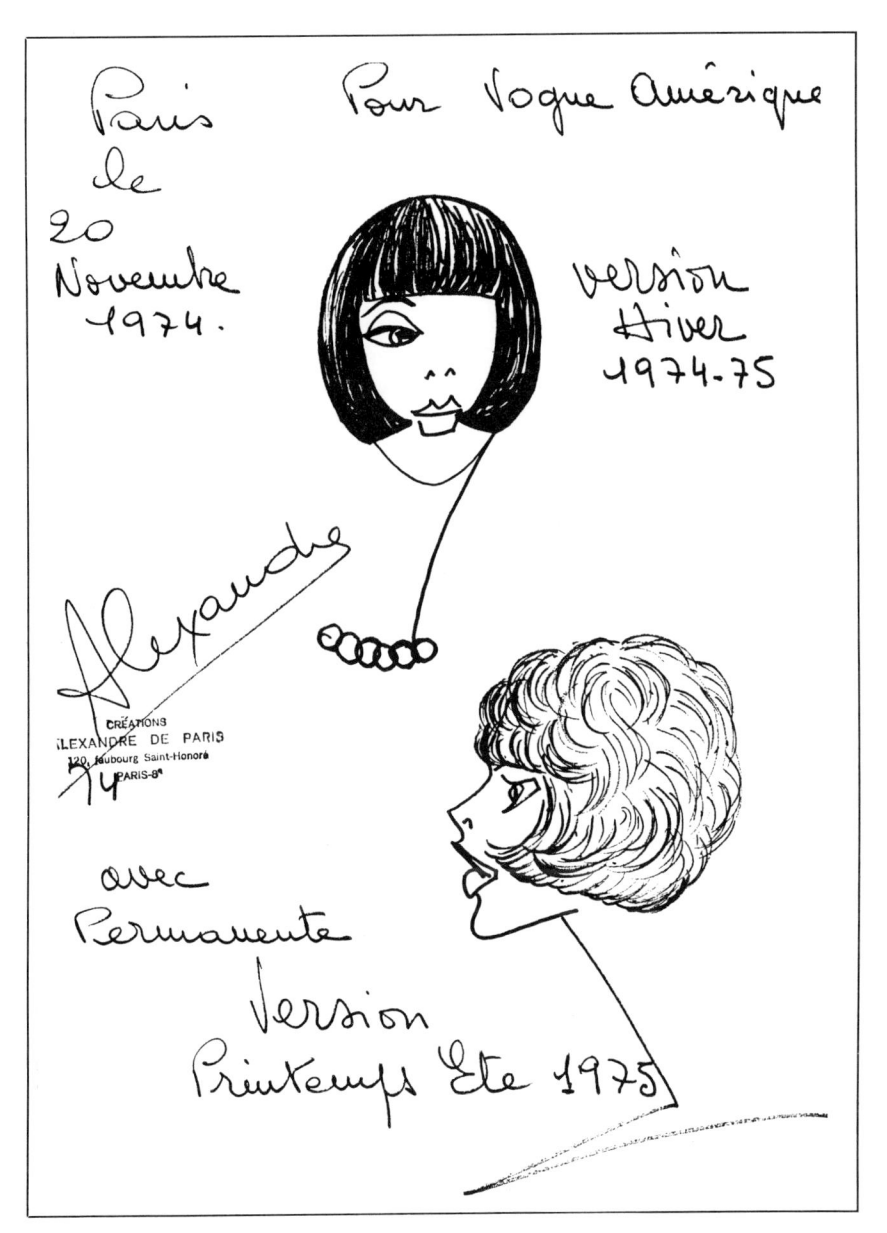

> Paris le 20 Novembre 1974.
> Pour Vogue Amérique
> version Hiver 1974-75
> Alexandre
> CRÉATIONS ALEXANDRE DE PARIS
> 120, faubourg Saint-Honoré
> PARIS-8ᵉ
> avec Permanente
> Version Printemps Été 1975

For Simone the cut was a risk that came off. She was right to think of it as a risk, for cutting very long hair into very short is certain to bring about a transformation, one that demands another set of rules to follow for style maintenance—and even a new makeup, too (see pages 67–68).

For the last few years we've been gritting our teeth, getting used to the males in the family playing early Samson, growing their hair to prove their strength or to prove their will anyway—son versus mother, son versus father, son versus girl friend.

The revolt is old hat now, and men's hair has settled down more or less just above the shoulder line for the revolutionaries, up back around the ears for those fed up with all the care a lengthy head of hair demands.

Woman's revolt against severe proscriptions on hairstyles antedated man's by about fifty years, when in that short-lived scuffle of the 1920s we won the right to wear our hair "bobbed" and our skirts short—in an attempt to help emancipation along.

Unlike men, however, we have been yo-yoing about hair length ever since—varying from the long (way past the shoulders) and romantic to the very short (remember Vidal Sassoon's first geometric cut of the early 1960s), back to long, and now, as international stylist Ara Gallant puts it, "All a woman wants is to be able to do her own hair—for no one wants to spend her life in the beauty salon anymore."

Ara's opinion happens to contain the truth as to what has really happened to *style* today.

When the test of a good set was its staying power, a salon visit took at least two or three hours. You expected to emerge combed and lacquered to the crisp consistency of cotton candy, and had every hope to live with this rigid work of art for at least three or four days before a teetering collapse necessitated another trip to the salon to hold up the remains. That torturous and tortured type of styling, hiding a multitude of sins, is out forever—thank goodness—and Vidal Sassoon is one stylist who can take a lot of the credit.

He swept into the hair headlines in 1963 when he delivered what was considered then a revolutionary idea—a cut that was longer in front than at the back. Vidal designed this for a Mary Quant fashion show—it was picked up by French designer Emmanuelle Khanh for her Paris show, and soon women all over the world were having themselves shorn like so many chic sheep. Nowadays Vidal hardly ever holds a pair of scissors in his hands, more likely an airline ticket as he zips from one continent to another watching over his empire of shops, but like all the top stylists, he firmly believes only beautiful hair can make beautiful styles. To release his first hair-care products in 1974, he said, "A basic haircut cannot fall properly or reflect its precision unless the hair has natural sheen and flexibility. It certainly will not hold any given shape without elasticity and tensile strength."

Now that hair's *style* is more or less sublimated to hair's *condition*, all stylists have to be on their mettle. They have better material to work with, but because the style is invariably simple, their work has to be more decisive.

To start where I came in, *length* is important, and the busier the woman, the more she veers these days to what can only be called *the perfect length of hair,* one that she can wear easily, curling it herself after shampoo and conditioner without any great struggle.

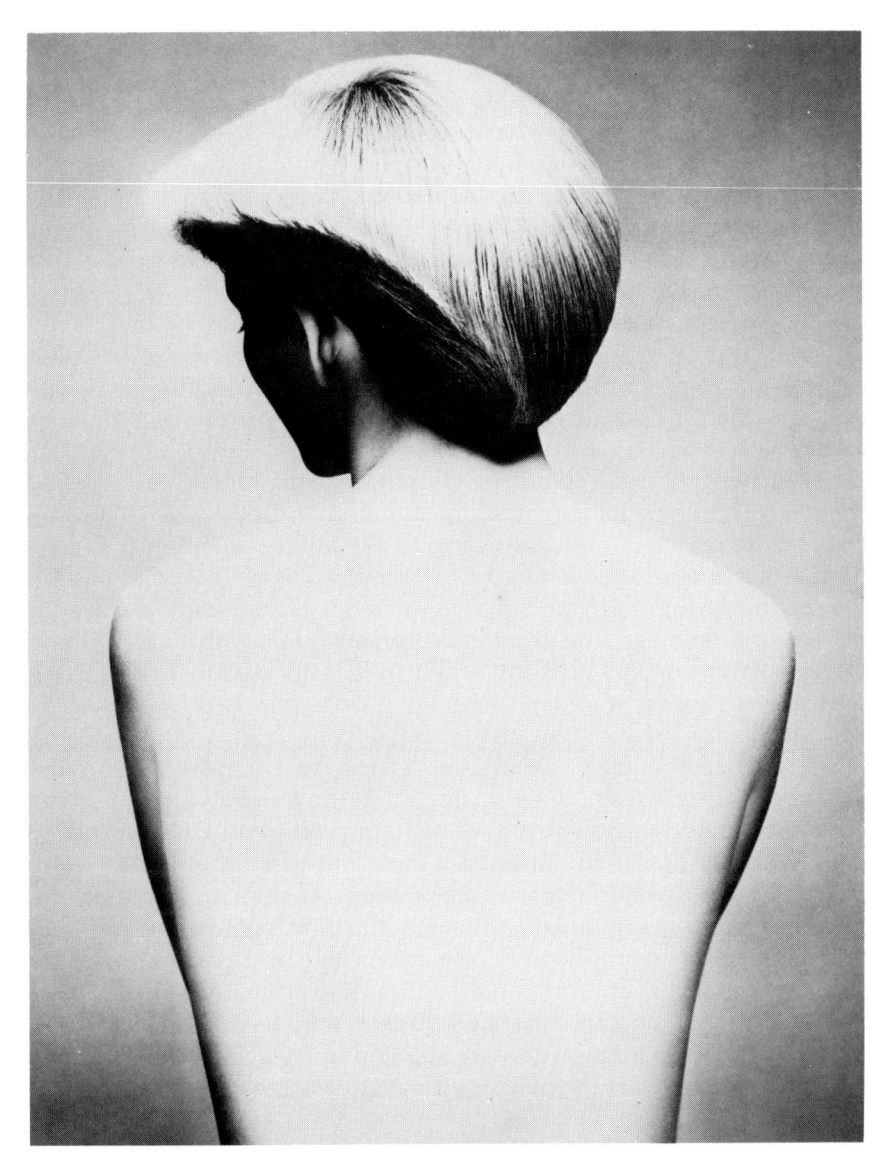

Hair draftsmanship by Vidal Sassoon, the man who started the Big Shear.

There Isn't a Set Length Like an Army Regulation

The perfect length of hair *for you* depends on a number of things. Everything a top stylist takes into consideration, *you* can take into consideration for yourself when tackling the job of finding the right length and so the right style.

When a new client comes into a salon, the best stylist mentally notes height, shape, the proportion of head to body, plus the way she walks.

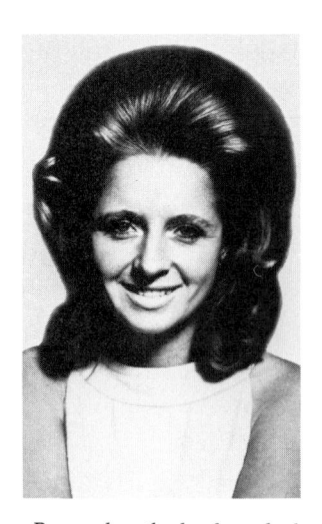

Remember the backcombed bouffant? The author had one in the mid-sixties.

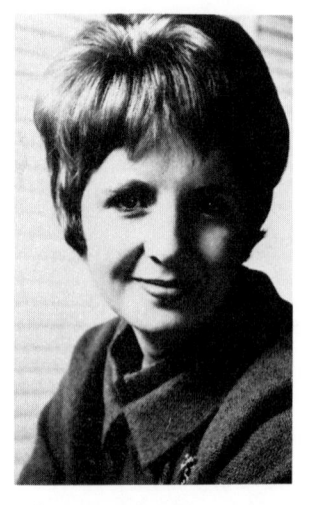

As woman's editor of London's Evening Standard *in 1960, a snappy businesslike short cut.*

When she sits down, he will next study face shape, head shape, and bone structure.

Next, if he really knows his rattail comb, he will ask the sort of questions that will show what sort of style will work with her life style, her environment, climate, and so on.

The hairstylist guesses his new client is probably sitting in his chair because she has either (a) read about his work or seen his styles in a magazine like *Vogue,* or (b) has admired a girl friend's new style and found out the name of her stylist.

But what *she* has in mind and what is *possible* may be two totally different things. "You can't fight nature," says New York stylist François. "Women expect too much of their hair; then they're disappointed when it doesn't work out to the mental picture they have of themselves."

The best stylists—"hairdressers with a conscience" as I labeled them in *Vogue*—never attempt the impossible. They will cut, style, color, and comb out only according to the ability of the hair to perform. Once the initial meeting has taken place, and the stylist has felt the texture of the hair, the way it grows out of the scalp, the way it falls around the head, the experienced one will follow through with no more worries—except possibly when he has to explain to the client why the style *she* wants just isn't possible but why the style *he* suggests instead is the right one for her.

Dina Azzolini from Milan, one of the best hairdressers in the world, puts it this way: "Obviously, haircutting and styling must fit a customer's personality which goes beyond prettiness. The style *has* to work with her life. If she lives on a farm and gets up at 6 A.M. every day, she will want her hair to work one way. If she's an actress in the theatre, who sleeps till noon and works till 1 A.M., she will need something else. Such psychological research is the best part of my work . . . my shop can't be compared to the conventional expensive hairdressing salon. You can come here from 9 A.M. to 7:30 P.M. to relax, lunch, bathe, take a massage, buy something from the boutique, and *discuss your hair*—even if this isn't the day to do anything about it."

New Looks for Old

The beguiling thought of a new image creeps into every woman's mind from time to time, hence the big snip that Mrs. Levitt gambled on and won, the long curly postiche that Princess Margaret used to pin to her natural crown, waiting for her own hair to grow to the same length (alas, it never did quite make it—hair growth varies a great deal from person to person, see pages 86–89), and the total change in Barbra Streisand's looks ever since at Jon Peters' insistence (her ex-stylist boyfriend) she grew her hair long and crimped it from crown to end. Hair can make or break our looks—whatever we put on our backs.

To go after a new image, a good haircut is the easiest route, for skillful cutting can make thin hair appear thicker, limp hair bouncier, thick hair more manageable, and long, long hair more graceful and contemporary.

Hair all one length is the easiest length to have, taking less time to maintain because it's easier to handle. If you want it graduated, then the best graduation is found in the new dimensional cutting, where working to a chosen perimeter, hair is graduated only by one sixty-fourth of an inch all around the head. Here, as length grows, so does shape. Out-of-shape does not happen.

A blunt cut is the safest cut, for it leaves a firm, steady all-the-way-round look that can be easily washed and blown dry, then worn as it falls, depending on the way it springs out of the scalp. Stylist Ara Gallant does a variation of the blunt cut on very fine hair when, "I cut with scissors and 'effilate,' that is, holding the scissors in an upright position, lightly feather the underneath hair so the outer layer turns under naturally. It looks like a blunt cut, but it is slightly different, leaving the ends more flexible. I have only one rule: let your hair dictate the way it's worn . . . if you go with the line nature gave you, it always looks the best."

Hair cut askew by a razor exposes more of the inner hair shaft, allowing valuable protein and moisture to escape. This is bad; remember the weakest part of your hair is at its ends, the only part not protected by the outer cuticle.

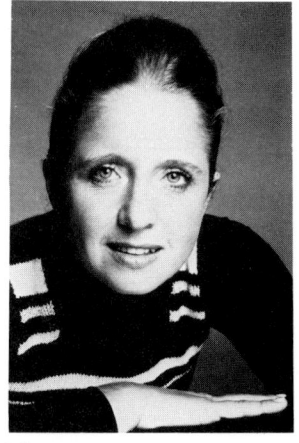

The author—a new look for Harper's Bazaar in 1970.

How to Be Your Own Expert

When the hairstylist takes that first look at you in the mirror, if he's one of the best, he will be trying to visualize you *without your hair,* trying to find "your outline," whether it's an oval, square, or diamond.

If there's no expert near at hand, you can still work out a new hairstyle for yourself, one you can ask your local stylist to carry out with no fears of making a mistake. First write down a self-portrait and check it out against the suggestions here:

If you have *an oval face,* you're lucky—you can wear almost any style, including the "not-for-everyone" side part, layered look with waves on both sides, hair tips lifted up with a hairpin to be light and fluffy.

Realize that *a round face* looks less round with a center part, hair gently falling across forehead and cheeks—so diminishing their size, pinned back at the ear lobes, just covering ears at the tops, spiralling out in two bunches on both sides, behind the ears, but lying close to the neck. This style makes the top of the face look smaller than the bottom.

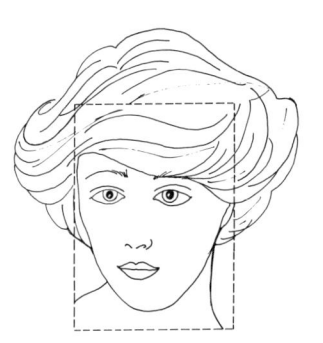

A long face can look prettier if delicate bangs trail over the forehead and hair is combed out *wider* at the top than the bottom, pinned back just below the ears to fall gently just above the shoulders.

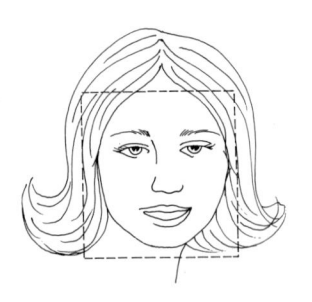

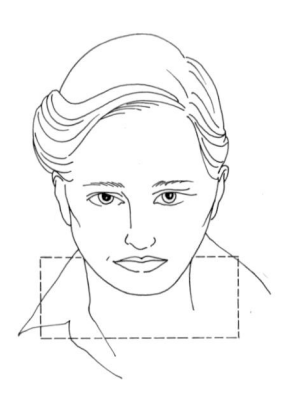

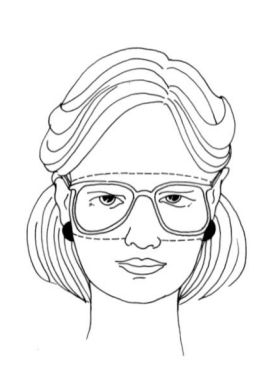

A square face needs a hairstyle to "round" it out, soften it with ends flipping up on both sides, and just the suggestion of a center part. To break up any hard angles, hair should be combed smoothly close to the head at the temples, brushing gently over the cheeks.

If face shape is *short, fat,* hair should be worn *high* above the ears, close, flat at the sides to brush over cheek and temple.

If nose is large, a curly or smooth ponytail diverts the eye with hair massed at the back of head, pinned high to fall down to midneck at the back. The length at the back of the head brings the nose into balance. Conversely, bangs help a *small nose* look more important.

If neck is short, hair should be given height on top, worn close to the head at back and sides to add a sense of length. Hair pulled back to create space behind the ears is neck-lengthening.

If a *jaw juts,* strands of hair curling in casually from below the ears on to the cheek, following jawline to just below the eyes, takes away the jutting effect.

For *girls who wear glasses,* an away-from-the-face style with hair lifted on top and full over the ears looks great. Hairstyles here should never be too severe or too fluffy and for the girl with glasses—earrings should be part of the look.

Hair swept up on top of the head adds *length* to any face.

Hair brought out in wings on either side of the ears adds *width*.

Hair brushed back, away from the face, or worn flat close to the head, makes face appear *larger*.

Hair brushed over forehead and across cheeks makes face appear *smaller*.

Hair massed on the crown or at the back of the crown takes away an impression of a *small chin*.

Hair massed low in a knot on the nape modifies a *long neck*.

Check Your Cut Against Your Hair Style

The important fact to remember about a cut and the way you wear it is that it must have *shape, fullness, movement*—easily obtained, if hair is straight but healthy, with a good perm, a good brush, care, and conditioning.

Really straight hair lies close to the head, and obstinately refuses to stay back or away from the face after it's been shampooed, dried, and set. Its natural movement is *down* and *forward*—the sort of hair that really deserves a good cut because it will benefit so much from it. The straighter the hair, the less it should be thinned out, for every bit of thickness helps natural curve at the ends, while the added weight helps the cut keep its shape. Although a layered cut takes a lot of maintenance, it looks great on really straight hair, cut while hair is wet, molded to head shape. After hair has been set in rollers and

HAIR
107

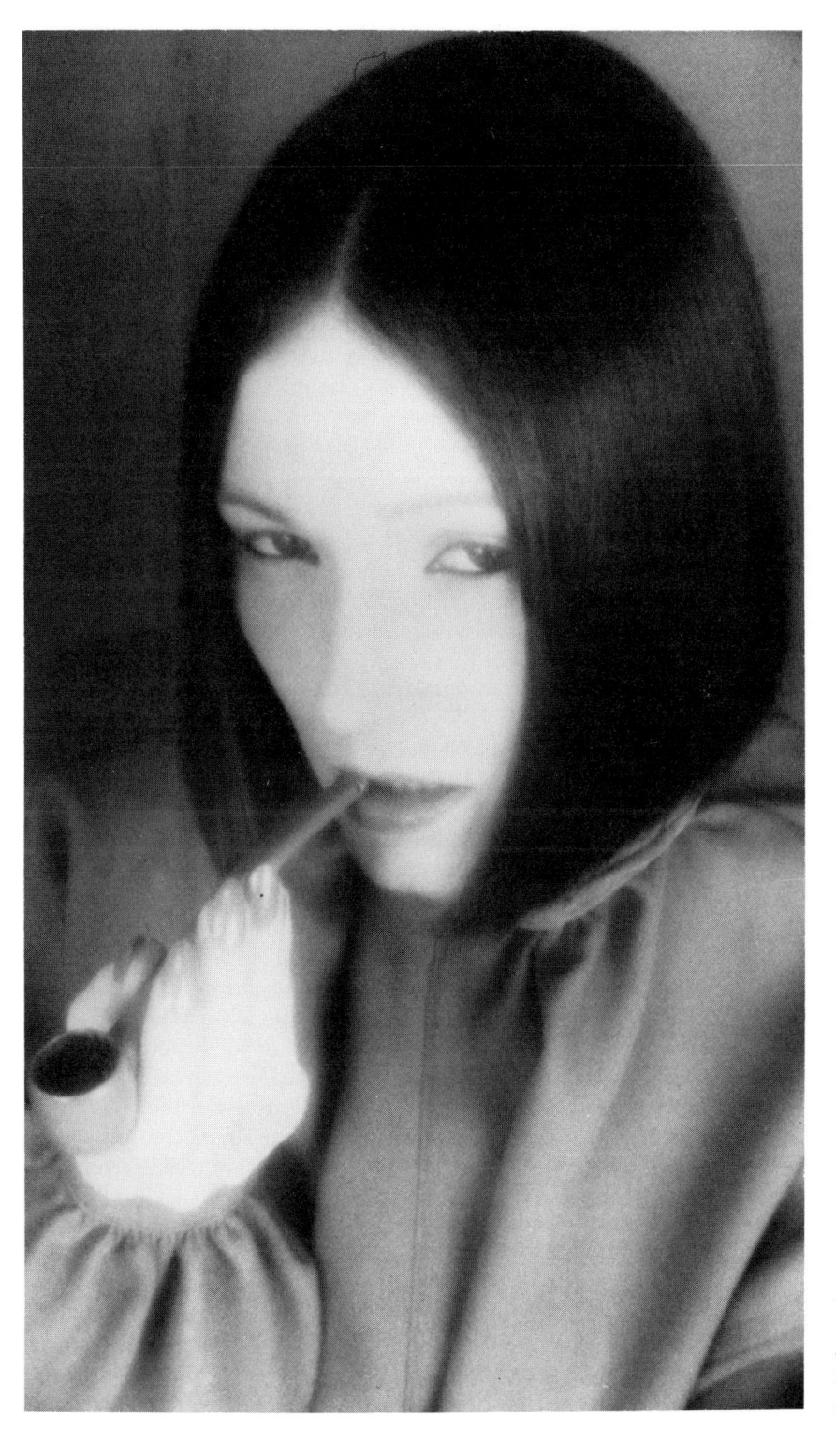

Really straight hair . . . is the sort of hair that deserves a good cut, because it will benefit so much from it.

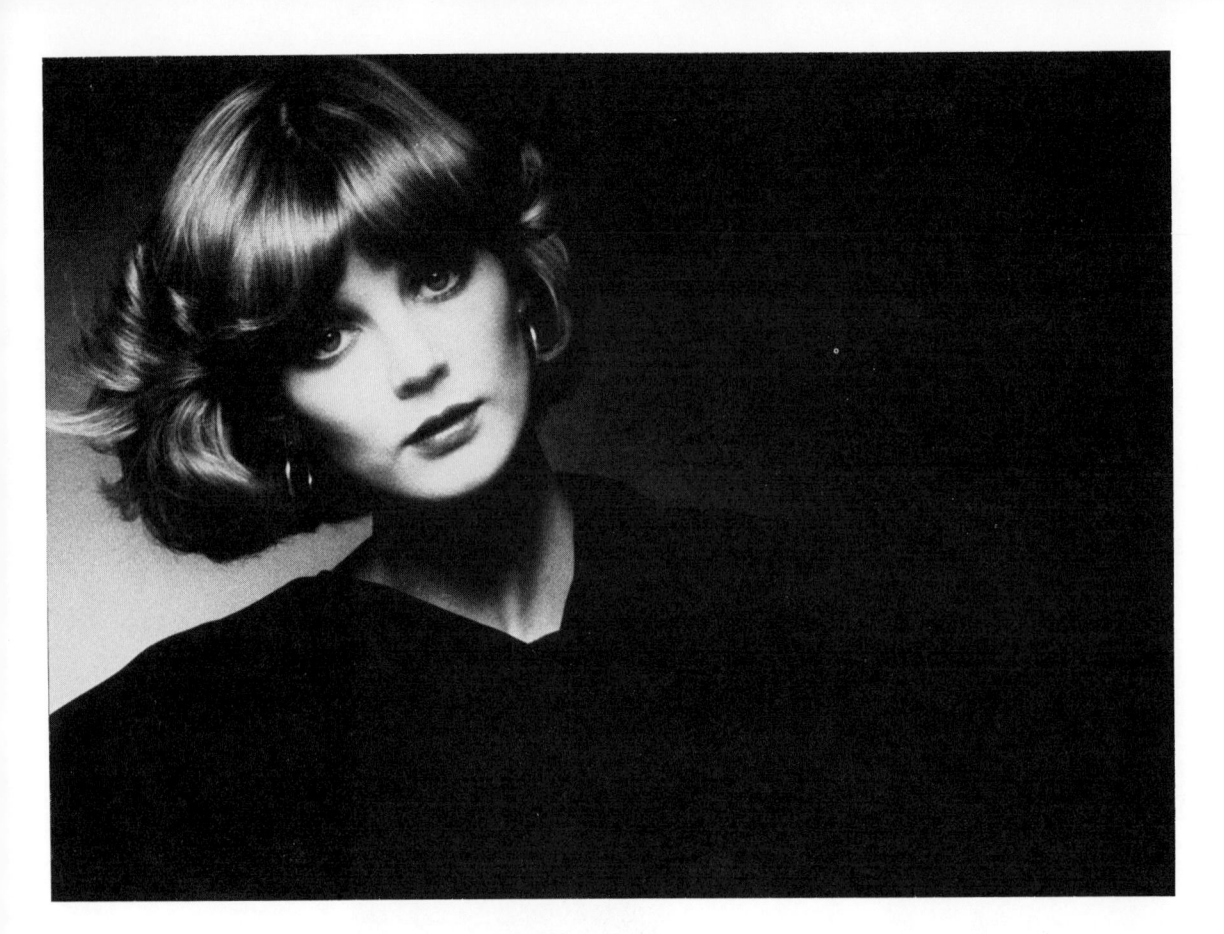

A wide face looks especially good with bangs and a layered look. . . .

dried, each "curl" is trimmed individually as it's combed, so that each layer knows its place, measuring about two and a half inches long except at the nape, where hair is tapered to an inch or less.

Bangs go well with a layered cut, either a full deep bang or a soft half bang, and all face shapes can be helped with bangs—varying shapes and sizes. A wide face looks especially good with bangs and a layered look, both cutting down on width, while a long face is "shortened" with a deep bang swept over to one side or the other. On a high forehead, bangs look best if they're long and wispy, while a low forehead should keep to a short bang that breaks into what looks like natural tendrils, lightly permed on straight hair—perhaps the only place on the head that's permed—with side hair cut so well, it remains straight but curves naturally up or under.

Perming no longer applies to the whole head only. It's a matter of "perming in the right places," according to face shape. The perms of today have little or no relationship with the permanent waves of yesterday that concentrated on delivering a baked-in immovable look. Today's perms are quick, need only put bend and body in the hair or soft curl at the ends.

Naturally curly hair or hair that's been on the perm route for years

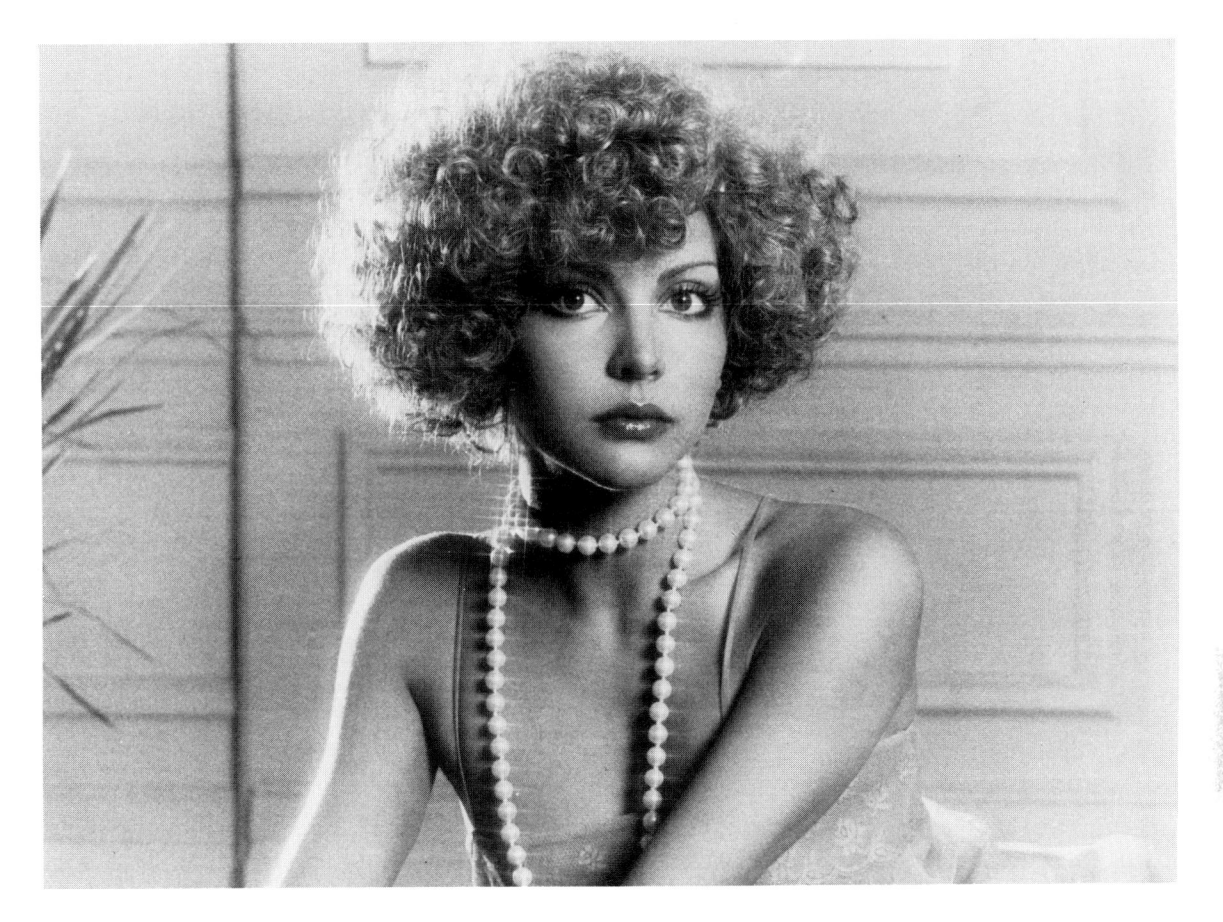

If hair is excessively curly, it should be kept one length, only tapered at the ends—or would you rather wear a wig?

can be groomed and maintained more easily than straight because curl adds life to the hair.

Curly hair needs a *blunt cut* to bring out maximum curl and good direction.

If hair is excessively curly, it should be kept one length, only tapered at the ends, and this is where measurement is important. If cut *too short,* coarse curly hair can end up looking like a brush; if left *too long,* it won't be easy to style.

For easy handling, curly hair works best with a setting-lotion type of conditioner, combed through hair while wet, before being rolled onto the largest size rollers. Once hair is dry and curlers are out, two brushes are better than one for brushing hair flat all around the head, holding the hair in place but still brushing until real wave pattern emerges, hair controlled by its session with the setting lotion. The only way to avoid overcurliness with perms, whether home variety or salon, is to ensure hair is in tip-top condition before the event.

If a natural overabundance of curls is getting you down, straightening is one answer, using a method that's similar to perming. Perming softens hair until it relaxes to take on the new shape applied to it; then a neutralizer *fixes* in the new shape, until the hair grows out.

Straightening works the same way—except when suitably softened, the hair is set to be straight, then neutralized into that position.

Fine hair is harder to straighten than coarse, and unfortunately, fine hair has more problems whichever way you look at it. However good the straightening agent, in damp weather a little frizz can rise to the fore, then that old standby, a hard-hold setting lotion, has to go into action.

Although straightening lasts as long as perming (depending on how fast hair grows), the problem of new growth is more tricky to deal with. A growing-out permanent stays curly to the end—where curl is needed most! The straightened head of hair grows in curly near the scalp—where curl is needed least. Very curly hair doesn't work so well if blown dry. It's best set conventionally with rollers, followed by root lifting with a curling iron to get maximum kinks out.

Sometimes there will be curl in some parts of the hair and not in others, or the hairstylist may decide to take curl out of one place to put in another, using a blow dryer to "brush out" natural curl to produce a smooth surface, putting curl back with a curling iron—but only at the ends.

If you find the style you like for your hair just doesn't stay, however hard you work and your hair is in good condition, it could be you're working *against* nature and the way your hair wants to go. It's always easier, as Ara Gallant says, to go *with nature* for the most successful result.

If you're letting your hair grow, a basic blunt cut, chin length at the front, a little longer at the back, can be maintained easily, inexpensively, as it only needs a slight trim about once in six weeks, the style growing the same way all the time. The best blunt cut starts at the nape, then works around to the front on both sides.

Editors are fond of this look for two reasons—time and money. A layered cut is the costliest—in time and money—needing reshaping and cutting often. Also it isn't easy to set oneself—mostly needs professional help.

If you feel you need height—and most people do, few being able to get away with just a flat crown—backcombing *without* teasing ("teasing" means the wrong sort of backcombing) is best carried out at the roots where hair is new and strong and where it isn't visible, hair being smoothed over the backcombing to give a light, airy look. Later, to comb out the backcomb, take each strand one at a time to work back through the length of the strand, inch by inch, until the comb moves freely. Tugging and pulling only break hair.

The no-set, blow-dry style depends more on hair condition for its good looks than any other. When hair looks like a cap of shining satin, cut sensationally, it puts any elaborate style really in the shade—but the shine must be one of *health*. The no-set, blown-dry style works best when front hair is short enough to be lifted by hand drying, holding its shape with plenty of thickness at the back. Hand drying—using only a moderate heat—can produce a look of vibrant, moving hair.

Model's Hair Takes a Beating

Lauren Hutton, probably the most individualistic of the world's famous faces, says she has thin, flyaway hair. Nevertheless it sometimes has to put up with at least four changes of hairstyle a day, involving hot rollers, combs, and plenty of hair spray.

To make up for this wear and tear, Lauren shampoos her hair every two days with a balsam herbal shampoo, followed up with a protein-rich conditioner. When she feels her hair is letting her down, she believes in homemade rinses of stinging nettle tea to strengthen it. Because her hair is so fine, the style she likes best—a tumble of what she calls "Scarlett O'Hara curls and waves"—is impossible away from the studio. "It gets combed that way by Ara Gallant so that it looks as if it grew that way." It actually takes the most precise setting and combing—and, alas, lasts only as long as the photo session.

Karen Graham, another top-flight model, also has what she considers unmanageable hair. To help a look last she believes in hair that's all one length—for her a length just above the shoulders, worn when she isn't working curled under in a simple pageboy. She, like Lauren, loves a "tumble of curls"—working best for her when hair is set damp on a myriad of very small rollers, the curl taking hold under the dryer. This is far better for Karen's hair than hot rollers, which she finds easily break her fine hair.

The Comb-out

The transition between set and finished look obviously depends on who is behind the hair and the rollers. Practice makes perfect, and if you follow the rules below—devised for me by Marc Sinclaire, one of the best and fastest comb-out experts in New York—you will get maximum results:

1. Don't move around while using rollers. Sit tight instead for the ten minutes necessary—five to curl and five to comb out. Once the hot rollers are installed, heat lasts about five minutes, all that's necessary to put in curl.
2. Choose roller size according to hair type. Hair that's colored absorbs heat faster than natural hair, so the largest rollers should be used here to avoid overtight curl. Fine hair also curls more easily than heavy, thick hair, so should concentrate on the large size.
3. Divide hair into sections, pinning it out of the way.
4. Start curling on the left-hand side in clockwise direction—unless left-handed, when you should start on the right.
5. Hold section of hair straight up from the root and angle it out sharply toward the face. Start winding roller in hair as if winding up a ribbon, being sure to keep the same angle to the face.

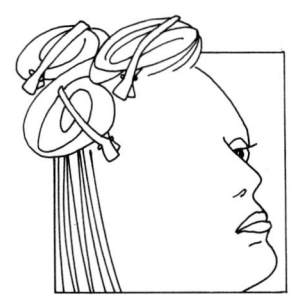

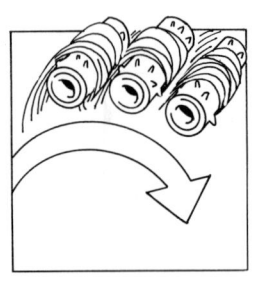

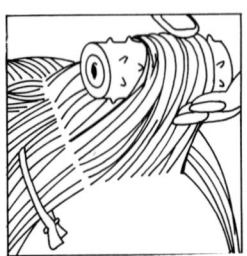

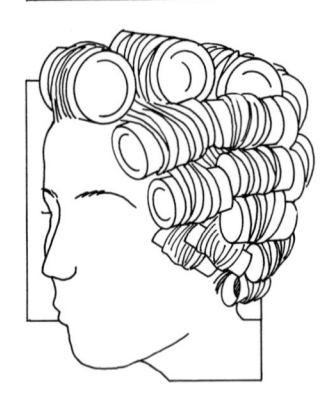

6. Use three large rollers on top which when unpinned give extra volume to any style. Remember to angle each piece of hair out toward face before winding. Don't have straggly ends. Use the smallest rollers at the nape.

7. Unrolling is as important as rolling. Do it slowly to avoid snarling.

8. Brush out all over with a bristle brush.

9. Backcomb with a fine-tooth comb near root, unless hair is very thick, when you can backcomb at the ends, too.

10. Don't use hot rollers every day. They dry hair and dirty it fast because direct heat on the scalp attracts oil to the surface, which in turn can create a pollutant buildup.

If you get good results curling your hair with hot rollers, you must check ends frequently. You may have to prune more often than usual.

Don't use heavy hair sprays in an attempt to keep comb-out going strong in humid weather. It makes hair droop all the more. Do as they do in humid Rio. Use only vegetal products or, if possible, no spray at all—it's too heavy for hair to bear in humidity.

For the comb-out following a shampoo and set at home with ordinary nonheated curlers, keep your dryer on moderate heat while you gently remove curlers. Let hair rest for a minute before brushing. Brushing actually helps the set last, not the reverse, and takes away any marks the rollers may have made.

Section hair according to the style you're after. If you want ends to flip up, place a hand firmly over bottom hair and brush hair up and around it. To turn under, place hand *under* bottom hair and brush down and around in a curve. Spray hair lightly, lifting side hair with brush, fluff it down over brush, then spray again to hold.

The Most Useful Accessory to Own

One way to try out new styles is with a wig—*once* you realize its potential and learn how to get the best out of it.

Wigs have come a long way, baby, from the heavy, unventilated "hard hats" of the past—worn mostly by those unendowed with a good crop of hair of their own. Now wigs are *fashion* accessories—easy, pretty, and *practical* to wear—once you've had some practice.

The most important thing to know is that a wig won't bite! You can comb it, brush it, just like your own hair. You can cut it if it's too long, curl it if it's too straight, and—with some fibers—even change its color, although there's hardly any point to that and a certain amount of luster may be lost.

As one wig manufacturer—a woman—puts it, a wig is a way to be *released* from the burden of coping every day with your own hair.

That's the way Arlene Dahl feels about wigs; Eva Gabor, Carol

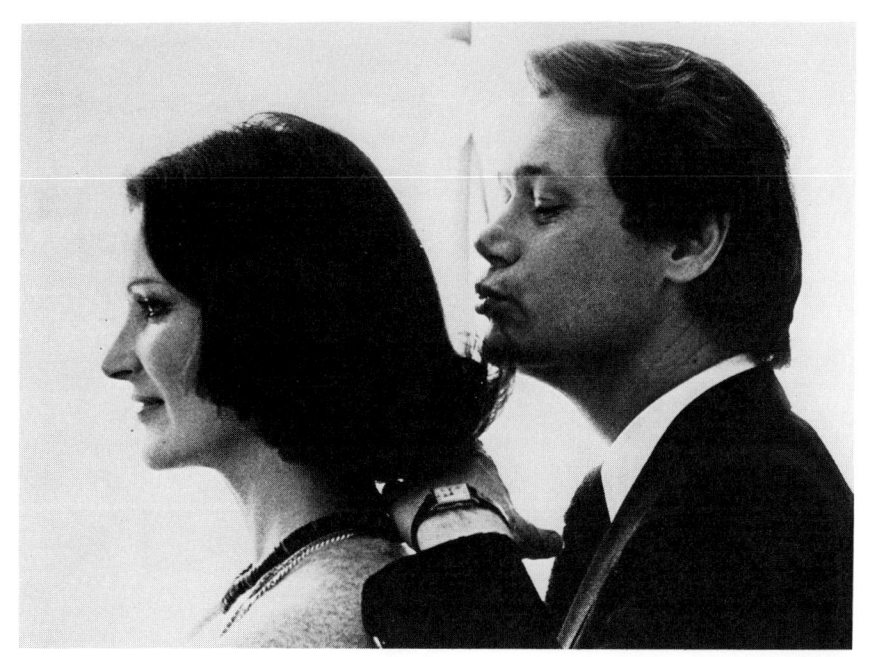

Marc Sinclaire, the man behind some of the best-looking hair in New York. Here, with Betsy Theodoracopulos, the finishing touch.

Channing, and Carol Burnett, too—all of whom can whisk a wig into perfect shape in no time at all.

The fiber people deserve the bouquets because it's the *fiber* that has made today's wig so versatile.

If you're wig shopping for the first time, look at the wig's base to check that it's well sewn and well ventilated. It should look lacy, and weigh no more than three ounces in your hand and on your head. Wigs made from real hair, ironically, gave them the "difficult" reputation in the first place. No wonder. To cope with *somebody else's hair* on your head when you can't cope with your own just doesn't make sense.

Take *time* choosing a wig—just as you would when choosing a dress, because *fit* is all important.

I think Kenneth, the grand hair master, has one of the best wig boutiques in the world located on one floor of his five-floor New York townhouse salon. Kenneth stresses the importance of always buying a wig or hairpiece that you feel is really you. Comfort doesn't only mean fit. It means something you wear so naturally, you forget you have it on. If you're always thinking, "I'm wearing a wig," it's a sure giveaway and, the more you think about it, the more you touch it, fuss with it, spoil it. Kenneth *knows* as a smart businessman, as well as a first-class stylist, that selling wigs isn't going to take any bread out of a hairdresser's mouth. On the contrary, the wig often gets taken along for a shampoo and set, too.

HAIR
114

The author wears a wig, the most useful accessory in the world for a busy woman—even the leading hairdressers surrounding her agree with this.

Unless you're contemplating a total color change and want to experiment first, a wig in a color close to your own—maybe one shade darker or lighter—makes more sense. Remember wigs are part of fashion, not fancy dress.

When you first try one on, don't be surprised if it doesn't fit 100 percent—unless it's custom-made, an unnecessary expense today. In most cases you have to maximize or minimize your own hair—*maximizing* by pinning hair into a flat knot or chignon on top of your head, *minimizing* by combing hair down completely flat around your head, with ends pinned into flat "rings" at the ends. If you have to do too much "minimizing," the wig is too tight. Too much "maximizing," it's too big. Choose again.

If you're timid about wearing a wig, try one with a bang, a slight fringe, or a hairline that curls over your own, so there's no need to use any of your own hair in front. When you're more practiced, for a really natural look, comb about one and a half inches of your own hair in front into a roller that you will completely merge later with the "test tube" hair.

Put your wig on front to back, like putting on a bathing cap. Pull it down on both sides at ear level, wiggling it into position, using large hairpins to pin it *securely* on the crown, on both sides above the ears and at center back. *Security is everything.*

If you're using your own hair, take out the front roller and brush your hair over the wig's hairline. Use a metal brush (no static) to add finishing touches, but above all, *don't be afraid to pull in order to move the wig into the shape and mood you want.*

Shake your head when it's on—gesticulate as you normally do to see that it moves when you move, effortlessly.

Wigs Need Care, Too

Wigs don't need as much washing as your own hair but at least after every ten to fifteen wearings. Swish through gentle warm suds, rinse, shake out. Today's wig dries as quickly as pantyhose, but unlike pantyhose, it *does* return to its original shape.

Never brush or comb a wet wig—it may stretch out of shape.

When dry, use a wide-toothed comb to get the most natural results.

Don't squash it while it's drying. Hang it on a doorknob or anywhere where air circulates, but not too near direct heat.

The best hairstylists plead, "Don't ask too much of your hair." I say don't ask too much of your wig, either. It's already been designed to do an efficient job, so doesn't need endless teasing—although cutting and shaping the right way never did any harm.

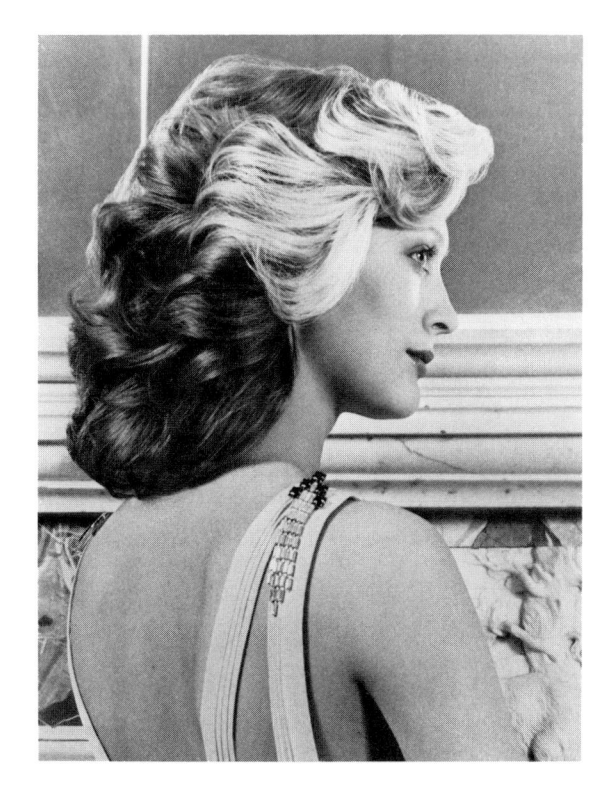

Quick change—from dark to light, from smooth to wavy—with the latest wig.

Examples of wig one-upmanship over real hair:

Wigs don't droop in dampness or humidity.

Wigs don't get sticky with pollution—the fiber is nonabsorbent and nonporous.

Wigs don't fade or oxidize in the sun or change color.

They don't get brittle in the cold.

They don't go up in flames.

They don't lose their hairs, go grey, get thinner or duller.

They don't take hours to wash and dry, however long the style.

Wigs *can* transform looks in a very short time, providing (1) the choice is right for head shape, skin tone, proportion; (2) plenty of practice is given to putting it on—not just twenty minutes before the big evening, but regularly every day.

Once it's second nature to put one on, you'll realize how a wig can be the most useful accessory you own.

Does She or Doesn't She Color Her Hair? Does Anybody Care Anymore?

A color change for hair isn't a secret anymore. On the contrary, exchanging colorists' names is a fairly common trade, while wearing a Leslie Blanchard color is as significant as wearing a Kenneth or Marc Sinclaire cut. Leslie plays color Merlin to a number of famous ladies, who look as if they were born beautifully blonde or brunette so skillfully does he match hair shade to skin—ladies like Barbara Walters, Alexis Smith, Peggy Cass, Joan Rivers, Joan Fontaine, Anna Moffo, and Helen Gurley Brown, all regular customers for color. Women may chat about their new "lights" or "brights," but men still rarely mention theirs.

Despite the colossal increase in expertise and product in the past decade, there's still a huge number of women out there—at least 70 percent of the female population to be precise—who don't *touch* the color of their hair, whether it's the color of yesterday's floor mop or the neglected family silver.

In this country the highest percentage of coloring is carried out in California—where you'd think the sun would be doing it naturally—while *disinterest* is at its height in New England—only 33 percent of the female population ever buy a hair-coloring product or service there.

Where Your Natural Color Comes from

Your natural hair color depends on two pigments—melanin (black-brown) and pheomelanin (red-orange-yellow). These pigments are present in the cortex of the hair (see page 95), and the amount you have of either determines the color you write down on your passport.

As we grow up, the cortex thickens, so our hair color appears deeper because pigment concentration is greater. This explains why although you may have been an ash-blonde baby, you now have medium-brown hair (commonly known as mousy). It's because your pigment deepened as the years went by. If you stayed ash blonde, it's because you had so little pigment in the cortex, only a small amount of concentration was possible.

The enzyme responsible for the production of pigment decreases in the body after forty, which explains every grey hair on your head—just a lack of new pigment.

Hiding grey was the first—and is still the major—reason for coloring hair. Next in line, the urge so many women have to go blonde, or at least to *lighten* their hair. There's still a subtle sexual reason for wanting to be blonde. As any brunette knows, it *seems* the blonde has more fun, and it's been that way since long before Anita Loos wrote the book! After all, who ever heard of a blonde wanting to change to brunette? It's a much easier coloring job, but it just doesn't happen—unless the lady's a spy!

Two Routes, Not Three

Although hair-coloring companies tell you there are three ways to color—temporary, semipermanent and permanent—there are essentially only two—those that wash out and those that don't. The washout variety includes those products labeled as temporary or semipermanent, the first washing out with the first shampoo, the semipermanent washing out far more slowly—color seeping away with each wash, usually completely out after six or seven shampoos.

Washouts

Washout products only *coat* hair, as makeup coats skin. They don't contain peroxide (an oxide containing a large proportion of oxygen), so in no way can they alter the *basic color* of hair. Depending on the color you were born with, they *can* considerably *enhance* it, adding "lights," and luster, making hair *look* more beautiful, because new shine gives a suggestion of *texture*.

If your hair is naturally light to medium brown, you can have a lot of fun with temporary products (usually called rinses). You can highlight, darken, tone down too much red or add it.

If your hair is dark, rinses don't have much color impact, except to leave a fleeting touch of red if you choose a bright-red rinse. They can add brightness, bringing out your own lurking highlights.

The Reason to Use a Semipermanent

Semipermanent products are more effective than temporary ones if you want a more intense effect. They contain organic derivatives (as do the "permanent real-color-change tints") but no peroxide, so can't *lighten* color, but can brighten, and darken or blend in grey, far more substantially than rinses.

The color in semipermanents forms a film on the cortex, "grabbing" hold more firmly than the temporary efforts.

If you've never touched your hair color and it's nondescript, even drab, it's time to start, and a semipermanent product is one way you can appreciate how a real color change would affect your looks. The built-in safety value is that if you don't like it, you know you're only a few shampoos away from your natural color.

This type of product usually offers side benefits today. Packed with conditioners, it's also easily applied, either shampooed in or foamed on to clean hair.

A lotion semipermanent is concentrated to give stronger color than the more popular sprayed-on version, which is full of air, and acts as an oxidizing agent, so that mixing is eliminated.

For the Best Results First Time Around

Stay within your own natural hair-color range, and choose either from the warm colors (all with a touch of red) if that's your hair type or cool colors (no red at all) if your hair tone is pale. Go lighter as you get older, *never* darker. If you choose a color that's near your own pigment type, you'll see results. If you don't, it's likely you'll see no evidence you ever went to the trouble.

One-Step Big Time

Hair-color language is confusing, although the companies do their best to translate the technicalities. The problem is a familiar one—the customer doesn't read the instructions; yet it's not only sensible to do so when contemplating a color change for your hair, *it's essential*.

Using a permanent hair color rather than a temporary one is, for instance, as different as renting is from buying, because a permanent product means you've made a *commitment,* one that involves constant maintenance.

A one-step permanent product (also known as a single process) can tint or lighten hair. You can darken it to any shade you want but only lighten it to a certain degree, depending on the color you already have.

A one-step permanent color job, as the name implies, can't be removed with a shampoo. With this process, hair color is really *changed*, not *coated*. The outer cuticle, which we can see, is softened enough with chemical ingredients for new color to penetrate right through to nature's paintbox, the cortex, where the new color is deposited to merge with whatever natural pigment is there.

Once natural pigment is removed to make hair lighter, or tinted to make hair darker and different, natural color will never return to the treated hair. Only new growth at the roots will change the picture, bringing back natural pigmentation, which has to be constantly lightened or tinted if you want to keep up on new color.

So *maintenance is key,* something to be considered before you make a move. Another thought is that because permanent processes work in an alkaline medium (first "unlocking" the hair cuticle to let new color in, a neutralizer then "shutting" it tight to *keep* new color in) seepage can occur through the use of highly alkaline shampoos. They don't *remove* color but can subtly *change* it, which is the main reason it's wiser for those with colored hair to use special products, shampoos, and conditioners formulated especially to *maintain* their color.

How to Choose the Right Color

The colors shown on the product charts relate to how they appear *on white hair,* which is why they're printed on white paper to show the shade in the truest way.

Unless your hair is the color of white paper—unlikely—the color you select on the chart will obviously be affected by the color you already have. A red tint, for instance, on medium-brown hair will result in reddish-brown hair, not true flaming red (who wants it?); on a blonde, it will be lighter; on a dark brunette, less apparent. Bear this in mind when you study the color chart and work out the effect your own color will have, diluting the color on the chart or strengthening it.

Don't automatically choose the color you remember you once were, either; skin tone fades as years go by, so hair color should never be in too much contrast. Very dark shades are aging for the over forty, and as Alexandre of Paris says: "Lighter is younger." If you were raven-haired at twenty, be content with chestnut at forty-five, even butterscotch at sixty.

Beware!

All permanent hair-color products contain peroxide or a similar substitute mixed with aniline derivative dyes—and that means strong chemicals, *strong enough* to penetrate the hair shaft in order to make a definite color switch. For this reason, a patch test to check on possible skin sensitivity is paramount (and law).

A patch test means mixing the color chosen with a developer and applying a tiny drop behind the ear. It should be left there for at least twenty-four hours before the hair is to be colored, so that if any irritation *at all* develops, the message is clear: Don't use the preparation. It's a warning that you are allergic to it.

Rubber or plastic gloves are sometimes included in hair-coloring kits, and they're there to be used *to protect fingernails*—for like the hair, nails are made of keratin, and so can absorb the color you want your hair to be—not the object of the exercise.

Obviously, any do-it-yourself hair coloring needs *great care*. Every label should be read and *totally* understood. Mishaps are costly. You can't wipe them away as you wipe away the wrong color lipstick.

Blonde Fever

A director of the leading hair-color company in the United States told me that approximately 1,500,000 *more* American women decide to go "blonde" each year—increasing the overall number of women who color their hair, but including a great many who after coloring their hair for years feel the first urge for a *blonde* fling.

Going beautifully blonde is a breeze if you can number yourself in the light-brown to midbrown family. If you're a raven-haired swinger, who feels she's a Dresden doll at heart, it isn't easy, although it's certainly possible. (I don't recommend it. Skin tone has to be considered, too!)

Double the Process for Big Color Changes

Black hair that wants to be pale blonde has to travel through *seven stages of lightening:* from black to dark brown, to brown, to red, red-gold, gold, yellow, and then pale, almost white yellow. The one-step color process just described can't cope with this exercise. This is where the two-step (or double) permanent coloring process enters the picture.

The first half of the double process goes toward making dark hair light, which really means hair loses its natural color.

The second half of the process concerns applying the right toner—for it's the toner that gives hair exactly the caliber of blonde color required, whether you've chosen to be the amber variety, strawberry, or even a silver of the subtlety of a Siamese cat.

The only way a toner can do its job properly and produce the color you've really set your heart on is when hair is paler than the toner chosen. Then when new hair starts breaking through, only the *lightener* is applied to the roots, not the toner.

This sort of operation *can* be carried out at home—there are several products on the market that achieve a double-process job superbly—but where there's any doubt (about hair condition, about the ability to achieve exactly the color required), expert advice is the answer. *Your hair deserves it.*

Hair coloring at home often falls down in this advanced category because the right timing is not observed. *Like everything in life, timing is all-important.* Double-process permanent color application is a delicate matter, balanced between time, mixing, and color choice.

After the lightening part of the process takes place—best on dry, ultraclean hair—the more time allowed to elapse, the paler the hair becomes.

If not enough time is given to this major step, the toner can't produce the color required, because it gets added to hair at the wrong stage of lightening—say gold instead of yellow. The lightening operation is there for another reason: to make hair sufficiently *porous*, for a toner also won't take properly unless hair is sufficiently porous.

As porous hair is weak hair, it needs *constant conditioning*—something that has to be stressed for hair that's regularly colored.

While an already light-haired person needs to leave on the lightener for a minimum of say thirty to forty-five minutes (that includes grey or white hair, too), a dark brunette may have to lighten twice to reach the right stage of light and correct porosity. There has to be twenty-four hours between each lightening trip. Very important!

Expert help shouldn't be ignored if hands aren't that steady—for lighteners vary in strength. If you're light-haired, you need only a mild one. If you're very dark, the strongest version has to be used.

A good reason for going to a color pro for all this is that he will keep a complete record, just like a doctor, as to what exactly has been put on your hair and when, not just for color preference but relating to its texture and strength. There are a multitude of colors to choose from, and a pro can make sure you pick the right one for your coloring immediately and avoid costly mistakes. On your "record," it will also state exactly how long it takes for your hair to achieve the right degree of lightness, plus any notes on texture and strength that have to be remembered. It obviously makes life easier, but then if you're diligent, you can always keep a record yourself.

Witches with Color

Hair coloring really comes into its own in the beauty salon, where customers tend to be as loyal to their colorist as they are to their doctor or dentist.

Faye Dunaway, for instance, wouldn't dream of letting anyone but colorist Rosemary keep her pale blonde looking exactly the same pale blonde around the clock, which means Rosemary, based in New York, has to make trips to the Coast to Faye's home for the sake of Faye's color.

HAIR
122

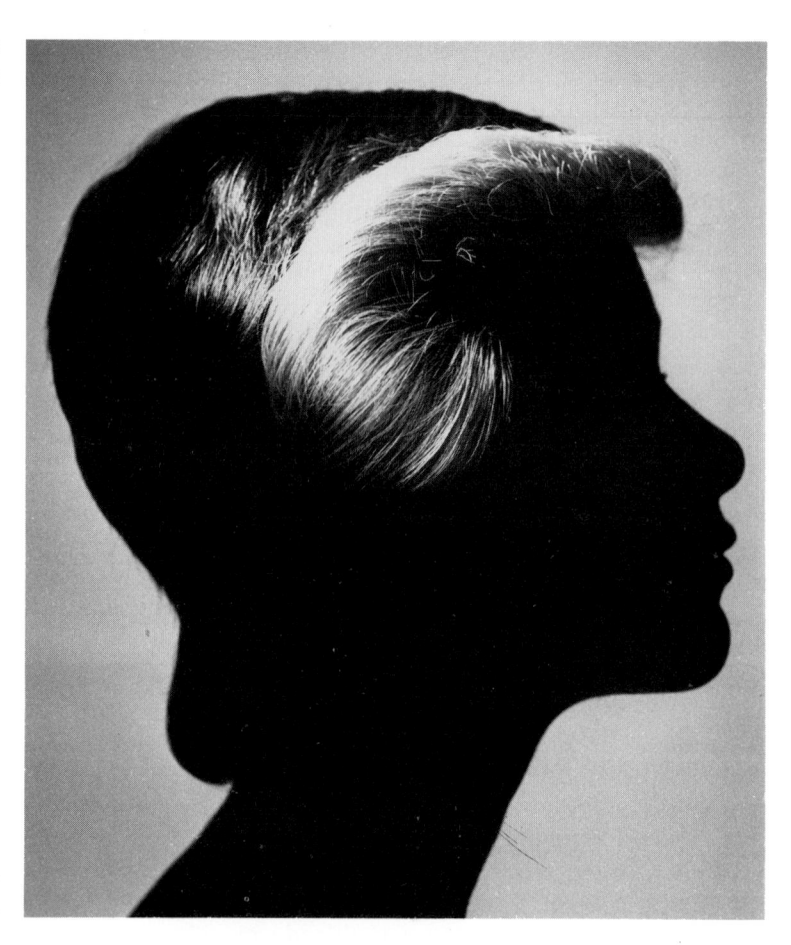

Flying colors—the new glow for hair.

Another witch with color is the Hungarian Rose Reti, who has been masterminding the hair-color changes of the stars for over thirty years. Joan Crawford gave Rose a pat on the back in her autobiography, *My Way of Life,* admitting her dependence on Rose for always achieving the right Crawford color.

Rose has helped many budding actresses become stars. Mia Farrow went to Rose for advice on her looks early in her career when she was testing for *Peyton Place*. Rose suggested heavy frosting to make her "ethereally blonde," and this certainly helped Mia's particular fragile appeal to show up on TV.

Cristina Ford's fairness is the result of Rose's alchemy, as is Luciana Avedon's, Dina Merrill's and the fair looks of Mrs. Angier Biddle Duke. Eileen Ford, head of the leading model agency in the world, wants to stay mid-brown, but well aware of the importance of a lit-up head of hair, regularly checks in with Rose for a new set of highlights.

Gloria Vanderbilt Cooper would be 95 percent grey if it weren't for her superb one-step permanent dark-brown coloring.

How much color, how often, and what to mix with what is where the top color craftsmen and women earn their reputations, showing skill by determining the amount and exact shade of color to be placed on each head. The biggest problem they face is to make sure color is accepted by the hair in a *level* fashion. This isn't as easy as it sounds, because hair does differ naturally in porosity. To get the same color in the root area as at the tip, plus uniformity instead of patches of color, colorists have to work like artists on a canvas, while still aiming above all for a natural look.

They are secretive about their formulas and the inimitable way they use brand names—and why not? Just as a chemist is known in the fragrance business for having a "nose," the antennae for selecting the right ingredients to make a good scent (there aren't many of them—see page 218), so the top colorists are known for their inventive approach to each head.

No wonder there's so much loyalty around in this business. There's a lot at stake when mistakes are so costly and time consuming to rectify.

Special Effects

Frosting, tipping, streaking, are all special effects for the hair, effects every woman can wear to advantage without looking in any way unnatural.

For frosting and tipping, hair is first lightened all over to the required level, then toned in certain places with a toner (the double-process method). A home kit will include a lightener, developer, color rinse, and perforated cap through which individual hairs are drawn to be "processed," hooked needle for drawing hairs through, a mixing spoon and bowl, plastic gloves and heat cap.

Streaking means lightening and coloring quarter to half an inch hair sections all over the head—not recommended for any hair that has already been treated or colored.

With *hair painting,* a flat brush skims over the hair, leaving behind light ribbons with a special lightening formula (one-step process). Left on for about twenty minutes, the formula is then shampooed out, for the longer it's left, the lighter—and so more unnatural—the "ribbons" look. Because of the peroxide, the lights can't be washed out and the result is shimmery and subtle. The extra beauty about hair painting is that it only has to be done every six months and can be carried out on hair that's already been treated (by either single or double processing) or virgin hair. Alas, it doesn't work so well for brunettes where the "ribbons" can resemble zebra stripes. The lighter the hair, the more effective the result, light- to medium-brown being about the darkest candidates.

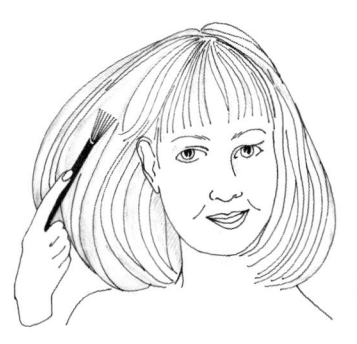

With all these effects, the object is to give a sense of light and airiness to the hair. Whenever you see "lights" in somebody's hair, it's because light itself strikes through the translucent outer cuticle and glances off the colored pigment deep inside the hair shaft. This "see-through color" is what gives hair its natural brightness, sense of life—and fascination. Modern hair colorings, whether used wholeheadedly or in tipping, streaking, or hair painting, help this reflection idea along. The special-effects department is really for those who don't want the bother of frequent retouchings, for although the processes are permanent, as color is not brought down to the roots where retouching takes place, you get more than your money's worth.

To recap, *tipped hair* involves bleaching the hair tips only. A *streaked head* is bleached in a few carefully planned sections. *Frosted hair* uses the specially designed cap described, lightening random strands all over the head. *Hair painting*—best on fair hair—lightens ribbons of hair with a flat brush.

Checkup at the Salon

Be sure on your first visit to a hair colorist that he or she examines your hair carefully, preferably in *daylight*. Artificial light can be misleading—you can end up with a shade you don't want to live with.

Make sure the colorist wraps your hair tightly around his finger—this way he can see nature's own coloring mix, the lightest to the medium to the dark. Make sure he also examines your roots for the same reason.

If you don't know what color you really want, ask the colorist to make a trial run on a test cutting for security.

Don't contemplate a change of color if you've just had a perm or straightening job. Too much chemistry in too short a time will damage hair. Leave at least two weeks between, preferably longer.

Remember that skin tone fades as you get older. Don't automatically choose the color you remember you once were, if you're trying to hide grey. It's ALWAYS safe to go a shade lighter.

If your skin is fair, stay with pale blonde shades, soft browns, even auburn. If you're under twenty-five, dark brown or even black can look stunning with pale skin—but only pale, *young* skin.

If your skin tends to be ruddy, it can look softer, paler, with the right hair color. Aim for beige lights. Discard anything red with a drabber, the product devised to get rid of too much red in the hair. (Every natural coloring except pale blonde has some red.)

Natural blondes or redheads should avoid reinforcing their natural color when they think it's fading—it can look too harsh. Instead they should reinstate their luck with two-tone effects—streaking or frosting. As kingpin colorist Leslie Blanchard puts it, "Think of it this way, hot face (pink, rosy), cool hair (ash blonde, light brown). Cool face (pale, white), hot hair (warm mahogany, even some traces of red).

Olive skin shouldn't try to be blonde, but should choose a brunette shade, and there are plenty of them."

Rose Reti, who once worked wonders for Mia Farrow, believes hair coloring can solve *face-shape problems*, too. She points out that a frame of light hair around the face "widens" a skinny shape, but is disaster for a round one, turning it into a real moon. A round face should choose random lights throughout the hair to take the eye away from the round effect.

The Top Colorists Agree

Colored hair must be protected from too much sun. It acts as an oxidizing agent, so that blonde becomes lighter but brassier; brunettes redder but harsher. Too much sun ruins the overall "natural" effect, making hair color patchy, taking away natural oils, and so the light and shine that hair color gives.

Colored hair needs regular scalp treatments, regular conditioning. Colored hair is far more porous than noncolored hair, therefore more vulnerable to every bad thing in the atmosphere.

Colored hair must use only those shampoos and conditioners formulated for it to ensure color is maintained correctly (no seepage—see page 117).

Do-it-yourself coloring is fine, providing directions are read as if it were a matter of life or death. It is—for the hair. Instructions are meant to be followed to the letter, and during an at-home hair-coloring session, there must be no interruptions. The right timing is key!

Henna is helpful to poor hair (see page 93) providing it's not used more than three times a year maximum. Henna changes color subtly, adding luster, and as it's a natural vegetable color, there's no risk of irritation. Natural light blondes, however, should never use it—it can turn their hair bright orange.

You Can Get Addicted

If you start off with a few highlights, move on to semipermanent color and finally decide on "the works" and make a complete color switch, with a double-process permanent color job, you have to realize you've taken on a big commitment. *Color maintenance has* to be part of your life, unless you intend to wear a cover-up hat for months or are willing to shave off your hair in order to start completely over. If there's any chance that you might move away from a big city where the experts are to an area without a pro in miles, delay any big color switch—especially if you've never taken the step before.

Hair coloring is a beautiful beauty treatment for hair, but for major recasting an expert must be behind it—at least the first time.

Quick-at-a-Glance Color Dictionary

ash: hair color without any red or gold tones, a natural blonde. *Drab* is the way professional colorists describe it.

basic color: hair's natural shade.

bleach: a lightener that removes natural pigment, moderately (by a few shades), drastically (10 to 20 shades), always employs peroxide.

blond on blonding: a blending of light and darker blonde shades, carried out with a one-process product on lighter hair, double-process on dark.

color filler: a product used on damaged hair or hair that's been so overcolored, it's too porous, needs "filling" in before any more color can be added.

color lift: a chemical that removes artificial color or tint.

color shampoo: devised for colored hair, to maintain true color as long as possible. Lower in alkaline content than most shampoos, it's designed to protect hair.

color test: a test to determine formula and timing, also called a strand test.

developer: the chemical used in "permanent" products, which mixes with the dye and then propels color to develop on the hair, sometimes hydrogen peroxide or a scientifically formulated substitute.

drabber: used to subdue undesirable red or harsh tones.

halo lighting: the crown hair is lightened; the underneath hair remains dark.

marble-izing: interlacing light and dark sections of shades.

oxidation: the development of color on the hair through the chemical union of oxygen with the coloring materials; also refers to an unwanted change in color due to exposure to strong sunlight.

patch test: a method to determine if a client is hypersensitive to a hair-coloring product (see page 120). A drop of the coloring product is applied behind the ear or in the elbow crease twenty-four hours before coloring takes place. This is required by law for any coloring that changes hair structure itself to effect a color change.

picture framing: a narrow section of hair lightened one or two shades around the face for 1½ to 2 inches.

plastic cap: used in semipermanent coloring treatments to help hold in heat for color development consistency, or with holes for use in "frosting" (see page 123).

porosity: hair condition enabling it to accept color changes. Porosity is increased by constant coloring, so overbleaching can eventually impair hair's texture. (Overperming and too much straightening can also damage hair through increasing porosity.)

resistant: hair condition that repels moisture or the action of chemicals—the opposite of porous—resists hair color, perming or straightening. May need medical help.

shampoo tint: a tint that cleanses as it colors.

strand test: the testing of a single strand of hair with a color product to see if the proposed color suits hair and skin tone.

three-dimensional shading: also called naturalizing, using three color tones in the same family, used on lightened to graded color.

tint: a permanent hair color that can cover grey and lighten or darken natural pigment.

tipping: lightening only the ends of selected strands throughout the head, seen to best advantage on short dark hair.

virgin hair: hair that has never had a tint, bleach, straightener, perm—has never been subject to chemicals of any kind.

white henna: a magnesium carbonate, highly alkaline, added to hydrogen peroxide in order to thicken and enrich the coloring solution.

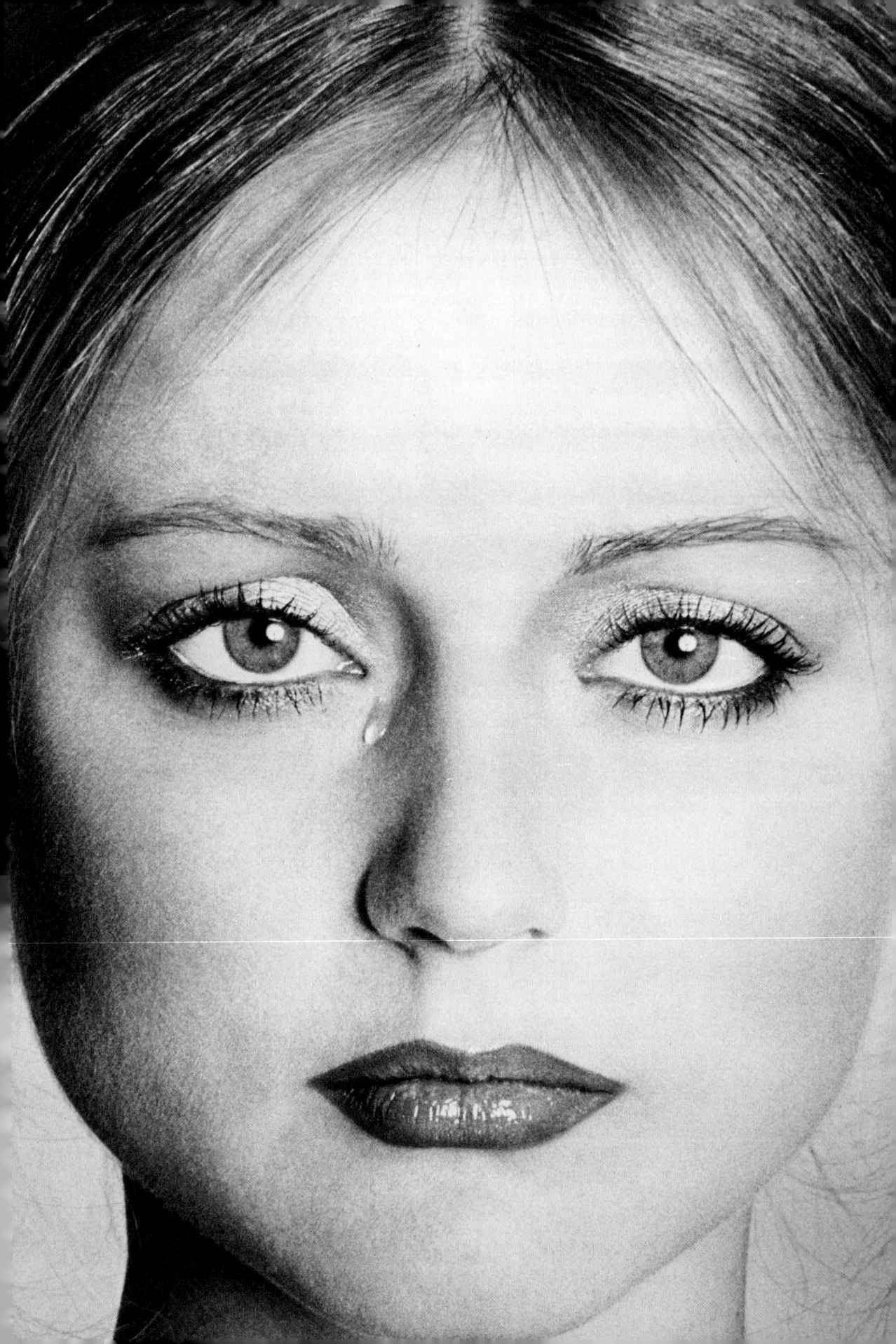

5

The Dieting Game

*Played by Martyrs
(165 Pounds Trying to be Size 10)
and Missionaries
(the Size-8 Girl Friends)*

Times change, and time changes us. Elizabeth Taylor was once a size 6, and a decade or so ago Sophia Loren could eat her way through three courses of pasta in one meal without a pang or a pound showing. Now Liz has doubled up on her size, and Sophia keeps pasta strictly for Sundays—once a month. They are both unwittingly—and unwillingly—representative of people living in well-developed countries (statisticians never see any puns), where one in three of the adult population is officially considered overweight.

The question is no longer to slim or not to slim, but *how*. In a single week across the country, it's possible to pick up at least a hundred different and apparently not too arduous ways to reduce in as

FACING PAGE
"I'm hungry . . ."

many magazines and newspapers. Few bear in mind, however, that while a hundred women may be fat, they will have a hundred different reasons for it.

Obesity is never due to one cause, although it's now been proved it can relate to the presence in the body of a greater percentage of fat cells than found in the generally lean. The body can regulate weight, so that whereas the normal person unconsciously maintains his or her weight at around 140 pounds, the abnormal and obese will reach 190 before starting to maintain. Further, experiments have shown that when the very obese (300 pounders) lost as much as 150 pounds, their number of fat cells remained the same, the weight loss deriving from each cell shrinking in size. The conclusion? Normal-weight people have less fat cells than fat people. A small comfort to those permanently on a diet. There is a genetic reason behind this, but—although in adult life, extra food only distends cells—it's thought fat cells can duplicate under the stimulus of extra food in infancy. Don't bring your daughter up to be a heavyweight, Mrs. Jones.

As Dr. Charles Read, Professor of Pediatrics at the University of Iowa, once advised, "I suggest to parents, throw away the scales. Tell your youngsters to look in the mirror and decide whether they like what they see. It's their 'mirror weight' which is important. A child who is self-motivated does lose weight and maintains the loss."

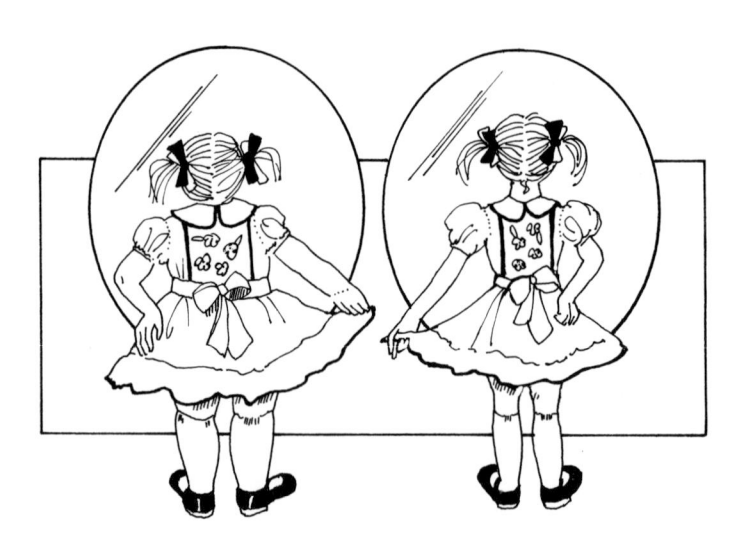

Deep in the brain is the part we have in common with all vertebrate animals, called the diencephalon. In man, this is the vital part from which the central nervous system controls all automatic animal functions of the body: breathing, sleep, sex, the urinary system, digestion and—via the pituitary gland—appetite. When it comes to the control of fat, its function can be—and has been—likened to that of a bank. When the body assimilates more food than it needs to live, the surplus is deposited in what may be compared to a "current account," easily withdrawn when needed. All normal-weight people carry their fat reserves in this "current account." When fat deposits grow rapidly with only a small number of withdrawals (in other words, the body is taking too much in and not spending enough), a point is reached when the "current account" becomes unmanageable.

Then the control system appears to set up a "fixed deposit" (of fat), no longer so easily withdrawn and burnt up in day-to-day activity.

This is the beginning of obesity.

Thereafter, normal fat reserves are held at a minimum, the majority of the surplus being put away in the "fixed deposit," and taken out of normal circulation.

So the chances are, the more you put on weight, the more risk you run of never being able to take it off—without a major and mighty shake-up of your whole system. "Tomorrow, I diet" just isn't the answer when the scales start creeping up. It isn't even a calculated risk, as the banker would say.

Admittedly luck does enter into it. If you were born with an abnormally low fat-banking capacity, it means your "current account" of normal fat reserve reaches its limit long before most people's, so a "fixed deposit," hard to move, soon takes over major banking of fat. This abnormal trait will show at an early age, in spite of normal feeding, explaining why in one family, eating the same food at the same table, one person becomes obese while the others do not.

Start Thinking Thin Early

From the day we're born, eating is one of our first activities, second only to breathing in importance. By the time we're forty, we've consumed about fifty thousand meals. Add between-meals snacks, and the total is up by many thousands. We have assumed a regular pattern of eating. Because there's such an outstanding difference in dieting success between people who became obese as children and those who became obese as adults—the former finding it infinitely more difficult to lose weight—it's obviously imperative to establish the right eating habits during childhood.

In our society it's the mother who teaches the child to overeat, in order to earn her approval. So every mother should reflect as to whether she's inflicting the penalty of a heavyweight life on her child, and work out the right pattern of eating for every member of the family. Audrey Hepburn and Twiggy, between sizes 4 and 5 all their adult lives, must have had very sensible mothers.

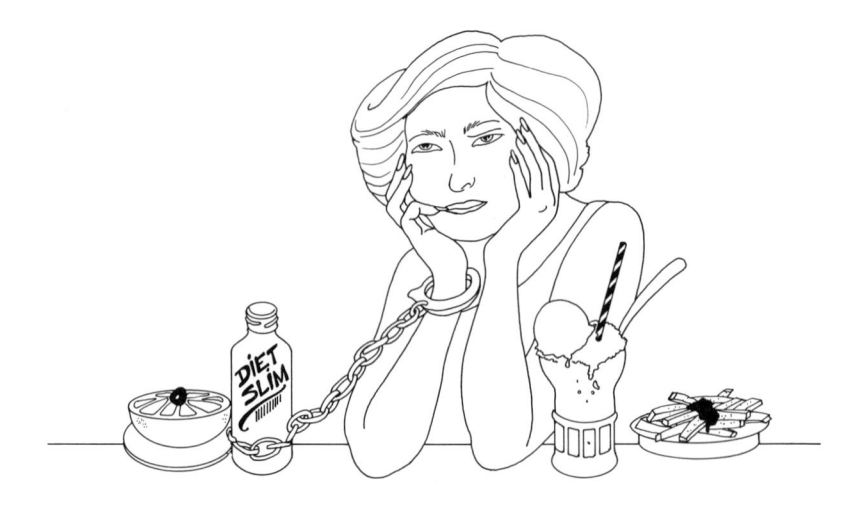

There's a well-established, all-male club in England called Saints and Sinners, and at the annual gourmet dinner, members—all distinguished in their various professions—choose either a white or red carnation for their buttonholes, denoting whether they consider themselves in the first or second category. It's interesting to note that most years, red carnations—the sinner's color—are in the majority.

When it comes to dieting, there aren't many saints around. Perhaps a better description for the ever-increasing members of the dieting club would be martyrs, for few people stay on a diet without indulging in long—and usually dreary—bouts of self-pity. This is reason enough to understand that, whether it's a desire for a size-8 dress or a fear of coronary thrombosis, there has to be *great motivation* before even thinking of life on a lettuce leaf.

A diet plan that doesn't take into consideration the psychological reasons behind a person's overeating habits—and remember fat means overeating—is doomed to failure.

One Hundred Pounds and Over Need to Be Lost: For Those Who've Almost Given Up Hope

The bigger the problem, the more drastic the remedy, which leads us to diets for marathon martyrs, who—in my opinion—deserve everybody's (quiet sympathy . . . for the first few weeks only. Afterward, as results begin to show, no self-pity should be tolerated.

One diet treatment which has had considerable success with co-

FACING PAGE
Motivation is the key—a size-6 dress is more appealing than a strawberry sundae.

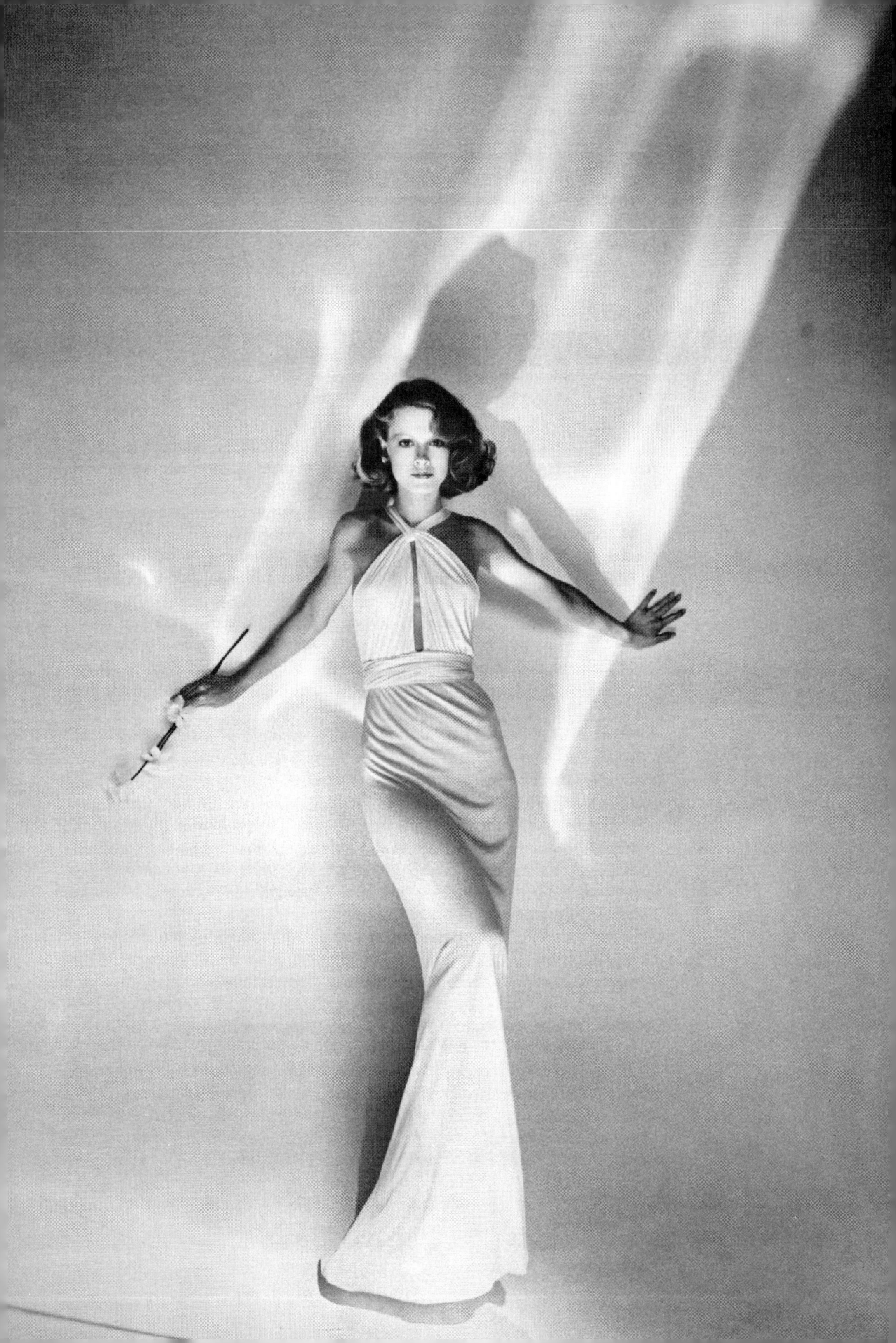

lossal heavyweights, those in the two-hundred-pound-and-up category, is the one usually known as Dr. Simeon's Diet, because a Dr. Simeon did indeed create it.

In 1954, while practising in Rome, Dr. A. T. W. Simeon created a worldwide cyclone of human interest with his paper printed in Britain's medical journal, *The Lancet,* on "The Action of Chorionic Gonadotrophin in the Obese." There he reported his findings of the past twenty years, during which time he had successfully treated over five hundred overweight patients during a forty-day course with a 500-calorie reducing diet (a more usual, but still stringent diet allows 1,000 calories a day) *plus* daily injections of 125 units of human chorionic gonadotrophin, the first course followed in many cases by others of the same duration. His findings gave more than faith, hope, and charity to the overweight world. They suggested a cure.

Dr. Simeon stated that although gonadotrophin alone did not reduce weight, it made a drastic curtailment of calories possible, rendering fat deposits long in residence in the body (the "fixed deposit" mentioned earlier) easily dispersable by transforming them to sugar and so easily burned up. By increasing the blood-sugar level in the body, the appetite became sharply depressed.

Equally, a 500-calorie diet *alone* would not necessarily effect the "fixed deposit," even if by some extraordinary quirk, a person on such a low food intake had enough *joie de vivre* left to get out of bed in the morning!

Since that first report appeared, the obese have not been put off by their early discovery that human chorionic gonadotrophin (now known as HCG) is a substance extracted from the urine of pregnant women. Today this method of treatment is eagerly sought throughout the Western world, and it's fair to say it is approved as being specifically concerned with the control of obesity and applicable to a large majority of cases. Courses are still held in Rome at the Salvator Mundi International Hospital and also are given by doctors all over the United States and at the Kennedy Clinic, 124 East Sixty-fourth Street, New York, where along with the daily injection, two meals are provided, ready packed, to be taken away for lunch and dinner to ensure the 500-calorie count is not exceeded.

Dr. Simeon subsequently pointed out that during pregnancy obese women found to their surprise they actually *lost* weight. This, the good doc explained, was because of the enormous amount of the hormone HCG circulating naturally in their bodies, which enabled the women to reduce their diets drastically without feeling hunger or in any way affecting the child in the womb. The "fixed deposit" of fat, generally impossible to get at, was being placed at the disposal of the growing fetus because of the HCG. In the treatment of obesity, with no embryo to feed, a severe dietary restriction had to take its place for the duration of treatment—for only when the body needed extra fuel, could more fat be withdrawn from the "fixed deposit."

Diet Letdowns

Where this treatment has fallen down is where other treatments have fallen down—a sufficient clinical, biochemical, and personality study of the patient has not been made. In other treatments, where low-calorie, salt-free, no-carbohydrate diets accompany injections, whether of vitamin B, appetite suppressant, liver stimulant, or diuretic (always under a doctor's guidance), a patient has occasionally produced side effects that have precluded her or him from continuing.

A person with good reflexes and general good health will obviously respond more quickly and with better long-term results than those with a sluggish temperament, often the outward sign of a poor constitution. As a doctor specializing in slimming says: "There is always factor x to consider. Money or family problems and most of all love problems." As far as the majority of his treatments are concerned, he goes on to say, "The purpose of the slimming injection is above all to speed up metabolism. It is the hormone balance of the body that controls its rate. Metabolism—and so digestion—is improved by getting a better blood output from the heart into the blood vessels and then into the alimentary tract where a greatly increased blood content should improve the digestive powers manifold."

Instant Cures?

Diuretic is a word often bandied about by laymen in connection with slimming treatments, but a diuretic is used solely to increase fluid output, which goes hand in glove with sodium output. Endocrinologists, nutritionists, and their medical colleagues know that salt and water retention is responsible for much body bulge and this retention is very much governed by the patient's pattern of eating over the years, the condition of various hormones in the body, the pituitary gland, suprarenal, cortical, thyroid, and sex glands—affected by age, exercise (or generally lack of it), and general posture.

A staggering piece of information in this category is that there is more weight fluid and salt loss *at rest* than when the patient is on the move. Many doctors are agreed that there's little validity in injecting diuretics. I quote: "Diuretics should only be given by injection for certain acute cardiac and other emergencies, and I cannot see any reason apart from a gimmick why they should be given by injection in the treatment of obesity. They increase fluid and sodium output from the renal route, but they also increase the output of potassium. If the blood level of potassium becomes too depleted, it can cause muscular weakness, kidney and liver damage, skin rashes, and bone-marrow cellular depression. Such injections are also said to have sometimes aggravated diabetes and to precipitate attacks of gout where this condition already exists. They would certainly not be given for 'tired kidneys' because a definite contradiction to their use would be renal disease."

On the other hand, there are many kinds of chemical compounds used for the purpose of slimming classified as diuretics, but widely different, not only in their effect on potassium levels, but also regarding the length of time in which they act. In some cases, the action lasts for a few hours. In others for as long as twenty-four hours. Again, there is another type which in some people could lead to potassium retention, extremely dangerous if supervision is not monitored by periodic blood biochemical analysis. Some diuretics have potassium incorporated in the pill in order to replace the potassium loss, which must occur with the majority of these compounds.

The amount of fluid loss daily varies with the amount of surplus in the body. A person some seventy or eighty pounds overweight could lose up to seven pounds a day, of which two pounds might be fluid, while a person only twelve pounds overweight, wouldn't lose more than half a pound daily.

The overweight girl in a hurry to regain some sort of shape is the one most in danger. Through taking too many pills against doctor's orders, cutting down too drastically on calories and particularly fluids, a potassium lack can result. She becomes nauseous, suffers a complete loss of appetite, which precludes her from eating at all, and frequently ends up with a kidney complaint to last a lifetime.

Appetite suppressors are often part of a weight-reducing program. When blood-sugar levels are depressed, hunger results. This can be done artificially by injecting small doses of insulin and naturally from starvation. Conversely, if blood-sugar levels are raised, so appetite diminishes. This is one of the effects of HCG as already described, but there are other methods, employing drugs with stimulant properties, essentially only used under medical supervision, accompanied by a medically approved diet. All doctors are against amphetamines, which while depressing appetite centers, also cause insomnia, pulse-rate rises, psychotic manifestations, and anxiety attacks.

When weight "sticks" at a certain spot, it is due to retention of water, but those who make a habit of dieting are hard, if not impossible, to convince that the amount of water they retain has nothing whatsoever to do with the amount they drink. On the contrary, if the fluid intake is insufficient to provide the water required, the kidneys are neglected and strained, and urine becomes scanty and highly concentrated. If more water is taken than the body requires, the surplus is easily eliminated, so to try to prevent the body retaining water by drinking less is not only futile but could be harmful.

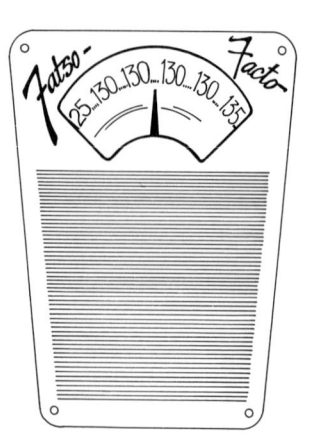

In a letter to *The Lancet* in 1962 Dr. Simeon wrote, "Whenever weight is lost rapidly, two not necessarily synchronised processes are involved. One is the utilisation of excess fat and the other the breakdown of adipose tissue. After a certain loss has been achieved, it seems as if the extraction of fat outruns the body's ability to break down the cellular tissue in which it was contained. It therefore replaces the fat it loses with water. As fat weighs less than water, the scales do not register any loss until the breakdown of the tissue catches up. I do not call the menstrual levelling-off a plateau (weight 'sticking'), because it occurs in almost every case and of this the patient has been forewarned. When a plateau lasts longer than five days, it is usually a sign a weight has been reached which the patient has held for several years before a further increase took place. Any plateau that is not due to careless dieting can be broken up by giving a single tablet of diuretic which relieves anxiety of those who cannot stand the strain of temporary disillusionment. . . ."

When it comes to the final moment of truth in a slimming program, the vitamin or hormone injection, the diuretic pill and/or appetite suppressant, all play the part of catalysts, triggering off the most vital aid to the treatment—the patient's own willpower to change the eating habits of years, to eat *less*—not just for a week or a month, but probably *forever. If willpower is not sufficiently engaged, no prescribed pill or injection is worth a fig.*

Reducing with Rice

Another doctor, Walter Kempner, M.D., of Duke University, North Carolina, has spent a great part of his life combating obesity on behalf of the obese. Frank Sinatra sent his mother to Dr. Kempner's Clinic one year, hoping to be able to say he'd given her "a new figure for Christmas," and Mrs. Sinatra was just one in a long line of celebrities who found themselves living primarily on rice, honest-to-goodness paddy field, unpolished stuff, two bowls of it a day, with or without chopsticks, accommmpanied by a variety of stewed, baked, canned, or fresh fruit.

During a three-week stay myself—in this instance as reporter-companion—I have to say I saw the most astonishing weight reductions of up to thirty pounds, following the rice diet under the all-seeing eagle eye of Dr. Kempner and his retinue of doctors—mostly female.

Dr. K. is a world authority on obesity, having spent years studying the metabolism of living cells, both healthy and diseased. He sought a diet that would not only deflate fat, but cure many of the ills associated with it—high blood pressure, diabetes, hardening of the arteries, heart disease. He eventually came up with what is now known as the Rice Diet.

Salt is the biggest enemy of the obese, says Dr. Kempner, and he stipulates it is part of our daily menu far more than we ever realize, so don't say immediately you never ever reach out for the salt cellar. Your salt intake is bound to be greater than you think.

To combine effective therapy with adequate nutrition in one diet,

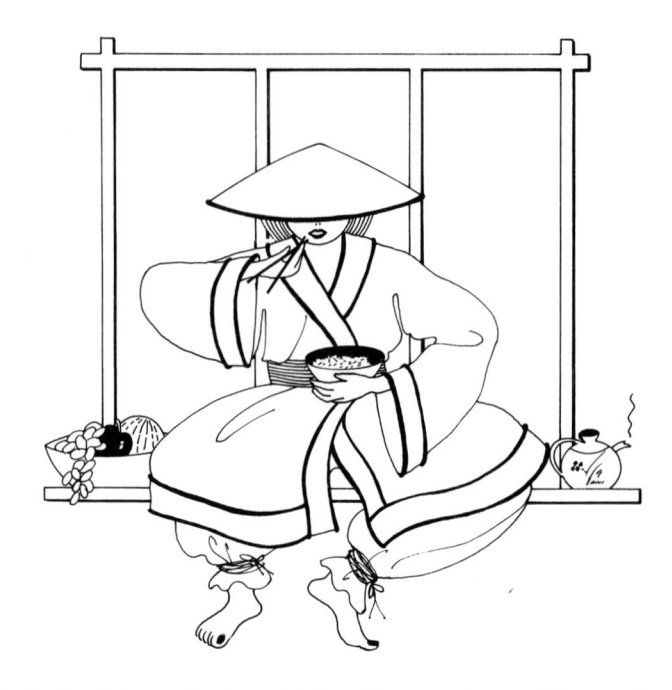

Dr. K. devised formulas in which salt, protein, and fat are kept as low as possible, while the body still receives the amino acids and fatty acids essential for life and growth. The combination of rice, fruit, and fruit juices completely fulfilled his requirements.

It's unique in that while it's low in protein, it's comparatively high in carbohydrate—usually a dirty word where diets are concerned. In fact, the Rice Diet contains almost twice as much carbohydrate as all other diets, only a fourth as much protein and less than one twentieth as much fat. As the carbo intake is tailor-made to provide the body's heat, light, and power, not one calorie left over to stay on the hips, the unusually low protein intake has been proved to be sufficient.

Why rice? Diets usually stress the importance of protein, but few go to the trouble of explaining that proteins, made up of various amino acids, differ from each other in type and in the proportion of amino acid they each contain.

Some are more useful to the body than others, and rice protein comes at the top of the list. It "approximates," as the good doc has said for years, "closely in biological value for man to that of beef, is easily assimilated by the body, and the amino acids compare exceptionally favorably with those contained in other proteins." He goes further: "So far as the metabolism of the kidney cells is concerned, rice protein can't be replaced at will by any other."

In other words, rice is good for you and better still for your figure.

Breakfast at the North Carolina Rice House consists of a piece of citrus fruit, some prune juice, a cup of tea (no milk, but sugar if you like) or Sanka. For lunch there is a big bowl of rice, cooked anyway you want, providing there's no salt or fat attached, together with two kinds of fruit—say half a can of peaches with a large piece of melon or stewed apples with a large bunch of grapes—tea or Sanka. At dinner there is again a big bowl of rice with other varied fruits, plus tea or Sanka.

Apples and pears are always peeled—there's salt in the skin—and fluid intake is restricted to between twenty-four to thirty-two ounces in each twenty-four-hour period, the fluid varying from milkless tea or Sanka to water or fresh lemonade.

Unless you have a doctor totally familiar and in agreement with Dr. Kempner's methods, it cannot be advised you try the Rice Diet at home, for medical checks are made every A.M. at both Rice Houses, where patients take their meals.

No pills, no injections, just rice, fruit, and fruit juices make up the menu, while rest after every meal is obligatory, as is exercise for half an hour six times a day. Most people walk, cycle, or play Ping Pong. If anyone cheats, they're out of the clinic at once—the waiting list's too long to bother with anyone who only wants to play at slimming.

Nearly Everyone I Know Wants to Lose Some Weight—Even the Skinny Ones—but Mostly It's The In-Betweens Who Want to Shed from Six to Twelve Pounds

The great law of life is replenishment. If we don't eat, we die. So our bodies depend on us for a fair deal, but often we eat and forget what the menu was. Our body has to remember *and* cope with whatever we put into it. Most fat people put a lot of carbohydrate into their bodies, mainly on the assumption that they're not going to lose weight, even if they do go without their English muffins at breakfast and their boeuf-en-croûte at dinner, so why should they suffer?

On the other hand, once a fatty sees the light however far away at the end of the tunnel, it's ten to one he or she may go for a low-carbo diet, because *everyone* knows although we need *some*, we don't need that *much* carbohydrate. Excess just turns the body into a great big warehouse.

Another growing body of opinion re the villain of the piece, carbohydrate, is that it is generally less hunger-satisfying than protein, which means one is able to consume more (and usually does) at any one sitting. There also seems to be evidence that carbohydrate helps the system retain natural moisture, thus filling out any curves the body happens to have.

The low-carbo diet has had many aliases, and new ones are always cropping up. Staying the course are the Drinking Man's Diet, the Air Force Diet (nothing to do with the boys in blue, says the Pentagon), the Mayo Clinic Diet (from which the Mayo Clinic in Rochester, Minnesota, completely disassociates itself), not forgetting the Grapefruit Diet, about which a top American nutritionist says, ". . . grapefruit . . . supposed to chew up and dissolve body fat is an asinine proposition. No food has such properties."

Chewing up or not, lurking underneath all that grapefruit at every meal is the oldy: no more than fifty to sixty grams of carbohydrate a day, which is put to work by the body, so never gets stored as fat (look for the carbo counter on pages 154–158).

For some people, there's no doubt this type of diet has worked miracles, because they have genuinely set out to find a new pattern of eating, eschewing the old and the bad, guided by nutritional values, which is what good dieting is all about.

Gimmicky titles take away from the fundamental purpose of the low-carbo theme—which is to enjoy an eating pattern that is (a) sociable, (b) nutritious, and (c) as palatable as possible. It's found in a low-carbo job, providing it isn't decked out with red herrings (no calories) to beautify the citrus industry's profits or the martini makers' balance sheets. If it's properly organized, it's sociable, because we can eat most of the same foods as the rest of the guests at the dinner party, only avoiding the bread, potatoes, and if possible, the dessert, without making a MGM production out of it. It's nutritious, containing meat, fish, eggs, some vegetables, and say half a pint of milk—foods rich in amino acids, vitamins, and essential mineral salts. Most important, it's palatable. Once we've quelled our addiction to sugary and starchy foods, we'll find much more subtle taste in our meat, fish, egg, and cheese dishes often swamped with extraneous flavors.

When one finally gets down to the nitty-gritty of losing pounds and inches, *every doctor concurs calories have to be counted.* Crash diets of bananas and pretzels every four hours or alfalfa sprouts on whole wheat every three may take away a few pounds, but they'll take a lot of the joy out of life, too—if you have any left after a while.

Worst of all, crash diets don't work. After the first thrilling plummet of the scales, the pointer inexorably creeps back up again.

For the majority of us, those who need to lose about twelve pounds, sensible dieting vis-à-vis the daily calorie count *has* to work, and I know from my own experience, it does—this time as an active participant, *not* as a reporter and/or companion. Whether you received A's or D's for arithmetic, everyone can work out this sum: a pound of fatty tissue equals in energy 3,500 calories. Every time you eat 3,500 calories less than you expend, you use up a pound of fatty tissue (out of that "current account," remember?). A deficit of 500 calories a day (eating 2,000 and using up 2,500 for instance) can lead to a loss of one pound a week—fifty-two pounds a year. Get down to 1,000 calories (the best number for a not-too-awesome eating program) and you can lose 104 pounds a year. Will you be able to see yourself in the mirror?

The reason calorie counting sometimes goes awry is the number of misconceptions connected with it. Too many believe there's a whole area of nonfattening food, where they can indulge their hunger pangs to their pituitary's delight. So they piously dive into steaks the size of Gulliver's shoe and gulp down king-size glasses of fresh orange juice, averting their eyes and their mouths scrupulously from all that "dreadful fattening food—bread, potatoes, bananas." They don't lose weight. They throw their calorie counter into a coconut-fudge sundae and bewail the injustice of it all.

The serious student of calories—and therefore serious dieter, too—has to study facts and learn that a three-ounce slice of roast beef, enough to cover a slice of rye bread, contains 260 calories. A tall glass of fresh orange juice, straight out of the peel, is 110; concentrated out of a can, it's 300. As for that coconut-fudge sundae—500 calories—is that spelled out enough?

Steak is a problem in itself, whatever its size. It's widely believed to be pure protein and therefore it can be consumed ad infinitum, allowing the consumer to emerge as skinny as Twiggy, but *all meat contains fat.* Three ounces of sirloin, for instance, or deboned rib roast contains an average twenty grams of protein (80 calories) and twenty grams of fat (180 calories). A three-ounce hamburger contains an average 20 grams of protein (80 calories) and 26 grams of fat (230 calories). Ham contains even more fat calories in relation to protein content.

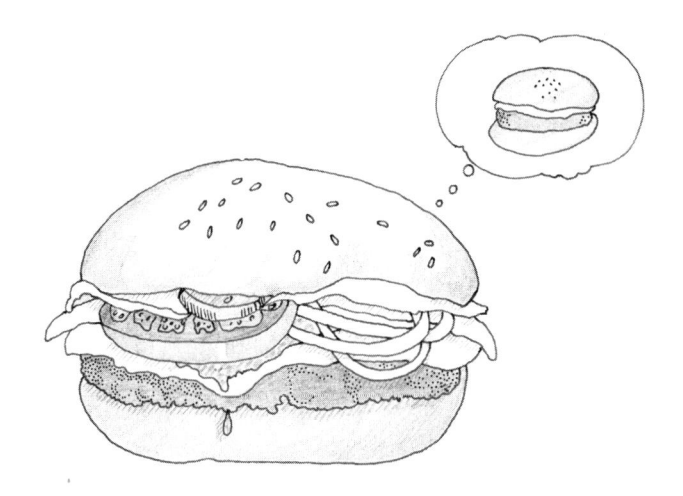

Size is just as important a factor as selection when it comes to choosing from a menu or cooking at home. Eating a large hamburger, but counting it as a small one will make the difference of two pounds of fat staying in place. Self-deception only leads to a hidden surtax which destroys the calorie budget just as effectively as the coconut-fudge sundae. Peanuts, you say? Sorry—850 calories for a couple of handfuls.

Millions of people are deluded by the word protein itself, thinking it is some magical panacea to diet and that if they stick to it only, pounds will fall off. Instead, with a carbohydrate and fat deficiency, health will suffer and pounds may not fall off, either. Protein contains about 120 calories an ounce, the same as carbohydrates (fats are more costly at about 280 an ounce), but when too much protein is eaten, and it is in the presence of carbohydrate, the protein is converted and stored in the body as fatty tissue. When there is no carbohydrate present (which is rare), excess can be absorbed and stored as muscle tissue. Depending on the type of protein and the type of person you are, the fatty tissue may or may not be reconverted into protein for the body's requirements. Where there is a tendency to obesity, the fat stays as fat.

It isn't easy to work out how many calories you personally burn up each day. As mentioned previously, factor x is at work governing the way you cope with life, apart from how you happen to spend it.

As a simple guide you can work out an approximate figure from the following:

1. Sleeping, the body burns up 11 to 13 calories per pound of body weight.
2. Sitting, relaxing, the body burns up from 13 to 16 calories per pound of body weight.
3. Sedentary work—secretarial or light housework—the body burns up from 18 to 20 calories per pound of body weight.
4. Hard work—exercise, making love—the body burns up from 28 to 35 calories per pound of body weight.

Let's say your ideal body weight for age (over thirty), height (5'5"), and body structure (medium) (see chart on page 160) is 136 pounds, and that you're an executive secretary, a fairly high-powered job which means you burn up the top rate of 20 calories per pound of body weight during much of the day. You simply multiply 136 × 20, which means to stay the same weight, you need to consume 2,720 calories each day; to lose weight, you must eat less.

The sad fact remains, as you get older, you'll need to eat still less to remain that curvy 136 pounds. Ask Liz and Sophia. Body functions slow down, exercise isn't so attractive, while food, for some unaccountable reason, gets more and more irresistible.

When you're on a conveyor belt of luncheons, cocktail parties, and dinners; when, if you're not going out, you take second helpings at home to encourage guests to appreciate the cook—then you can be in trouble, particularly as this usually happens a little later on in life when your husband and sometimes you yourself have become successful.

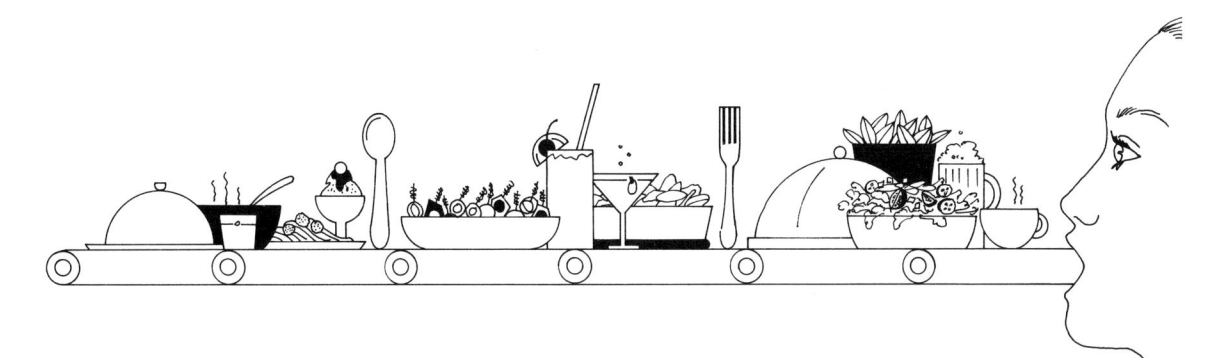

When you're in the social boat, it takes more than motivation, more than diuretic pills, to break through the food barrier and win back measurements. It takes cunning not to be boring (and so fall easy victim to an over-eager hostess anxious to break your diet rules—why *will* women do that?) and not to be bored with an everlasting eating syndrome of grapefruit and steak—diet by courtesy of your youngest daughter, you know the sort of thing.

To keep your bounce and social nounce, certain foods, low in calories, ought always to be on the menu to equip the body naturally in its diet endeavor. Lettuce, onions, celery, and spinach all contain silicone, which is a natural body brightener, helping prevent nervous exhaustion and mental fatigue. Oysters, clams, raisins, and leeks are natural sources of sodium, aiding endurance, clearing sinuses, diluting moodiness, while seafood is always good for you if you can take it, containing as it does complete protein, which supplies the essential amino acids the body can't manufacture and must get from food. Milk is important, because with other dairy products it provides nearly two thirds of the body's calcium demands. If there's a lack, it shows up most in nervous tension. Whether taken straight or used in a low-cal soup, sauce, or shake recipe, one eight-ounce glass of skim or buttermilk should be taken every day. Eggs, chief source of protein, are tricky because of their cholesterol value. Four or five a week is a safe margin, providing you don't lose count when using one in a recipe.

Best Food for Dieters

One of the most underrated—and in some cases wrongly accused—foods is the avocado. It's underrated because it's a beauty armory, containing eleven vitamins and seventeen minerals (just to start with), and wrongly accused of being fattening because it isn't when you compare it to a multitude of other far less deserving chow. One average-size half contains 132 calories, less than a cup of plain gelatin or two ounces of the dieter's perpetual lunch—broiled hamburger. It's head and stalk above so many other fruits because of its numerous nutritional qualities: the protein content is of equal status to many kinds of meat. It contains little starch and practically no sugar (both devils to diets as we know); it offers generous quantities of calcium, magnesium, potassium, sodium, copper, phosphates, manganese, and iron, and is even more valuable because of its high percentage of polyunsaturated fatty acid, which gives the fruit its mellow texture and nutlike flavor. The Mexicans call it "butter growing on trees," and they use it like that, too, spreading the pulp on their tortillas. It's an amazingly complete meal in itself, and if you lunched on one half every day, you'd find it a great incentive to losing the last few obstinate pounds that refuse to budge.

Vitamins are Vital, Yet Easy to Forget

Vitamin A, great for getting a flawless skin, is found in all green—especially leafy—vegetables, yellow ones, too, plus yellow fruits, chicken, liver, egg yolks, and cheese.

Vitamin B Complex includes all members of the Vitamin B family, which must be present before any living organism can burn glucose, the fuel that keeps us on the move. It helps supply oxygen to the vital areas of the body—especially the brain. Eat it in liver, kidney, oysters, all grains.

Vitamin B12 is an energizer, fighting disease, age, nervousness. Eat it in broccoli, crab, mushrooms, skim milk.

Vitamin C (ascorbic acid) is the body's way of making the "cement" that holds the cells together. A poor vitamin C intake leads to tooth decay and longer-lasting bruises. Bean sprouts, oranges, peppers, and persimmon are all rich sources.

Vitamin D is a body builder and a slimmer in that it helps the body burn off sugar more efficiently. Sunshine is a beautiful source (watch that ultra violet, though. See pages 28–31), so is milk.

Vitamin E increases hormone production, to do wonders for your sex life, improving the health of your glands, so shaping up shape and also doing the deepest cleansing job on skin—from the inside. Fish, apples, liver, some cheeses, eggs provide E.

Vitamin P fights illness through acting on the capillaries. Spinach, parsley, lettuce, and all citrus fruits are fine for P.

Minerals are a Must, Too

Check that you're mobilizing the right ones for health, strength, and shape:

Calcium for good bones and teeth, relaxed nerves and muscles. Drink milk, eat yogurt, and clams, kale, and cheese.

Phosphorus is calcium's running mate; brain tissues are rich with it. Nearly all vegetables and fruit provide phosphorus.

Potassium is a directing force, sending the right nourishment out of the bloodstream to the cells. If there's a deficiency, constipation is the result. Leafy green vegetables and fruit for you.

Sulphur suits your blood, promoting the liver to absorb what's good for it. Brussels sprouts are sweet with sulphur.

Iron provides oxygen. When there's a short supply, anemia's the result, Parsley, kidney, and fresh fruit for iron eaters.

Iodine is a gland fuel, helping produce the hormones that control many of life's processes, metabolism and other timings for the body. Garlic may be antisocial, but it's high in iodine; so is seafood. Langouste Catalan, anyone?

The following are psychological aids—don't knock them. They're as important as weights and measures—to remind you about your great shape crusade.

1. Sit near a mirror at mealtimes, so you can see how you've bloated the shape nature gave you.
2. Wear a tight girdle about the house, but not when you're going out. Then, a tight girdle can "show on your face" like tight shoes.
3. Before a gala, weigh and write your weight down to glance at when you powder your nose.
4. Eat very slowly. Chew well, and eat from a smaller plate.
5. Take the edge off hunger before a meal with snacks of bouillon, a heart of lettuce, a handful of raisins, a spoonful of yogurt.
6. Season food with spice or herbs or tart fruit juices. Sprinkle sunflower seeds on salads, or soups; coconut meal on vegetables—all to add variety to your willpower.
7. Cut down dramatically on alcohol by asking for something you don't like. If you've been on martinis for years, ask for scotch-on-the-rocks. Hate rye? Ask for a long one. You may grow to like it eventually, but you'll have consumed a lot less liquid in the indocrination period.
8. Pamper yourself in other ways. If breakfast in bed is your idea of heaven, indulge yourself. Make a good start to your diet with an ideal A.M. break of orange slices, one poached egg on whole wheat bread, coffee with skim milk. Then put a makeup mirror on your bed tray and take your mind off your weight by looking at your face. Experiment for fifteen to twenty minutes with colors or face packs or anything you fancy.
9. Rest more anyway.
10. Exercise more, too, not enough to frighten the neighbors, but in a relaxed, pleasant way. Don't bend your knees when you retrieve the glove you dropped or put the lead on Fido (buying a dog is one way to exercise more). Stretch up to reach for something—even if it's out of reach, stretch anyway. Climb a couple of flights for a couple of days. See how the pavement feels under your heels. Walk if you can for at least fifteen minutes each day, Fido or no Fido.

There's no doubt about it. If the only muscles you ever move are the chewing muscles, it makes the whole slimming-down process far more difficult.

The No-Nonsense Low-Carbo Diet

Rule 1. Before embarking on any diet, have a checkup and talk it over with your doctor.

Rule 2. No more than 50 to 60 grams of carbohydrate every day.

Rule 3. No large or second helpings (probably ever again).

Rule 4. No more than one alcoholic drink per meal (before, during, *or* after—and never, ever, between).

All numbers in brackets refer to grams of carbohydrate, not caloric content.

Breakfast: Choose from poached egg (0) or medium size haddock (4) or 2 pieces of lean grilled bacon (0) with grilled tomato (6), plus 2 slices of diet bread (8) or 1 piece of rye or white (12) or whole wheat (11), 1 pat butter (0), coffee or tea, dash of milk if required (4), sugar substitute (0).

Lunch: Choose from grilled trout or plaice or sole, sliced tomato salad with French dressing, 1 ounce cheese, 2 water biscuits, coffee (13); *or* ½ cup soft-shelled crab (8) with asparagus on the side (½ cup, 3) plus butter sauce (0), coffee or 1 serving baked, boiled or deviled ham (0) with 1 ounce zucchini (1) plus ½ medium cantaloupe (9), coffee.

Dinner: Choose from onion soup (4) plus filet mignon (0), brussels sprouts (½ cup 6), 1 fresh plum (7), coffee, or 1 medium artichoke (5) with butter sauce (0) plus baked or canned salmon (0) with cucumber salad (2), french dressing (2), ½ cup jello (18); or oyster cocktail (8), spareribs (0) barbecue sauce (2), 1 ounce camembert (½), 1 cracker (5), coffee.

Add a Manhattan before dinner, you add 7 more grams of carbohydrate to your daily total. Add a martini before lunch, and it's another 1. If you're a wine drinker, the tax is heavier: 12 for most medium dry to sweet white wines, 14 for red—but you can celebrate occasionally with a glass of Champagne. 3 ounces totals 2 grams of carbo only.

Count 1,000 Calories to Lose the Weight You Need

Rule 1. Before embarking, have a checkup and talk it over with your doctor.

Rule 2. Count every calorie you consume (see calorie-counter on pages 154–159).

Breakfast every day (and don't skip it, breakfast whips the metabolism awake to keep in tune throughout the day): orange juice, 1 small

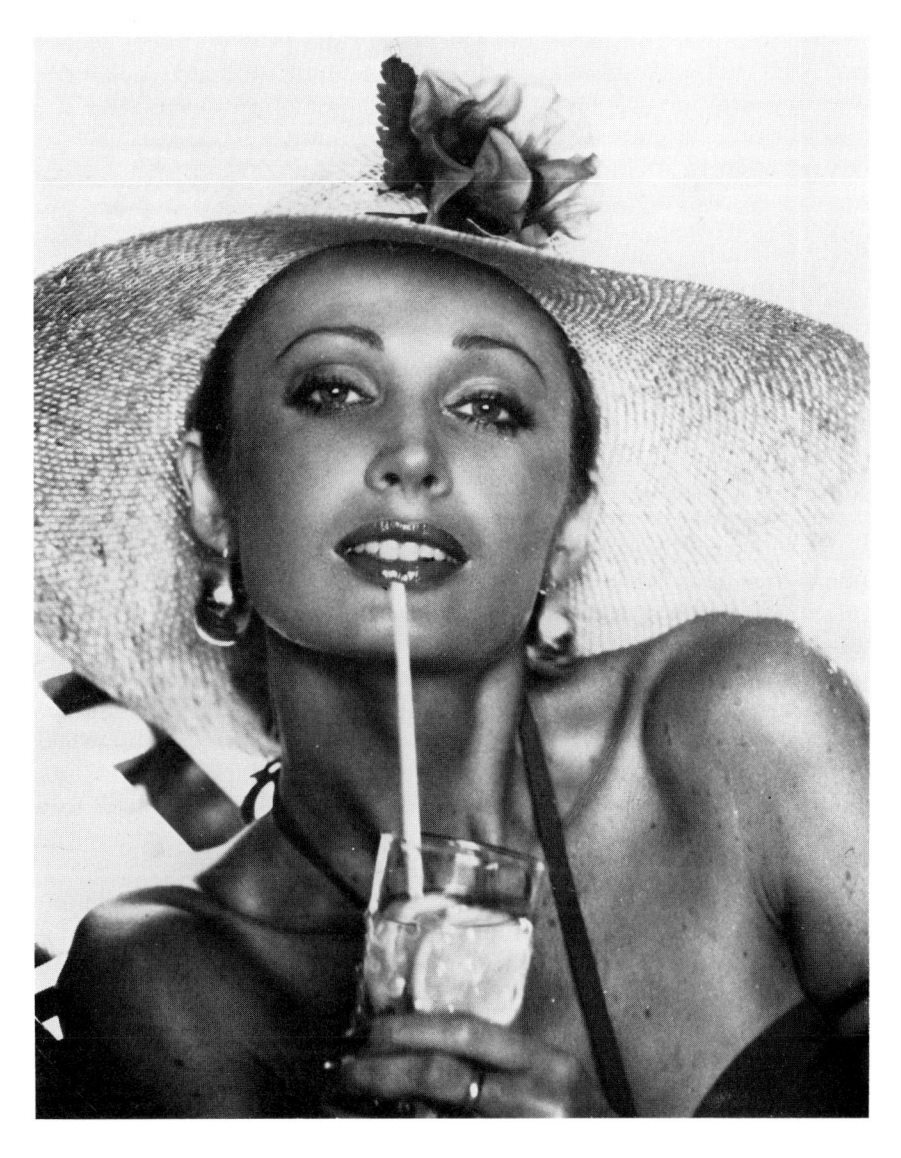

Alcohol is no help on a diet. Ask for something you don't like, to learn to do without it.

glass; 1 poached egg, whole wheat bread—1 slice, coffee with skim milk.

Lunch: Choose from (1) frankfurter, asparagus (6 spears), 1 yogurt, coffee with skim milk or tea with lemon; **or** (2) 3 ounces crab meat with lettuce and tomato, 1 cup canned cherries, coffee or tea; **or** (3) tomato juice, turkey or peanut butter, lettuce and tomato sandwich, coffee or tea; **or** (4) clear soup, salmon salad, with little mayonnaise, lettuce and 1 tomato, coffee or tea.

Dinner: Choose from (1) broiled lean lamb chop, peas and carrots, 1 slice white bread, coffee or tea; **or** (2) 1 medium slice roast beef,

½ cup rice, tossed salad with lemon juice, 1 slice pound cake, coffee or tea; **or** (3) broiled flounder with cabbage, 1 raw tomato, 1 flavored yogurt, coffee or tea; **or** (4) broiled scallops, 1 baked potato, 1 cup cooked beets, ½ grapefruit with spoonful of honey, coffee or tea.

Adds up to about one thousand calories a day.

Happy Counting!

Group Therapy

Most people have heard of Weight Watchers. The founder, Jean Nidetch, is anxious to point out that WW, as it's now familiarly called, is a program, *not* a diet. Once a fat lady herself, Jean created WW out of her personal experience, realizing she had become thin through a sense of competition entering into her slimming campaign—when she exchanged progress reports with her friends.

Based on the old theory it always helps resolve when you know others are suffering the same pangs, WW grew into a nationwide business through a reeducation program of eating habits.

At the weekly classes and lectures, everyone is weighed and publicly congratulated or otherwise. Everyone receives their weekly menu, which may include a potato or even spaghetti, but it is all compensated for in the overall program. Of course, the meals are planned around a calorie count—they have to be—but the caloric content is not discussed because WW believes that counting calories can lead to a person "saving" them and eating a piece of chocolate layer cake in the happy assumption they are well within their limits. The overall philosophy is that anyone can go on a diet and lose weight—momentarily—but it means nothing if *food habits have not been basically changed* to a program of well-balanced, healthy, nutritional meals. To WW—and anyone who has any sense—*nutrition* is the most important aspect of dieting—and eating.

How to Get Fatter When You've Been Too Thin All Your Life

Maria Beatrice de Savoia, daughter of ex-King Umberto of Italy, is a member of the most envied minority group in the world—the skinny people, around or less than one hundred pounds, size 3 to 4 variety; other members of the group are Gloria Vanderbilt Cooper, Audrey Hepburn, and Mia Farrow—even when she's pregnant she only looks as if she's swallowed an olive.

Medically speaking, the lightweights are way ahead of the heavyweights in the lifespan race, but the line between lightweight and underweight is, understandably, a thin one. *Underweight* can also mean under-nutrition, which calls for a diet just as urgently as any case of obesity—a diet which would seem delightful to most people, obviously being based on a high-calorie intake.

It's practically impossible to get thin people to admit to liking their shape. They always say they want to gain but can't, just as fat people say, "But I eat like everybody else." The fact is they don't. They only think they do. Just see your thinnest friend eat—it resembles a sparrow at work.

Why They Stay Thin

Unless there's a medical dysfunction, a chronic infection, a hormonal imbalance, an underactive adrenal gland, or an overactive thyroid—all of which obviously need medical attention—the forever slim and willowy or underfed and skinny (depending on how you look at it and whether they know how to dress or not) stay that way because there's rarely any feeling of acute hunger in the body. A low-calorie intake maintains the status quo.

Dr. Rachmiel Levine, executive medical director of the City of Hope, California, has related details of experiments that prove habit factors greatly affect our shape. When a fat and a lean person were put into a room furnished only with a table, a chair and a clock, the fat person called for food when the clock told him it was lunchtime, while the thin person showed no reaction. In fact the clock was rigged to go twice as fast as normal, but one look at the time was enough to send hunger signals fast from the hyperthalmic appetite-regulating portion of the fat person's brain, producing reactions of saliva and even stomachache from hunger.

A lack of appetite is frequently behind a lack of measurements, and this in turn can be caused by anorexia, a nervous condition which dissipates any interest in food. Some doctors with a number of too-skinny patients observe that a minuscule appetite can be stimulated artificially with medical help, but as these patients are likely to have some sort of blood disturbance (diabetes or the reverse, low blood sugar), a glucose tolerance test is a wise course of action before embarking on any gain-weight program.

Even if there's no medical explanation behind an obstinate inability to gain pounds and inches, doctors maintain excessive sugar intake is a mistake. With a correct blood-sugar level, appetite *can* be regained more easily and maintained. To that end ironically, *diet* sodas, weak tea and sugar substitutes are sometimes recommended even when trying to gain.

The Easiest Mistake to Make

The most common pitfall is to think a gain-weight diet is the opposite of a reducing one. Gulping down rich ice-cream sodas, eating extra cheese cake, sugar, and sweets won't help the picture, for these foods deliver the "empty" kinds of calories, the ones that *fill you up* without *building up* nutrition.

The best gain-weight plan is obviously to increase calorie intake with the *building kind of foods.* As 3,500 calories is roughly equivalent to one pound of body weight, it really means consuming about 1,000 calories a day more than your body uses up for fuel. To add to average eating habits, it's best to choose portions of unrefined carbohydrate—potatoes (from 95 to 230 calories, depending on cooking method), peas (105), corn (165), wild rice (395), olives (40), avocados (260), bananas (175), lima (150) and chili beans (320). In fact, most types of Mexican food are great for putting on the curves. Carbohydrates are less satisfying than proteins, so one can consume more. There's also evidence carbohydrates help the system retain natural moisture, plumping out the figure in the bleak spots, but it's still best to choose more of the unrefined type than the refined (foods that are heavy with sugar, flour, or cornstarch). If you smoke and/or drink more than moderately, cutting down or, best of all, giving cigarettes up can only help spur the appetite.

Vitamins Are Vital

Whatever vitamins you're taking now, there should be an increase in vitamin E and B complex intake, plus more concentration on foods already packed with them naturally, like liver (85 calories), whole grain (56 calories) and enriched cereals (from 95 to 310 calories), bread (from 30 to 190 calories), and nuts (95 calories). It's been proved the fastest method of gaining weight is the snack, which is why nibbling is taboo to the other more ordinary kind of dieter. Three or four snacks taken throughout the day can add an amazing number of extra calories.

For instance, by adding a cup of skim-milk powder to a cup of soup, custard, or hot drink, you immediately gain an extra 435 calories. By adding an instant-food mix to an eight-ounce glass of milk (160), you add 290 calories; while adding three tablespoons of malted milk powder, too, increases the total by 405. These tricks make it easy to add 1,000 extra calories a day—which will eventually show on the scales—and curves.

Hypnosis—Can IT Help and How?

FACING PAGE
She is not asleep, not awake; she is hypnotized for her health's sake.

She is hypnotized, not like Trilby by Svengali, or Walter Scott's Lady of the Lake, not asleep, not awake, not unconscious, but to quote Dr. Herbert Spiegel, Associate Clinical Professor of the Department of

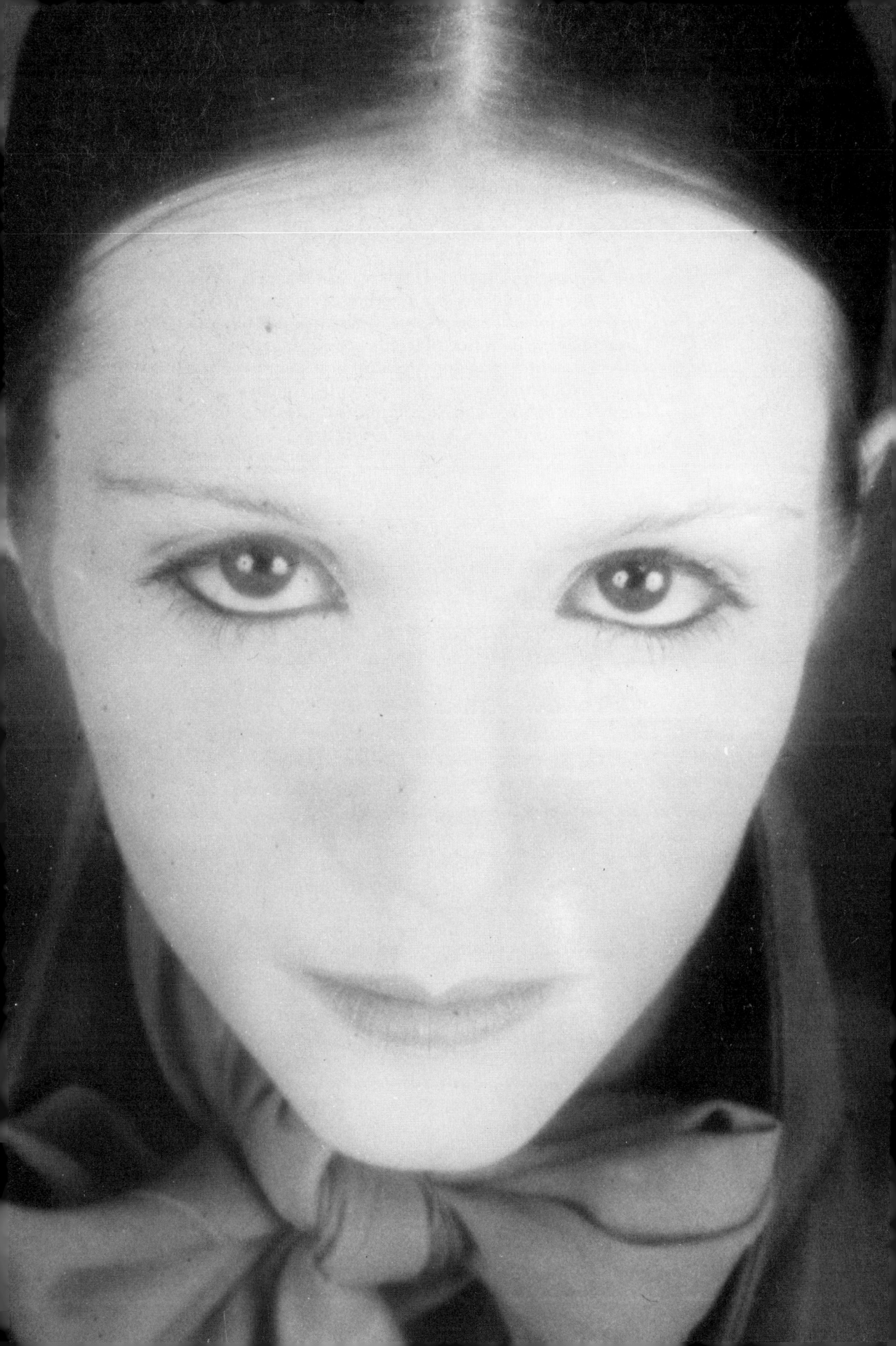

Psychiatry at Columbia University, "She is in a form of *intense aroused attentive concentration. Responsive concentration.*"

To use other words, Dr. Spiegel is describing the hypnotic state as it really is, not mystic, frightening, or hocus-pocus, either, but a condition induced by many doctors today to help in the treatment of a number of self-inflicted sicknesses—brought about by overeating, overdrinking, or smoking.

Hypnosis is also used as a valuable ancillary to treatments working toward overcoming a number of phobias (fear of flying, fear of heights, crowds, cats or dogs), plus helping to assuage grief, shock, and relieving pain in childbirth—pain generally.

Today both the American Medical Association and the American Psychiatric Association have accepted hypnosis as *aiding treatment* providing it takes place under the auspices of skilled doctors.

Obviously such august medical bodies would only recognize qualified treatment, but actually most laymen can be taught to hypnotize others.

What distinguishes the skilled practitioner from the layman is *knowing what to do once hypnosis is induced and having the ability to recognize who is hypnotizable and who is not.*

According to Dr. Spiegel about 70 percent of the population can be hypnotized, which means 70 percent have the ability *to concentrate well.*

"It's a complete fallacy," he says "that only the weak-minded can be hypnotized, for it is the weak-minded who are unable to concentrate for any length of time and so discipline their thoughts. The lower the intelligence, the poorer the subject for hypnotherapy."

What Does It Feel Like to be Hypnotized?

Patients have described it as a totally relaxed languid feeling of tranquility, pleasant, peaceful, a sensation of floating. People who sleep deeply may even doze momentarily, while light sleepers feel completely awake.

Physicians describe it as a state that occurs *normally* somewhere between the diurnal rhythm of being asleep and being awake. This midway state is deliberately extended by the doctor, so that treatment can be carried out within its bounds.

Once hypnotizability is established, the entire emphasis in treatment is on replacing or superceding negative ways of thinking, feeling, acting (ingrained over the years as habits) with totally new *positive* ways, rather like using a projector on the mind, focusing on a new slide, giving the patient a different aspect of the situation.

The human mind, one ninth conscious, eight ninths subconscious, is extremely suggestible and becomes more so under hypnosis—"the state of receptive attention" as practitioners often call it.

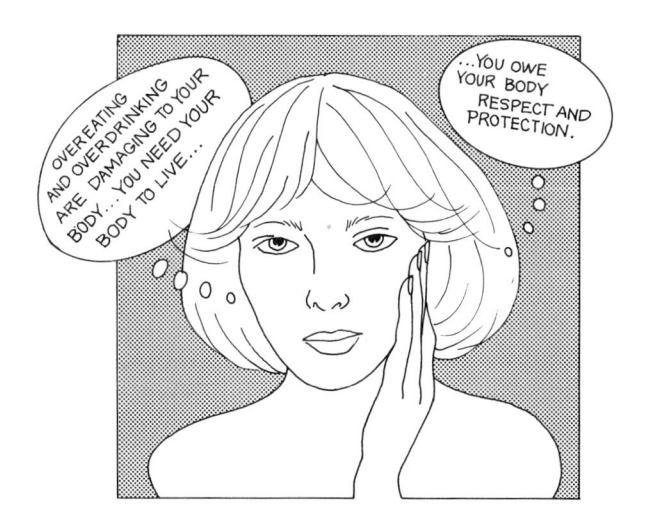

Their object is to put forward a view that the patient is *for* rather than against. For example, the unsuccessful dieter on a permanent on-and-off diet syndrome is helped to be positive and so more successful in her weight campaign by the doctor putting deep into her mind three basic but forceful facts: (1) overeating and overdrinking are damaging to your body. (2) You need your body to live. It is the precious physical plant through which you experience life. (3) You owe your body respect and protection.

These facts are put there to distract her attention completely away from her constant urge to eat the foods she knows defeat her objective. *Like all urges, if repeatedly not satisfied by being ignored, it eventually withers away.*

In trying to cut down or stop anything one knows is detrimental to health and spirit, the most frequent mistake is to put all emphasis on *not doing so:* I must not eat cheesecake; I should not eat cheesecake; I will not eat cheesecake.

As Dr. Spiegel reiterates: "This kind of thinking is dead wrong. It makes about as much sense as if you concentrate on not having an itching sensation on your nose. What happens if you concentrate on *not* having that itch? You have it all the more."

The same thing happens when you concentrate merely on avoiding fattening foods. You end up more preoccupied with them than ever. The person accustomed to freedom is not helped with permanent sanctions against the urge that is uppermost in her mind, but she can affiliate with and arouse her compassion for a worthwhile and obviously self-preserving goal—*respecting the body, protecting it.*

Critics of hypnotism bring up the fact that it takes up so much time. The fact is, it doesn't. Today most significant progress relates to the success of self-hypnosis, taught by the physician after only the first session. The patient using twenty seconds ten times a day is taught to float into his own island of awareness, and there to *reimprint* the new positive aspect for living already shown demonstrated under hypnosis.

Hypnotism can't be forced on anyone who doesn't want it and neither can hypnotism induce anybody to act totally out of character. In other words, a basically moral person cannot be made to behave immorally, or vice versa. On the contrary, hypnotism frees people of inhibitions and their surface "personality," allowing them to behave as they really are.

There are already programs in existence that had their basis in hypnotism such as the rerouting of consciousness used in Dr. Grantley Dick-Read's method of natural childbirth where the mind is distracted, led away from pain, and directed with programmed breathing

BEVERAGES	Calories	Carbohydrates
Beer (12 oz.)	170	18
Brandy	120	0
Carbonated beverages—Cola	107	20
Champagne (3 oz.)	80	2
Chocolate beverages with milk (8 oz.)	205	18
Coffee, black	0	0
Cordials	121	6
Gin, dry	120	0
Rum	105	0
Sherry	85	10
Tea	0	½
Whiskey	110	0
Wines, dry (3 oz.)	85	5
Wines, sweet (3 oz.)	160	12

BREAD AND CEREALS		
Bran flakes	145	21
Bread, raisin (one slice)	65	13
Bread, rye, dark (one slice)	57	12
Bread, wheat, cracked (one slice)	60	12
Bread, white enriched (one slice)	64	12
Bread, whole wheat (one slice)	55	11
Corn Flakes (one bowl)	96	18
Crackers, graham (one)	30	5
Crackers, saltines (one)	15	3
Doughnut	125	17
Macaroni, cooked (4 oz.)	209	80
Noodles, egg, cooked (4 oz.)	200	49

toward a specific job in helping the child be born. Programmed Motivation, developed by Dr. Frederick Wright, is also related—tape systems helping one become more receptive to new thoughts—"diet without drugs," "listen and stop smoking,"—working in the way one learns a language through repeated sessions with cassettes or recordings.

Research carried out in universities and medical schools across the country (through grants given by the National Institutes of Health) has revealed that the shifting of awareness into another health-based, self-preservative category in response to a signal from another permits more intensive concentration upon a designated goal and, in this way, is of enormous benefit to medicine.

This means only one thing: *hypnosis.* You can't underrate it.

	Calories	*Carbohydrates*
BREAD AND CEREALS (cont.)		
Popcorn (1 cup)	54	10
Potato chips (10)	108	10
Pretzel (5 small sticks)	18	1
Rice, cooked, white (3 oz.)	160	30
Rice, puffed	55	13
Roll, plain	118	20
Roll, sweet	178	20
Shredded wheat	85	18
Spaghetti, plain, cooked (3 oz.)	165	35
Waffle	216	30
Wheat flakes	125	23
DAIRY PRODUCTS		
Butter (one pat.)	50	0
Cheese, bleu (one piece)	104	½
Cheese, Camembert (one piece)	85	½
Cheese, Cheddar (one piece)	113	½
Cheese, cottage	225	3
Cheese, cream	106	½
Cheese, Swiss, natural	105	1
Cream, light	30	1
Cream, heavy	49	2
Ice Cream	120–260	15
Sherbert	236	28
Milk, chocolate flavored	205	18
Milk, half and half	320	1
Milk, whole	166	10
Sour cream, light	455	1
Yogurt, plain	120	5

DESSERTS AND SWEETS

	Calories	Carbohydrates
Cake, plain	180	31
Cake, pound	130	15
Cake, sponge	75	22
Candies, bar	175–295 (small to large)	40
Chocolate, syrup	42	11
Cocoa	21	12
Cookie, plain	109	9
Cup cake, iced	161	31
Custard, baked	283	14
Fig bars, commercial	55	12
Gelatin, dessert	80	18
Gelatin with fruit	140	21
Honey (tablespoon)	62	17
Jams, marmalades, preserves (1 dessert spoon)	55	14
Jellies	50	14
Molasses, medium	46	13
Sugar, brown (1 teaspoon)	45	12
Sugar, granulated (1 teaspoon)	45	12

FRUIT

	Calories	Carbohydrates
Apple, fresh	90	18
Applesauce, sweetened (1 tablespoon)	184	25
Apricots, raw, 1	18	13½
Avocados, raw, ½	160	6
Banana	175	23
Blackberries, raw, ½ cup	41	10
Blackberries, syrup pack, ½ cup	85	12
Blueberries, raw, 1 cup	85	20
Blueberries, syrup pack, 1 cup	225	24
Cantaloupe, ½	60	9
Cherries, fresh, 1 cup	65	16
Cherries, canned, 1 cup	122	8
Dates, dried, pitted, 1 cup	490	7
Figs, canned in syrup, 3	85	36
Figs, dried, 1	40	15
Fruit cocktail, 1 cup	110	50
Grapefruit, fresh, ½	40	14
Grapefruit, canned, 1 cup	140	42
Grapefruit juice, sweetened (6 oz.)	175	18
Grapes, American, 1 cup	105	16
Grape juice, 1 cup (4 oz.)	145	21
Honeydew melon, ¼	49	10
Lemon, fresh	25	6

FRUIT (cont.)

	Calories	Carbohydrates
Lemon, juice (1 tablespoon)	4	1
Lime, fresh	5	10
Olives, 10	220	2
Orange, 1	75	16
Orange juice, fresh, one 6 oz. glass	110	18
Peaches, fresh, 1	35	10
Peaches, canned, 2 halves	79	24
Pears, fresh, 1	40	25
Pears, canned, 2 halves	79	23
Pineapple, raw, 1 cup	65	20
Pineapple, canned, crushed, 1 cup	204	54
Pineapple juice, 1 cup (4 oz.)	140	15
Plums, raw, 1	29	7
Plums, canned	186	25
Prunes, dry, 4 uncooked	73	20
Prunes, cooked, unsweetened (5)	120	22
Prune juice, 1 cup (4 oz.)	190	22
Raisin, dry, 1 tbsp.	30	30
Rhubarb, stewed, sweetened, 1 cup	375	96
Strawberries, raw, 1 cup	54	13
Strawberries, frozen (3 oz.)	90	25
Tangerine, 1	45	10
Watermelon, 1 wedge	235	29

MEAT, FISH, POULTRY, EGGS

Bacon, 2 slices	97	1
Beef, hamburger chuck	316	0
Beef, rib roast, boneless	266	0
Beef, steak	257	0
Bluefish (baked)	180	0
Bologna, 1½" slice	467	½
Caviar (1 teaspoon)	24	0
Chicken, canned	180	0
Chicken, fryer, breast	210	5
Clams	92	2
Cod, dried	106	½
Egg	77	0
Flounder (baked)	200	0
Frankfurter	124	1
Haddock, fried	165	4
Halibut, broiled	215	0
Ham, fresh or smoked, cooked	338	0
Herring, smoked, kippered	210	0
Lamb chop	356	0

	Calories	Carbohydrates
MEAT (cont.)		
Lamb, leg, roasted	230	0
Liver	75–85	8
Liverwurst	80	1
Lobster, canned	78	0
Mackerel (small to large)	190–305	0
Oysters, six	200	8
Pork, loin	240	0
Salmon	180	0
Sardines, drained	171	1
Sausage, pork, uncooked	150	0
Scallops, uncooked	89	11
Shrimps, canned, drained	115	0
Tuna, canned, drained	135	0
Turkey, uncooked	304	0
Veal, uncooked	184	0
NUTS		
Almonds, 18	130	7
Peanut Butter	92	3
Peanuts, 1 cup	840	28
Pecans, 1 cup	700	16
Walnuts, 1 cup	654	20
SANDWICHES		
Chicken Salad	245	19
Egg Salad	280	18
Ham	280	18
Roast Beef	400	20
SAUCES AND FATS		
Chili sauce (1 tablespoon)	17	4
French dressing (1 tablespoon)	59	2
Margarine, 1 pat	50	0
Mayonnaise (1 tablespoon)	110	0
Oils (1 tablespoon)	124	0
Tomato Catsup	20	4
SOUPS (all 1-cup portions)		
Bean	191	19
Bouillon, cube	2	0
Bouillon, ready to serve	9	0
Chicken	75	7
Clam Chowder	86	10

SOUPS (cont.)

	Calories	Carbohydrates
Creamed soups (vichyssoise)	201	10
Noodle soups	117	6
Pea	120	23
Tomato	75	16
Vegetable	65	13

VEGETABLES

	Calories	Carbohydrates
Asparagus (1 portion)	22	3
Beans, canned, baked, 1 cup	310	48
Beans, kidney, 1 cup	230	42
Beans, lima, 1 cup	152	30
Beans, Navy, 1 cup	642	30
Beans, snap green, 1 cup	27	10
Beets, 1 cup	68	16
Broccoli, 1 cup	44	8
Brussels Sprouts, 1 cup	60	12
Cabbage, 1 cup	40	10
Carrots, raw, 1 cup	21	10
Carrots, canned, 1 cup	44	10
Cauliflower, cooked	30	6
Celery (1 stalk)	18	1
Cole Slaw	102	12
Corn, sweet, fresh (1 ear)	100	16
Corn, sweet, canned	165	40
Cucumber	15	2
Lettuce, 2 leaves	7	1
Mushrooms, 1 cup	35	10
Onions, raw, 1	40	11
Peas, canned, 1 cup	100	32
Peppers, green, 1	16	3
Pickles, sweet, 1	150	5
Pickles, dill, 1	15	2
Potatoes, baked (large)	140	21
Potatoes, French fries, 10	140	16
Potatoes, mashed (½ cup)	95	30
Radishes, raw, 5	10	2
Sauerkraut, 1 cup	25	6
Spinach, 1 cup	40	6
Squash, summer, 1 cup	30	8
Sweet potatoes, baked, 1	140	36
Sweet potatoes, candied, 1	115	60
Tomato, raw, 1	35	6
Tomato, canned or cooked, 1 cup	46	10
Tomato, juice (4 oz.)	50	5
Turnip, 1 cup	30	10

Height-Weight Table

For Women

height with shoes, 2-inch heel	small frame under 30	small frame over 30	medium frame under 30	medium frame over 30	large frame under 30	large frame over 30
4'10"	92–95	95–98	96–101	101–107	104–111	111–119
4'11"	94–99	99–101	98–104	104–110	106–114	114–122
5' 0"	96–100	100–104	101–108	108–113	109–117	117–125
5' 1"	99–103	103–107	104–110	110–116	112–120	120–128
5' 2"	102–106	106–110	107–113	113–119	115–122	122–131
5' 3"	105–109	109–113	110–116	116–122	118–126	126–134
5' 4"	108–112	112–116	113–119	119–126	121–129	129–138
5' 5"	111–115	115–119	116–123	123–130	125–134	134–142
5' 6"	114–118	118–123	120–127	127–135	129–138	138–146
5' 7"	118–123	123–127	124–131	131–139	133–141	141–150
5' 8"	122–127	127–131	128–135	135–143	137–146	146–154
5' 9"	126–130	130–135	132–140	140–147	141–150	150–158
5'10"	130–135	135–140	136–144	144–151	145–155	155–163
5'11"	134–138	138–144	140–147	147–155	149–159	159–168
6' 0"	138–143	143–148	144–152	152–159	153–163	163–173

For Men

height with shoes, 1-inch heel	small frame under 30	small frame over 30	medium frame under 30	medium frame over 30	large frame under 30	large frame over 30
5' 2"	112–116	116–120	118–123	123–129	126–133	133–141
5' 3"	115–119	119–123	121–127	127–133	129–137	137–144
5' 4"	118–122	122–126	124–130	130–136	132–140	140–148
5' 5"	121–125	125–129	127–133	133–139	135–144	144–152
5' 6"	124–129	129–133	130–140	140–143	138–146	146–156
5' 7"	128–132	132–137	134–140	140–147	142–152	152–161
5' 8"	132–137	137–141	138–146	146–152	147–157	157–166
5' 9"	136–140	140–145	142–149	149–156	151–160	160–170
5'10"	140–145	145–150	146–152	152–160	155–165	165–174
5'11"	144–149	149–154	150–157	157–165	159–165	165–179
6' 0"	148–153	153–158	154–162	162–170	164–174	174–184
6' 1"	152–157	157–162	158–167	167–175	168–179	179–189
6' 2"	156–162	162–167	162–170	170–180	173–183	183–194
6' 3"	160–165	165–171	167–176	176–185	178–188	188–199
6' 4"	164–170	170–175	172–181	181–190	182–193	193–204

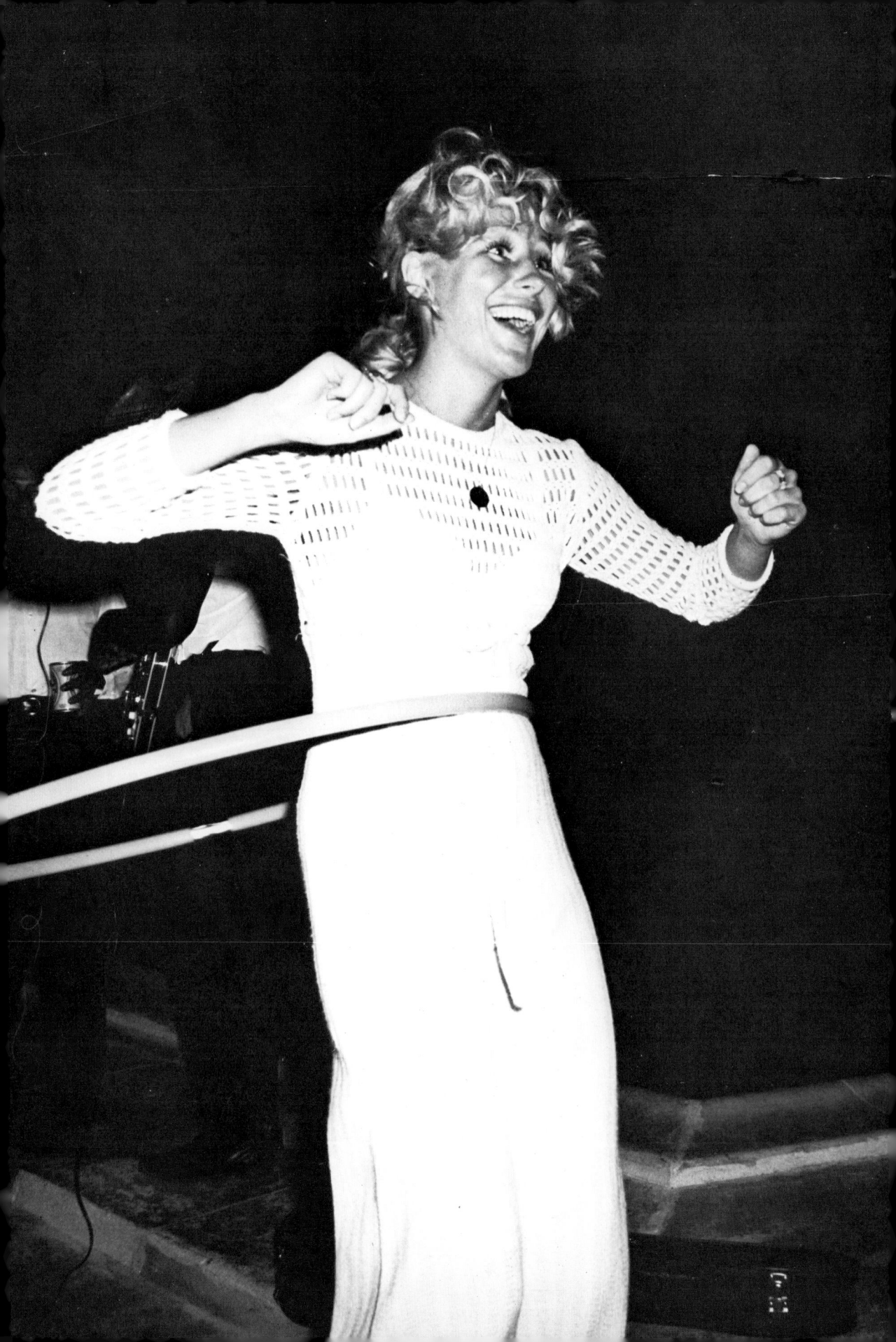

6

How to Fall in Love with Exercise

and

Everything You Ever Wanted to Know About the Subject

Nobody owns up about exercise, owns up to the fact that it bores the leotards off most of us, unless it's attached to a favorite sport. Tennis anybody?

While exercise teachers, gymnasts, calisthenic tutors, and yogi gurus seem to grow in number every year, pupils mostly come and go—admittedly always to be replaced by more pupils, who, alas, also come—but then go. Staying the course is really the exception rather than the rule, which is another reason, statistically speaking, we are so out of shape as a nation (see Chapter 5, page 132).

Psychoanalysts point out that the relationship between posture and mental attitude is illustrated for all to see in paintings and sculp-

FACING PAGE
A few minutes each day . . . a little exercise never hurt anybody.

ture dating back hundreds of years. The man who is depressed is crouching there on the canvas. The man or woman who is confident and happy *stretches* out with exuberance, which, as every exercise-happy psychoanalyst will tell you, is the first and most fundamental exercise, one that starts every worthwhile exercise class.

The fact is we know that stretching and much more are good for us. We know we should carry out our exercises every day as diligently as we brush our teeth, and, as I've written myself at least two thousand times, "only a few minutes every day will help."

We also know that for some reason exercise is like daily medicine, something that we tend to pretend we forget to take. We're too busy. We work too hard, so we're too exhausted. It's too cold in the morning —too tiring at night.

The truth is for most of us WE DON'T LIKE IT, except as far as I'm concerned I *used* not to like it, but I've learned to. How? Through being brainwashed by so many experts, and through seeing with my own eyes, *the end results.*

That Few Minutes Each Day

What isn't boring about exercise is undoubtedly the beautiful end results, as many can testify like ex-Governor Ronald Reagan, for instance, David Janssen, Tina Sinatra, Barbra Streisand, and Vidal's now extraordinarily svelte wife, Beverly Sassoon.

All of these neat people *loathed* exercise, until they came under the influence of a body shaper—in the first four instances, a well-known one in Hollywood called Marvin Hart; in the case of Beverly Sassoon, a guru named Bikram Choudhury. They were all quickly gratified to discover that *supervision* from someone you respect is the best way to beat man's ancient enemy, lack of self-discipline.

Marvin Hart, whose beat-your-body exercises I'll tell you about later (see page 190) has transformed more sluggish shapes than Darryl Zanuck transformed starlets into stars. And because of *results* people like Ronnie, Dave, Tina, and Barbra keep at it, believing Marvin when he says, like all exercise experts, *"To be effective exercise has to become as much part of a lifestyle as eating and sleeping."*

This brings us right back to those "few minutes every day." It's a fact that has to be faced: those few minutes just *have to* be devoted to daily practice.

Curiously enough, the right set of movements carried out every day *does* eventually lead to a feeling of well-being and, best of all, better looks. Unfortunately, nothing is achieved if exercise is a once-a-month or a once-a-week act of martyrdom.

The right mental attitude has to be there, as important as the exercise itself. The trim, must-be-slim-at-all-costs set—from Jackie O. to

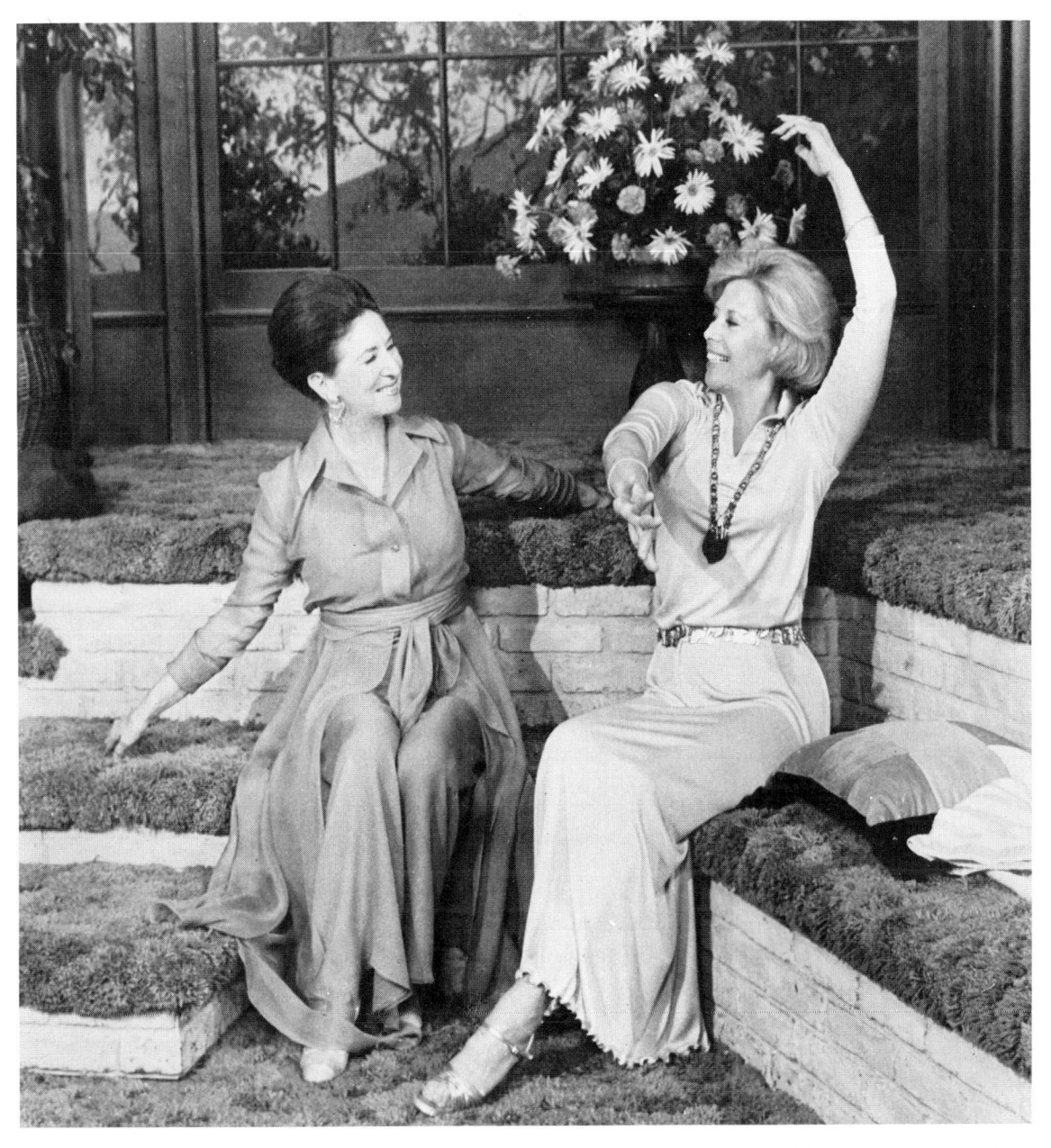

Two's company when it comes to exercise. Here Dinah Shore and Mala Rubinstein go through their paces on TV.

Farah Diba, the Shah's wife—work at it with tenacious concentration wherever they happen to be, and as far as Jackie and Farah Diba are concerned, they happen to believe in jogging, rain or shine.

Going It Alone Is Doomed to Failure

To begin, for the totally out of shape to *get* in shape, outside help is needed. Even a TV tutor or radio pacemaker is better than no one, for direction—and supervision if possible—is *vital* initially whatever exercise method is chosen. . . . I'm going to cover them all.

Ideally, the exercise program should start with at least a twice-weekly date with an instructor, plus a daily practice of ten to fifteen minutes at home.

Learn How to Breathe

No instructor worth his exercise mat will start anyone moving a muscle without first teaching and preaching correct breathing. Yes, *breathing*. It's a curious fact that generally without realizing it, beginners tend to *hold* their breath when attempting their first exercises, hoping that way they'll achieve more, because they're used to tensing up that way whenever they have to *achieve!*

Double breathing is the way to break the holding habit. This means a combination of inhaling and exhaling at given times during the exercise.

1. At the beginning you should concentrate on *inhaling* through the nose. This guarantees that more oxygen will flood the lungs to move on to your bloodstream to give extra life and energy to your body.
2. Toward the middle of the movement *exhale explosively*. This rids the body of carbon dioxide and waste matters filtered from the bloodstream.
3. *Inhale* deeply once more (more oxygen).
4. Finally *exhale* just as noisily as before.

If you learn to be *conscious* of your breathing, when you start to exercise, inhaling and exhaling as described, this will also develop the diaphragm, enlarge the rib cage, and strengthen all muscles connected with the breathing apparatus—very useful in just keeping up with life's hustle and bustle without getting breathless.

Jack LaLanne, a TV tutor for more than a decade and the owner of a number of keep-and-get-fit health spas around the country, always asks his TV audience to keep inhaling when touching their toes and coming back up erect, exhaling only when finishing the exercise by flinging their arms up wide and back, lifting and expanding the rib cage. As Jack says, "Creating life's bellows, forcing out dirty old air."

There's more power behind this simple breathing exercise than most people realize. On inhaling, for instance, nature uses built-in filters to strain out impurities in the air, allowing only pure oxygen through, also changing it to body temperature before it reaches the lungs. On exhaling, the smoker, for example, gets rid of cigarette smoke as well as carbon dioxide and other wastes from the body.

Whenever you're frazzled, carry out the inhale-and-exhale "exercise." You'll be surprised how refreshed you'll feel.

Which Method Is for You?

Men and women have turned mental somersaults, searching for exercise methods that would not only bring about results, but might be fun, too. Perhaps it's no wonder that in cities like Stockholm, Hamburg, San Francisco, and Copenhagen, sex is suggested as part of the exercise manual, with positions, gyrations, and gymnastics based on the supposition that as muscles begin to shrink from about twenty onwards, stretching them back can be accomplished with a member of the opposite sex. Nobody—yet—has suggested, however, that sex helps achieve a well-articulated pelvis.

The dance method of exercise, however, does do this—if carried out correctly—so do calisthenics (exercises using only the body, no real "equipment"), gym (with equipment), yoga (with guru). Now where to start and what to choose?

Contrast is really the key thing to look for in any exercise plan—look for one that's in direct *contrast* to your usual life.

For example, if you're a desk-bound, typewriter-trapped, sedentary secretary, join a gym where you can work off buttock boredom on a vast array of equipment or join a club with a swimming pool, so that water can help deliver results.

If you're a house-bound, child-tied, husband-happy housewife, get introduced to yoga—to grab some contemplative moments along with shape-making movements.

If you're a happy, horsey, hippy, jolly hockey-sticks of a lady, try a svelter form of exercise, and join a dance class with mirrored walls and evocative music to help you move more sinuously.

Three things to remember:

1. If you laugh at yourself or others while exercising, you'll accomplish nothing. Laughter means you're too relaxed. Your movements can't have the necessary thrust.

2. Pain means the exercise isn't working properly—and exhaustion isn't the object of the exercise either. Move but don't over-exert yourself.

3. Girdles can inhibit exercise, particularly restricting the flow of fresh blood circulation to and from the area being exercised. Girdles are a deceptive crutch anyway, for apart from restricting the blood flow to the lower part of the body (the part most put upon by flab), they don't allow lazy muscles any chance to work. Imagine every time you wanted to lift your arm, someone lifted it for you. It wouldn't be long before the arm muscles became so flabby and weak, you wouldn't be able to lift it yourself. So the girdle encourages muscles to be lazy in just the area where flab likes to sit and do nothing. Girdles should be "sometimes" occasions, never always, and buttocks should practice contracting several times a day to act as nature's own girdle. Try it now as you read the next section.

Who Wants to Dance Her Way to Shape?

Not since Fred Astaire made every girl want to Ginger up has the dance method of exercise (dance classes for nondancers) been so in demand. Ballet, modern jazz, Afro, West Indian Limbo—it's been proved that all these movements correctly taught and practiced bring as much tone to the body as the hula hoop.

Plent of plié (knee bends) in the morning and some relevé (stretching) at night appeal to some far more than jogging or, as the disenchanted call it, "dreary exercise."

Since few people have even a smidgen of Margot Fonteyn, the beginners' dance-exercise class can seem downright ordinary, because the most conscientious teachers set out to prove in slow motion how each dance movement can tone various parts of the body, rather like swimming on dry land. (Swimming and exercising in wet water are another story, see page 50. Even plain ordinary swimming exercises every part of you, providing your feet are off the bottom.)

Most dance-exercise classes start with a standing or sitting warm-up—swinging arms vigorously back and forth, head down, head up—to eliminate "all tension." Then, there's a lot of lateral movement involved because, as is usually pointed out, "We don't move from side to side in daily life—so this movement wakes up muscles that rarely get used."

Contrast Is All

When lying down, students may be asked to flex their muscles in time to music or the teacher's finger-snapping tempo. Each area is moved separately—head, neck, shoulders, rib cage, pelvis, ankles, stomach, buttocks, and thighs—hopefully in time to get tuned up.

If the dance class is classically oriented, this means *barré* work—the ballet way of describing movements carried out at a bar attached to a (usually) mirrored wall. The bar is great to anchor those unused to deep knee bends and sideway leg stretching, with shoulders kept *back*, the head *up* in as lofty a manner as possible. Ballet movements help people with problem legs, whereas jazz exercises—stretching and shaking—affect the body all over, *if* carried out *consistently*.

There are teachers who believe that in the early stages of the game pupils should work with their eyes closed, so they're not conscious of what they look like (!) but—hopefully—start reflecting on what's happening *inside* as movements get more and more away from the movements of daily life.

In the modern-dance exercise classes, initial workouts can be tough when to rock music, students are expected to bend and flex in time to the rhythm with beach balls wedged between their knees.

Later, trained by the beach-ball technique, they move on to waist trimming with music, undulating on bended knee to tone the pelvic area.

The Harem Act Can Help

Belly dancing has reared its solar plexus aggressively in the last few years—offered not as a titillating Turkish treat, but as a direct method of decreasing flab without increasing the size of the belly. It's claimed there are over 450 different steps and combinations (dance-steps combined) to belly dancing. When carried out to Middle Eastern music, under the stern eyes of a lady who gives no indication of ever having been near a harem, poise, grace, stamina, and shape *can* improve. As a way of bringing young mothers back to prepregnancy shape, belly dancing has been given the once-over by hospital physiotherapists and pronounced OK for toning stomach muscles.

Yoga for Constant Youth

The relationship between dancing and yoga is distant, yet definite, says the guru: "Dance movements loosen the muscles, strengthen the body, *and relax the mind and spirit.*"

This is key, because yoga, one of the most popular yet not altogether understood forms of exercise in the United States, relates as much to the mind as to the body.

In California, Beverly Sassoon has improved her shape as she says, "Out of all recognition." She sleeps better, her skin is better, but most important of all she is more able to cope with a very hectic lifestyle, three young children, a full social program, plus traveling the world with husband Vidal to help him with his hairdressing empire. Beverly says she owes her new equilibrium and everything else to yoga, taught to her six days a week by guru Bikram Choudhury, a graduate of the Yoga College of India in Calcutta. As he says succinctly about his "science," "Yoga psychology recognizes mind and body as interdependent. Just as the mind cannot function perfectly when the body is suffering, so the body is in trouble when there are mental disturbances."

At his yoga class, or at any given by a true yogi, you start learning how to achieve control over your body to further self-discipline.

The majority of students who turn to yoga as a means of maintaining, attaining, or retrieving a beautiful shape learn about forty exercise movements fundamental to yoga, along with vital breathing techniques that enable them, if necessary, to be able to go through life practicing satisfactorily alone.

The main accomplishment of hatha (physical) yoga is toning and firming the body by releasing muscle tension and learning to utilize breathing, literally, in the most refreshing way. *Ha breathing* is a positive exercise devised to help cope with the negative aspects of life. Providing there's privacy to ensure concentration, it can be practiced anywhere at any time. The extra beauty about yoga is that it is a time-honored system of physical culture that allows anyone of any age or condition to exercise according to capacity and at his or her own pace.

To Breathe the Ha Way

Standing with feet well apart, arms at sides, breathe *out, out, out,* as if to lose every breath in your body. Slowly raise arms up over your head, and inhale through the nose. As you lower your arms s-l-o-w-l-y to the sides, exhale once more.

Ha breathing is part of hatha yoga, the discipline or science concerned with perfect health that's most generally taught in the West. Because there are *sixteen systems of yoga,* not surprisingly there's often confusion, even fear in the Western mind about this complex but fascinating Indian philosophy.

The sixteen systems were first recorded by Patanjali, who lived three centuries after Buddha and greatly admired his teachings. The Yoga wheel developed by Patanjali was largely inspired by the Buddhist wheel of life, and comprises sixteen spokes, eight outer ones concerned with the *physical* world, eight inner ones concerned with the *spiritual* world. Significantly the wheel collapses without one of its spokes.

When a mere mortal has complete grasp and control over all sixteen spokes, the final step is called *raja yoga.* You will find practitioners among the Eastern mystics who can feel heat or cold at will, sleep on a bed of nails, or go without sleep or any apparent food and, it's said, can control the act of self-levitation. There are no Western raja yogi—enough comment on the serenity to be gained in this part of the world—but hatha yoga has many practitioners here. The contemporary Western man and woman gain a sense of peace through these particular exercises that rely on mind and body working together, exercise and thought.

An Elementary Yoga Class

This is the sort of thing that might happen at your first yoga class.

You will be asked to kneel to listen to slow rhythmic music, your head folded onto your crossed arms.

As you listen, you will be asked to show you love the music by hugging your arms to your body, all the time inhaling deeply, and to relate the music to nature and the nature of things by enacting a scene, following the yogi, but thinking your own thoughts. You stretch back still on your knees, moving your arms as far back as you possibly can. Then, like the yogi, you fall forward into the "earth" and are told to imagine rain pouring down to make things grow, stretching forward with your arms, following your arms with your body, pressing your head down, "becoming a seed." Outstretched you keep down, exhaling, holding that position until you maintain retention of breath. Again you will be asked to think only of nature as you listen to the music. This time, stretching back up, you inhale fresh oxygen from life's power—air—using stretching as a tranquilizer used by man and nature alike. You will shake and sway, imagining the wind blowing, flowers quivering; then you will be asked to fold down gently, slowly as seeds do, relaxing completely, back to your first position on your knees, head folded into your arms . . . as if to sleep till next spring.

Elementary but surprisingly effective, and, of course, that's just the beginning.

Show-Business Yoga

Two favorite yoga exercises for actors and actresses are called the Lion and the Gargoyle, both aimed at developing a supple spine *and* spirit.

In the Lion position, you kneel, hands on knees, with buttocks resting on heels. The Lion springs into action as you lean torso forward, tensing all muscles, making even your hands tense as your fingers spread apart to touch thumbs while your fingertips brush the floor. Stick out your tongue as far as you can and feel your face and neck muscles tense. Slowly roll the tongue back until the underneath side of its tip presses against the roof of the mouth. Relax, return to your kneeling position, and repeat ten times. Singers say this exercise relieves tired, even sore, throats.

From the Lion position, more advanced students move on to the Gargoyle, retracting the tongue but with the head still down. Then the mouth should be opened as wide as possible, bending the head back as far on the neck as it will go. The last movement is to clench the teeth—not the lips—three times. I'm told this is a sure-fire preventative for grinding one's teeth in one's sleep, while both the Lion and Gargoyle are exercises that are anti double chin, crepe neck, and jowls.

Still quoting show-business sources, opera singers have told me they love a triple breathing exercise from yoga, stating that as it strengthens the neck, it strengthens the voice, giving it new quality. When they carry out this breathing exercise before an appearance in public, it's said to give the face extra radiance.

Inhale and exhale through the nose with a "bellows effect," making neck veins stand out. When inhaling, try to blow out the stomach deliberately as if it were a balloon filling with air—it isn't easy, as it feels as if you're working at cross-purposes, but that's the object.

When exhaling, try to draw in the stomach. Yogis say it's necessary to do it at least twenty-five times in the beginning to be able to get the rhythm, then it comes easily after only seven or eight times.

Deep breathing helps your skin, too. By taking in more oxygen, you take in more water molecules that form moisture in the body, vital ally to skin texture (see page 15).

Surprising as it may seem, even if you've never seen the world the other way up, you probably will be encouraged to try a headstand at your first yoga class. Yogis and gurus believe in it—so do all exercise experts in the know—because the headstand (or even a near miss) sends fresh blood to nourish the brain structure, *benefiting every other part of the body* and also increasing coordination. The brain and heart receive stimulation from the change of gravity and the increase in oxygen and blood. Every muscle and organ benefits. The aorta, caratida, and arteries receive the bonus blood that finally reaches the entire body, spinal cord, and central nervous system, so sharpening intellect and memory, relieving asthmatic discomfort, headaches, and dizziness. High-wire workers often do a headstand before getting on the trapeze. They find they have less accidents that way.

Upside Down Do-It-Yourself

To get that way up, first practice kneeling with weight resting on your arms, hands on mat, fingers interlocked, cupping head to keep it steady. Rise on your toes and with relaxed knees move slowly forward until you feel the weight of your body balanced on your arms. Practice until you feel in control and comfortable, then slowly raise legs, remembering your weight is being held by your arms resting on the floor, while your hands hold your head steady, stomach muscles and spine assisting.

Everything about yoga requires *thinking*, so that a tedious job becomes an exercise for improving your muscles—and so your shape. Yoga is a continuous process—as thousands have discovered, the more body and mind become one in endeavor, the fitter, shapelier, and happier they become.

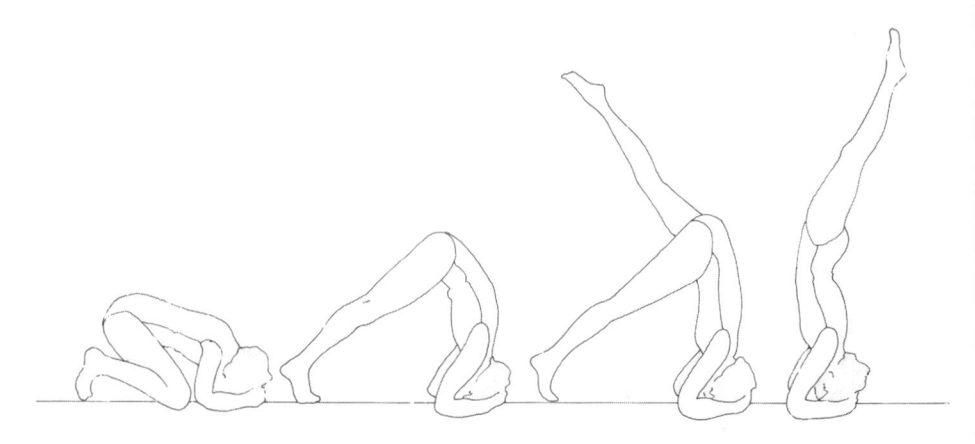

Physiotherapy—You May Not Know You Need It

The physiotherapist's job is to help you mobilize your muscles, although you may not always know your muscles need mobilizing! Here the expert helps you educate or reeducate the muscles that control posture and movement, so that they perform their tasks with the ease and symmetry Nature intended.

In the medical and surgical world, physiotherapy is a vital ancillary science, aiding recovery from illness or accident. In the world of beauty, it offers a scientific route toward elegance and shape.

Whether you go through life burying your head in the sand or are known for your remarkable stiff upper lip, the wear and tear on your lily-white neck is tremendous. This is where much back trouble can stem from, and the pun is deliberate.

Take five seconds off to think about *how much* depends upon the neck's state of health—its ability to move freely—not only the larynx, the thyroid and lymphatic glands, and various nerve roots, but the large blood vessels that supply the brain.

The neck muscles, that ensure we keep a steady head on our shoulders, not only fight a constant battle against the downward pull of gravity, but are easily dispirited by emotional upset, tension, worry, fret and fuss—and whoever knew a female who was never subject to any of those?

Yet the neck is neglected, frequently left out when it comes to the daily and/or nightly beauty ritual—when skin care so often stops short at the chin—and it's rarely if ever *exercised.*

It's a pity, the physiotherapist tells me often enough, because the right set of neck exercises can relieve *all* feelings of congestion and pressure inside the head and generally contribute well-being to the whole body. *Practiced regularly* like the pianoforte, neck exercises can even improve public appearances, cutting down to the right proportion the ancient problem of how-to-win-friends-and/or-influence-the-right-people.

The following do-it-yourself exercises were originally devised by an eminent British physiotherapist, Norman Sandieson, DO, MRO, but only for those *not* under medical care for any spinal complaints. Used as part of an overall exercise program at the leading British spa, Forest Mere, although they may appear to affect only the neck, you will *feel* they affect back muscles, too, which they are meant to do, hence the medical warning.

Basically there are four movements to concentrate on for homework:

Side bending: Keeping the face to the front throughout, bend the head first to one side, then to the other, trying to bring the ear as close to the shoulder as possible.

Forward and backward bending: Bring the head slowly forward until

HOW TO FALL IN LOVE
WITH EXERCISE

SIDE BENDING

FORWARD AND
BACKWARD BENDING

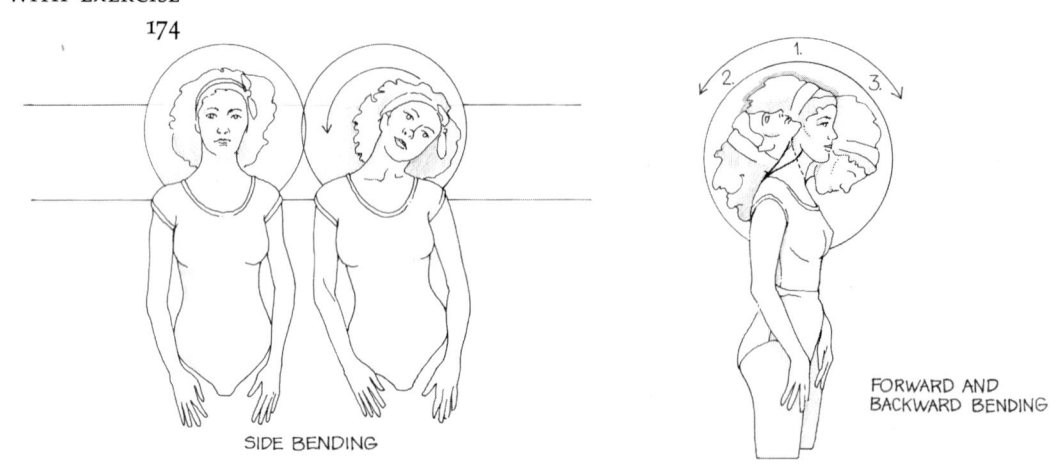

the chin is pressing on the chest, then up and back as far as possible, keeping the mouth open slightly so that the lower jaw is relaxed and doesn't retard movement.

Head rolling: Start with the side bending movement, then continue trying to "roll" the head as far as it will go around to the back, then move slowly forward again to the opposite side, before reversing the entire movement. Another "rolling" exercise involves turning the head s-l-o-w-l-y, trying to peep over your own shoulder, stretching so that by glancing down you can almost see your heels—first to one side, then the other.

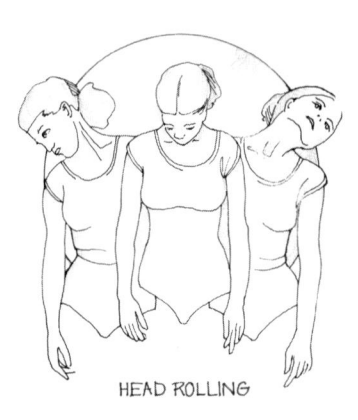

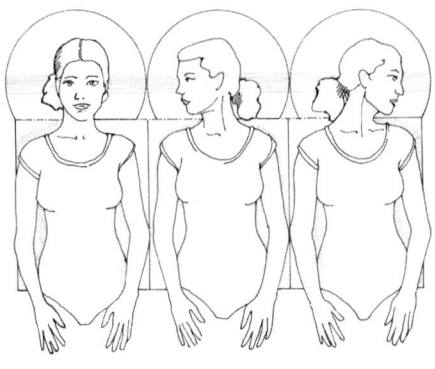

HEAD ROLLING

SLOW HEAD ROLLING

Carried out tortoise-slow in front of a mirror twice a day, the best results come through patient practice, gradually pressing a little harder each time so that the muscles really get stretched. Creaking and cracking may go on, especially in neck rolling, but do not worry—it merely shows how much the exercises are needed. The physiotherapist always employs massage, along with special exercises, during her treatment. Bending legs back, "cracking" arm muscles, alternating muscle workouts with soothing, stroking movements. Everyone should make a point of checking over their muscles with an expert physiotherapist once a year—whether they "hurt" or not.

Pool Work

To give muscles the perfect chance to play exhibitionist, the physiotherapist likes to put you in a swimming pool—or at least enough deep water in which to swim.

Swimming exercises *all* the muscles, providing you don't rely on the dog paddle once out of your depth, for as any expert worth her diploma would say, "Underwater exercises are the telling kind." You're not cheating if you keep your head above the surface.

For the benefit of neck, stomach, arms, and legs, try this: Holding head erect, start to breast stroke, then move into reverse—first pushing water *back* with your arms, *then* pushing it *forward*. At the same time, move one leg straight up and down underwater with a slow scissors movement. After thirty kicks, move the other leg. It isn't easy, but—just like riding a bike—once you've mastered it, you wonder what all the fuss was about.

Keeping one foot flat against the side of the pool, stand on the other foot. Bend from the waist, arms out, thumbs locked. Inhale. Hold breath as you push away from wall. Glide relaxed for as long or as little as you can. Exhale slowly before you regain footing. Repeat twenty times.

Another good exercise for the whole body is to kick from the hips with relaxed legs, holding onto the wall if you can't swim. Better still, if you can, do it without a prop. Slap down on the surface of the water with the instep of the foot. Short, quick strokes are faster and less tiring.

If you haven't enough water around to get out of your depth, work out in your bath. Loofah legs, thighs, buttocks *underwater,* moving *upward* all the time, keeping first one side taut, then the other.

Out of the bath, massage with a loofah sprinkled with surgical spirit—it can ignite circulation as fast as a four-minute mile, and it's a great way to banish gooseflesh.

As physiotherapists the world over reiterate: "Movement is life; stiffness is death"—which is the obvious reason physiotherapy plays such a vital part in the back-to-shape-and-health plan on land and in the water.

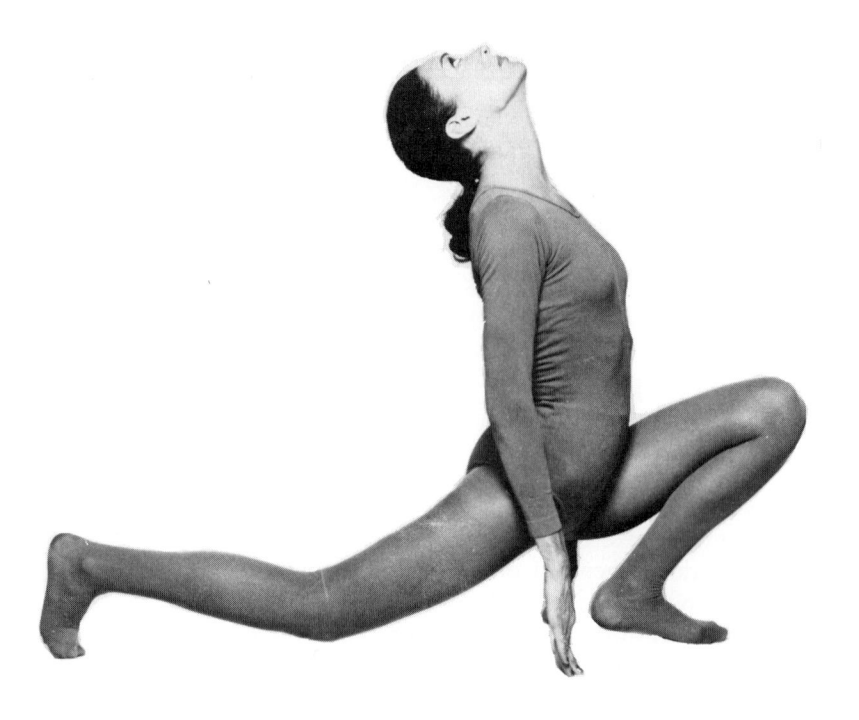

The professionals' slogan is, You can't put the tent pole up until the guy ropes are slack. This comes about with *neuromuscular techniques:* deep specialized massage slackens the guy ropes—in other words, relaxes the muscles—by *manipulation, mobilizing,* or *articulating* the joints (especially the spine), *correcting* or *adjusting* the vertebrae.

Calisthenics—Instant Exercises That Work

Calisthenics is a clumsy word to describe the simplest exercises—those we can do without apparatus—or, with only the minimum, like barbells.

Some American women excel at calisthenics, leading the slipshod world with daily examples of warm-ups carried out as a natural part of their life.

As one physical-education professor puts it, "Exercise is the hydraulic fluid of the gears of activity. When done properly, it will move every muscle, bone, and ligament from head to toe, including the face. Exercise can counteract the lack of activity forced upon us by the increased mechanization of modern living . . . should be organized to overcome the effect of fat, fatigue, and the constant pull of gravity on the body."

To this end, a whole army of dedicated women carry out what is

HOW TO FALL IN LOVE
WITH EXERCISE
177

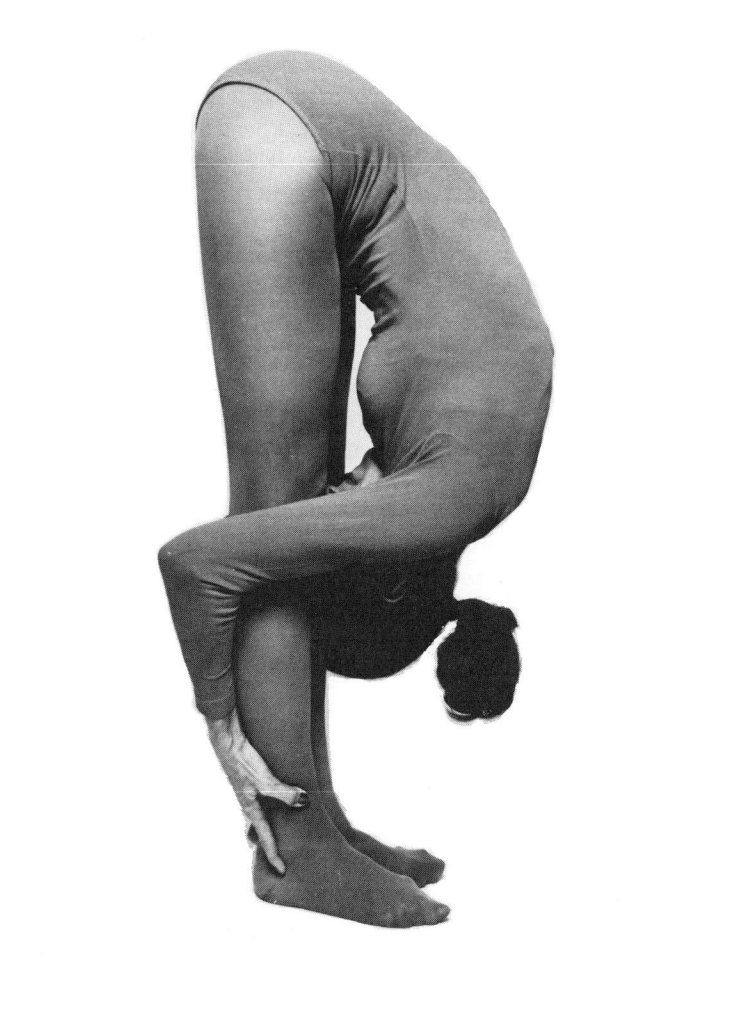

LEFT AND
FACING PAGE
"You don't need to do anything strenuous," says actress and singer Julie Wilson, who admits to her fifty-one years of age. *"Simple limbering-up exercises are fine if you do them every day."*

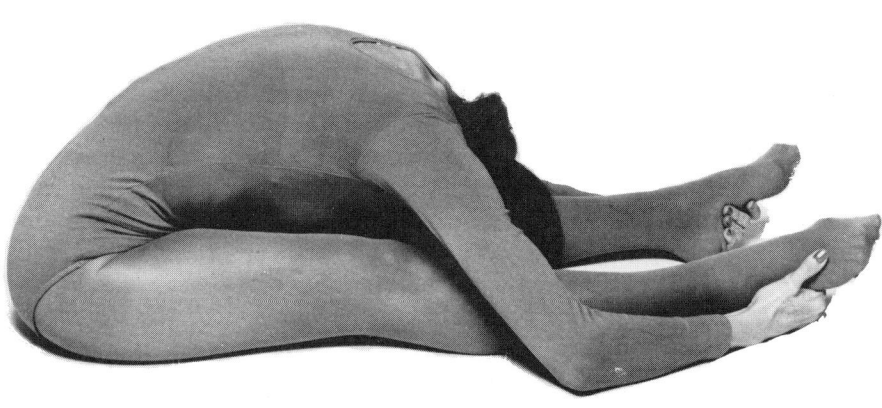

generally known as "instant exercise"—movements they can, and do, do anywhere at anytime with the one aim of keeping the body in great shape.

Eileen Ford, the name behind one of the biggest model agencies in the world (Karen Graham, Lauren Hutton, are recent names from her big game stable; Suzy Parker was one of yesterday's), starts her day rolling—literally—out of bed onto the floor where she immediately starts her exercises.

"Exercising is a part of life—my life anyway." While brushing her teeth, she puts her foot on top of the basin and flexes her knee, first the right, then the left—very good for inner thighs.

"I do my chin exercises driving to work. People think I'm sticking my tongue out, but it's all part of my shape-up program. My office is my world, so I sometimes do leg lifts while talking on the phone or dictating to my secretary." Instant exercise, in other words.

Tall girls like model Betsy Theodoracopulos and actress Vanessa Redgrave know they have to think about exercise more than short girls. Without good posture they know they don't look so good, but bent and older. The good girls *think* tall because they are tall. Mrs. Kissinger should learn from this; she's too round-shouldered through years of thinking "short."

When the rib cage is up, better posture results automatically. Because shoulders are lowered, the neck feels longer—try it, you'll like it.

Short snappy exercises help. Such as . . .

turning the knob of the next door you open with your left hand (if you're left-handed, do it with your right).

picking up something from the floor without bending your knees, then using your left hand to do it.

going upstairs two at a time.

lying down to put on pantyhose, extending legs up in the air, pointing toes while pulling stockings up.

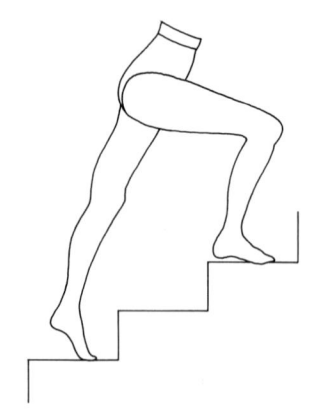

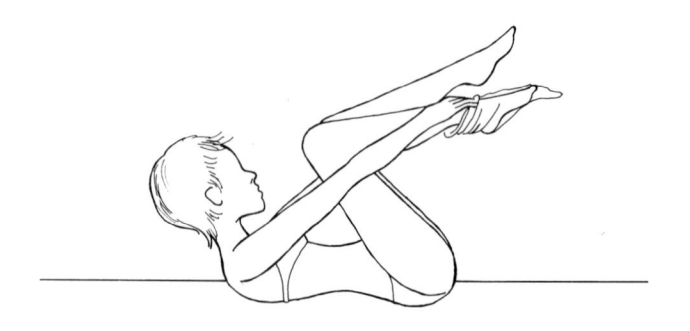

walking downstairs toes first, then lowering the heel—good for foot and leg.

reaching up for something on a top shelf, standing on your toes to do it—stretching first with the left, then with the right hand.

jogging whenever you want to get from one room to another—for at least part of the day.

Reducing Each Spot

For some people, general exercise may not give them what they really want, that is *spot reducing on the one spot that defies trimming.* In the Western world, it's the thigh area that's the number one trouble zone—hard to tackle mainly because we're all too *sedentary* by habit and so inclination.

Calisthenics can be broken down to direct the action to one trouble area—but like every other exercise, at least fifteen to twenty minutes should be spent carrying out the movement—A.M. and P.M.—not too near bedtime. Too much exertion can bring on insomnia.

Marjorie Craig is a name (and a gorgeous shape) that will bring several illustrious ladies out of the chaise longue to rush to the wall bar. Her influence over exercise has been felt for many years because of the most logical reason: results.

For Waist, Abdomen and Upper Hips

Miss Craig's favorites are the following:

1. Lie on the floor on your back, arms out at shoulder level with palms up. Bend knees to chest, then drop both knees to the floor directly out from hips to one side. Keep knees close to the floor, pull them up towards elbows. Hold, then roll knees back over chest. Hold. Repeat exercise on the other side. Do this ten times.

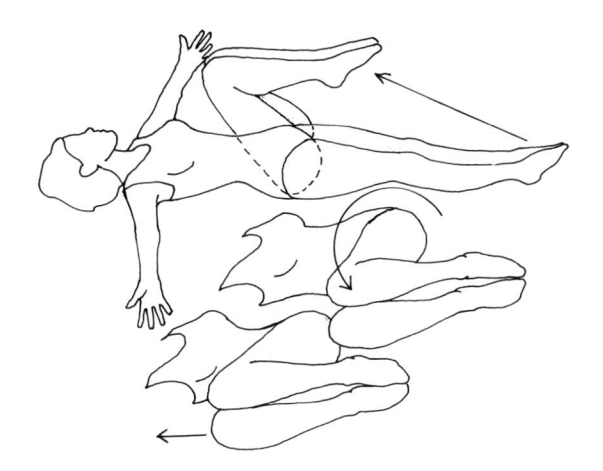

HOW TO FALL IN LOVE
WITH EXERCISE
180

2. This exercise is a good attack on thighs and on a fatty back too. Stand with legs apart. Bend knees slightly and pull hips under you. Raise both arms over head, hands clasped, palms turned up. Keeping hands joined, bend to touch floor in front of right toes. Bend knees as you bend down. Come up, bringing arms up over head, again pulling stomach in and up. Repeat movement, this time touching floor between feet . . . come up, arms back over head. Bend again, knees bent, to touch hands to left toes . . . and so it goes on . . . ten times.

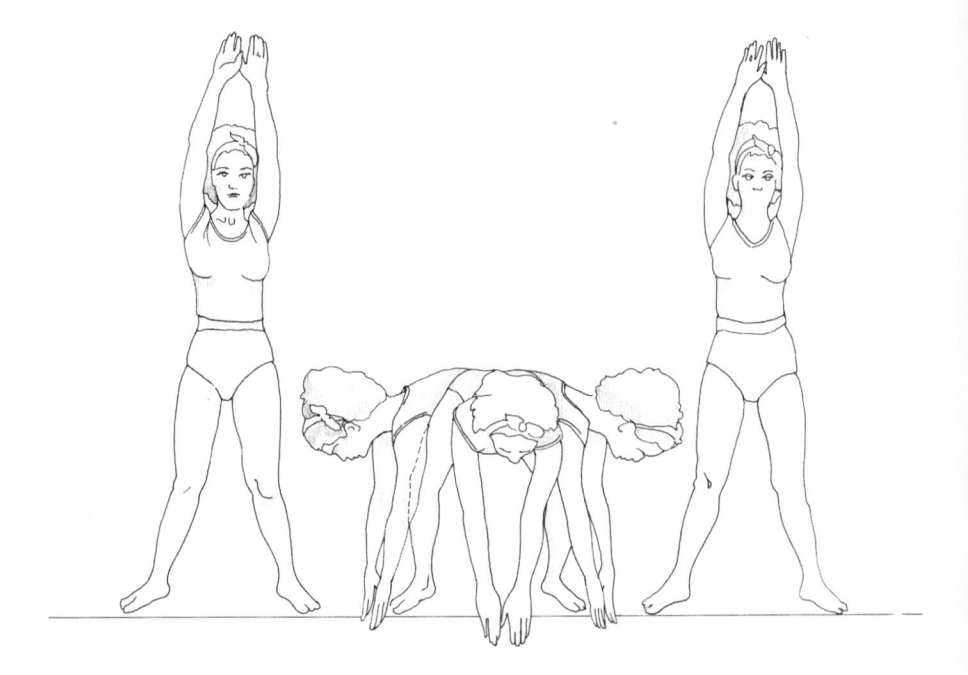

Arlene Dahl, not just a lovely face, but a worker for better looks, sought out several exercise experts before releasing her *Slim-Down for Thighs Movement:*

Lie on left side with body in a straight line, left arm extended under head, right hand placed in front for balance. Raise the right leg as high as possible at a 45-degree angle with the floor, contract buttocks, hold, then lower slowly to the floor. Repeat six times before rolling over to do the same for the left leg.

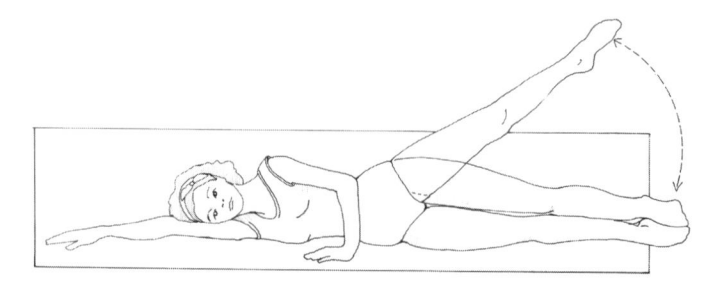

At the Greenhouse Spa in Dallas where comfort and luxury go hand in hand with a rigid streamlining program (see pages 55 and 60) the thigh exercise that brings results is the following:

Lie on your back with hands beneath buttocks, head relaxed, feet flexed. Lift legs straight toward ceiling, then open legs wide and close, inhaling as you open legs, exhaling as you close them. Do this twenty times.

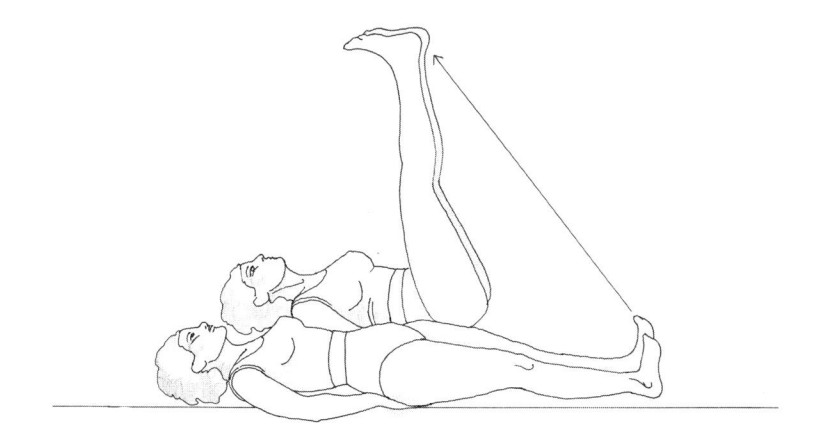

Also from the Greenhouse:

Lie on back with hands under buttocks. Keeping spine flat on floor, raise legs and cycle in large circles, inhaling as you lift right leg, exhaling on the left. Forty times medium fast.

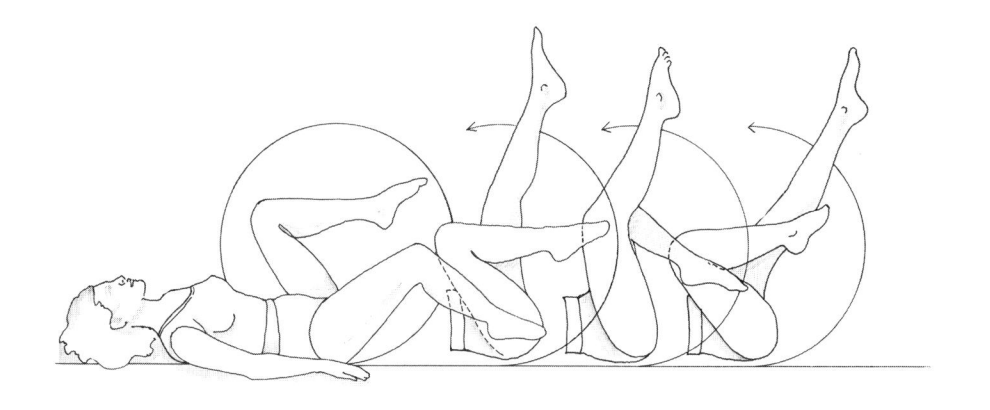

For the Hips and Waist

Stand upright with good posture, lift arms overhead and bend torso eight times to the right, eight times to the left. Next, bend knees eight times, keeping buttocks tight, abdomen pulled in. Drop upper body from the waist, arms and knees relaxed, eight times. Repeat all these movements in the same order eight times.

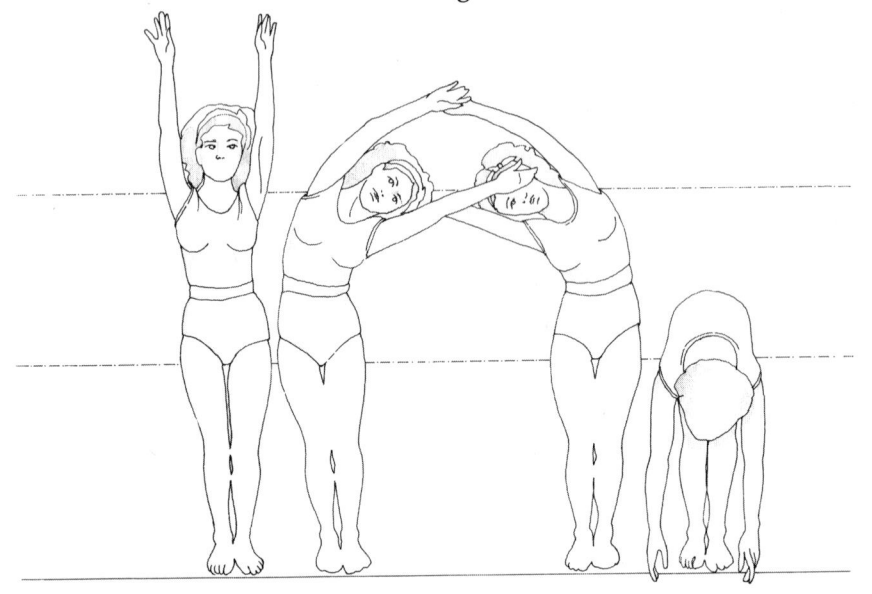

One more for hips and waist: Place hands on hips, then swing torso to the right, forward, left, and up—then reverse. Sixteen times.

For Upper Arms

1. Towel exercises are helpful because seeing a towel can jog your memory to get going in the early A.M. Stand upright with legs apart

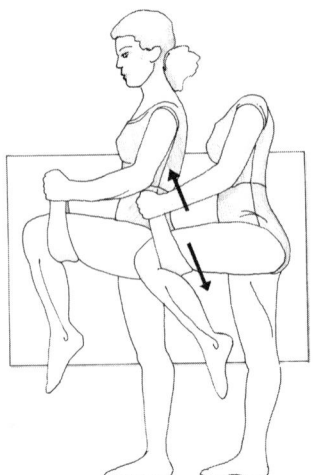

and hold a towel in both hands, behind your left knee with thumbs facing upward. Attempt to push backward with leg but *resist* with the towel held taut, using arms only. Switch towel to behind your right knee and again attempt to thwart leg movement. Alternate legs.

2. Standing upright, grasp a book in each hand or use a pair of dumbbells, keeping thumbs down, arms at sides. Curl arms up to shoulder level, without moving upper arms. Lower to sides, then repeat. Always stand erect.

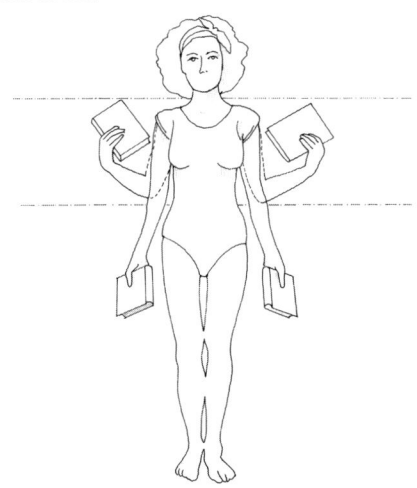

3. Grasp a book or weight in each hand and lean out and forward from the waist, keeping upper body in parallel position to floor. To work upper arm muscles, extend arms back and as high as possible without moving body. Return arms to sides, bending elbows, attempting to point books toward ceiling. Continue exercise as many times as possible. *Don't* get exhausted.

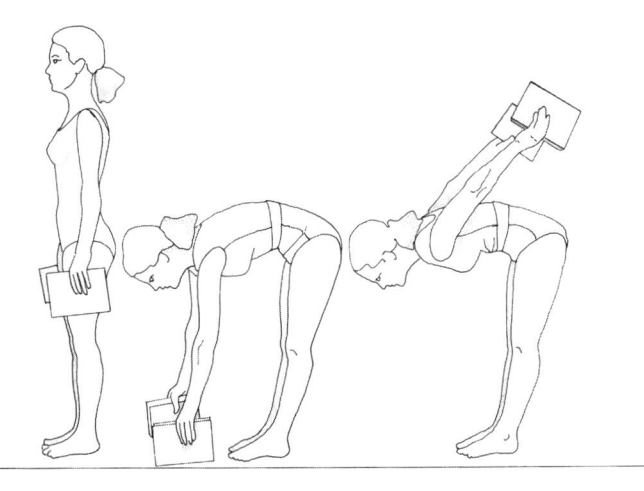

The Nonboring Approach to Exercise

At the Golden Door in California—where deep thinking is as much part of the curriculum as deep moving—the experts advise:

Always begin any exercise session standing very tall. Close eyes. Inhale deeply and hold for a count of six. Exhale deeply. During breathing exercises think about and visualize air entering and leaving body. Repeat ten times."

For Hips and Waist

At the Golden Door, successful exercises for these two most tiresome parts of the body are the following:

1. Stand tall, tucking stomach in well. Raise arms perpendicular to torso and hold palms up as if stopping the traffic. Push out with right hand as far as possible in a horizontal and steady direction. Repeat eight to ten times with alternate hands.

2. With legs wide apart, stand tall, head up. Raise elbows to horizontal position with palms down, pelvis forward. Twist body to left side; pause, face forward; twist to right side. Repeat eight to ten times each side.

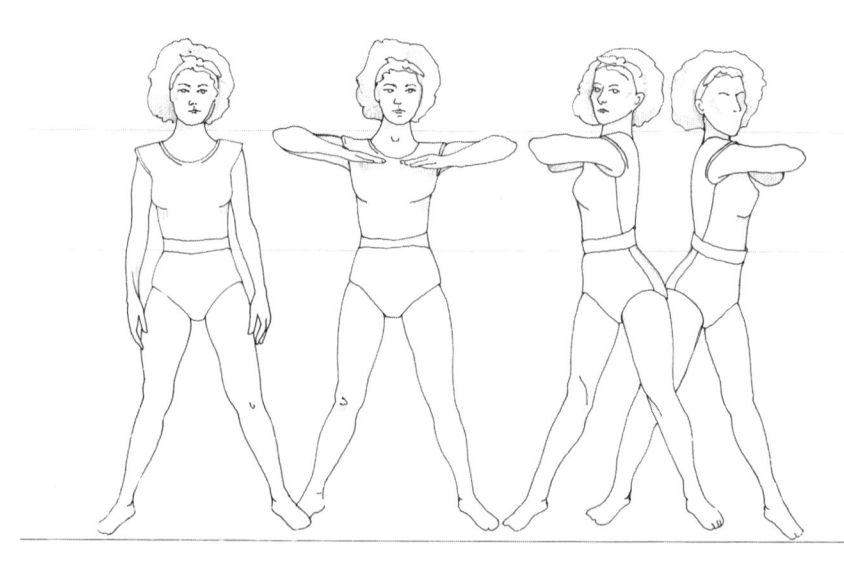

3. When a waist really becomes *tiresome* with emphasis on the spare *tire*, stand, raising arms above head, and in a sweeping motion twist body from the waist to the right, sweep down to the toes, around to the left, and back up to the original position—always keep-

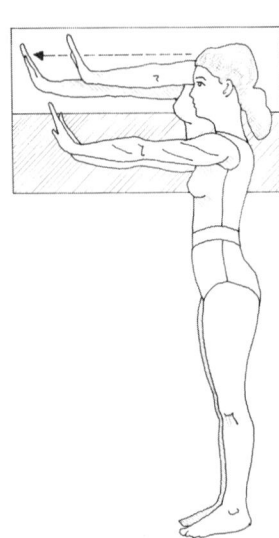

ing arms above the head. This is really acting out a windmill. Repeat twice to the right; then reverse. Move from the waist only. The lower part of the body should face *forward* all the time.

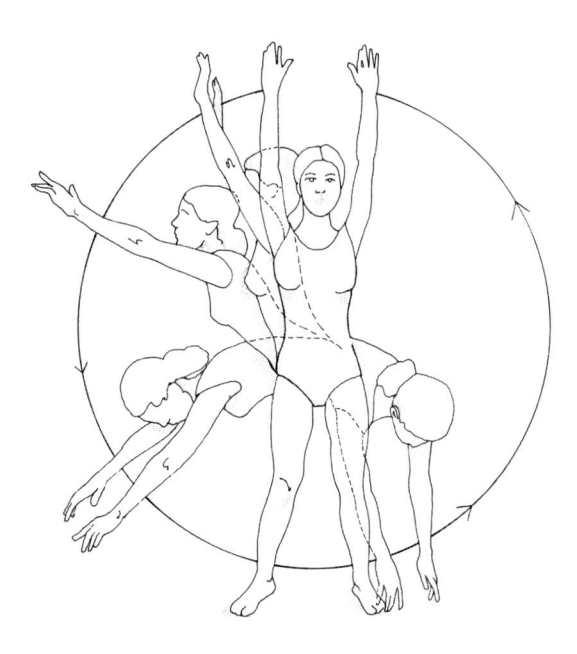

4. This exercise works well for me if carried out with that old military discipline: Lie flat on back with arms extended wide at shoulder level. Bend knees and roll from side to side, keeping shoulders flat as you roll. The more you bend your knees, the higher you will roll. If thighs and lower hips need the most work, bend knees only slightly. If higher hip and waist are in trouble, bring knees to chest. Roll five times to each side, working up to twenty.

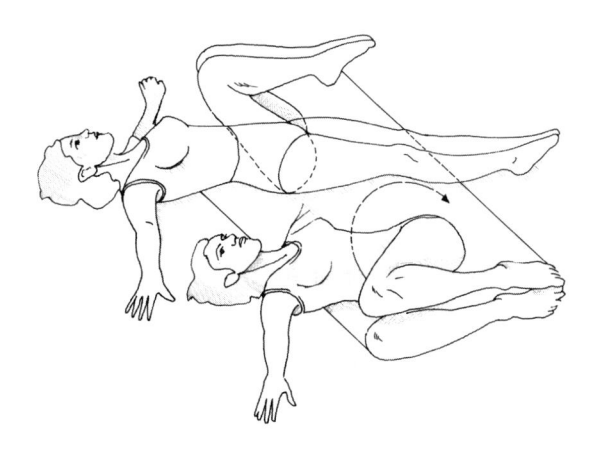

HOW TO FALL IN LOVE WITH EXERCISE

Another person to influence exercise for the better—encouraging the likes of Lee Radziwill, Lady Whitmore, and novelist Edna O'Brien to *follow* instead of trying to *lead* their own brand of shape making—is Lotte Berk (her special brand of exercise can now be found on both sides of the Atlantic). A lady, whose age is difficult to assess, she has the shape and vigor of an eighteen year old, yet the experience and knowledge of someone three times older.

Lotte's exercise for the *Stomach and Waist region* is an easy one to follow:

Lie flat, tucking feet under sofa or bed. Press small of back into floor. Slowly pull yourself up from waist into half-sitting position. Keep small of back straight while reaching forward with hands, bounce backward and forward from waist, then slowly return to lie flat on floor. Relax, repeat. Take it slowly. It's difficult, but it gets a little easier each time.

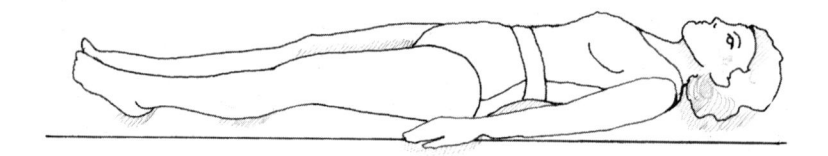

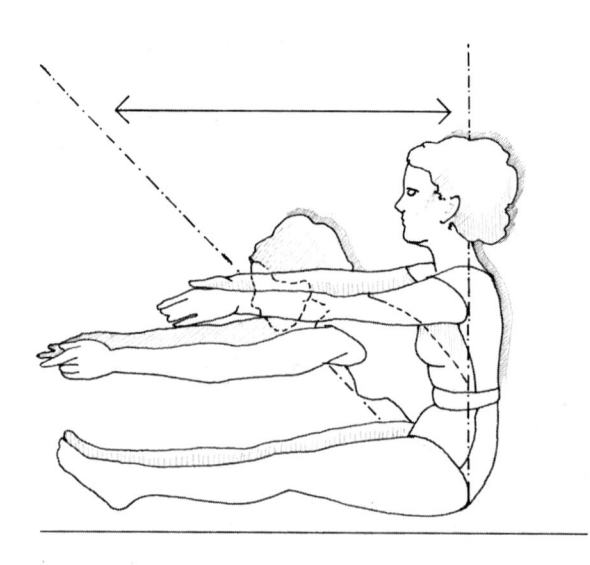

HOW TO FALL IN LOVE
WITH EXERCISE
187

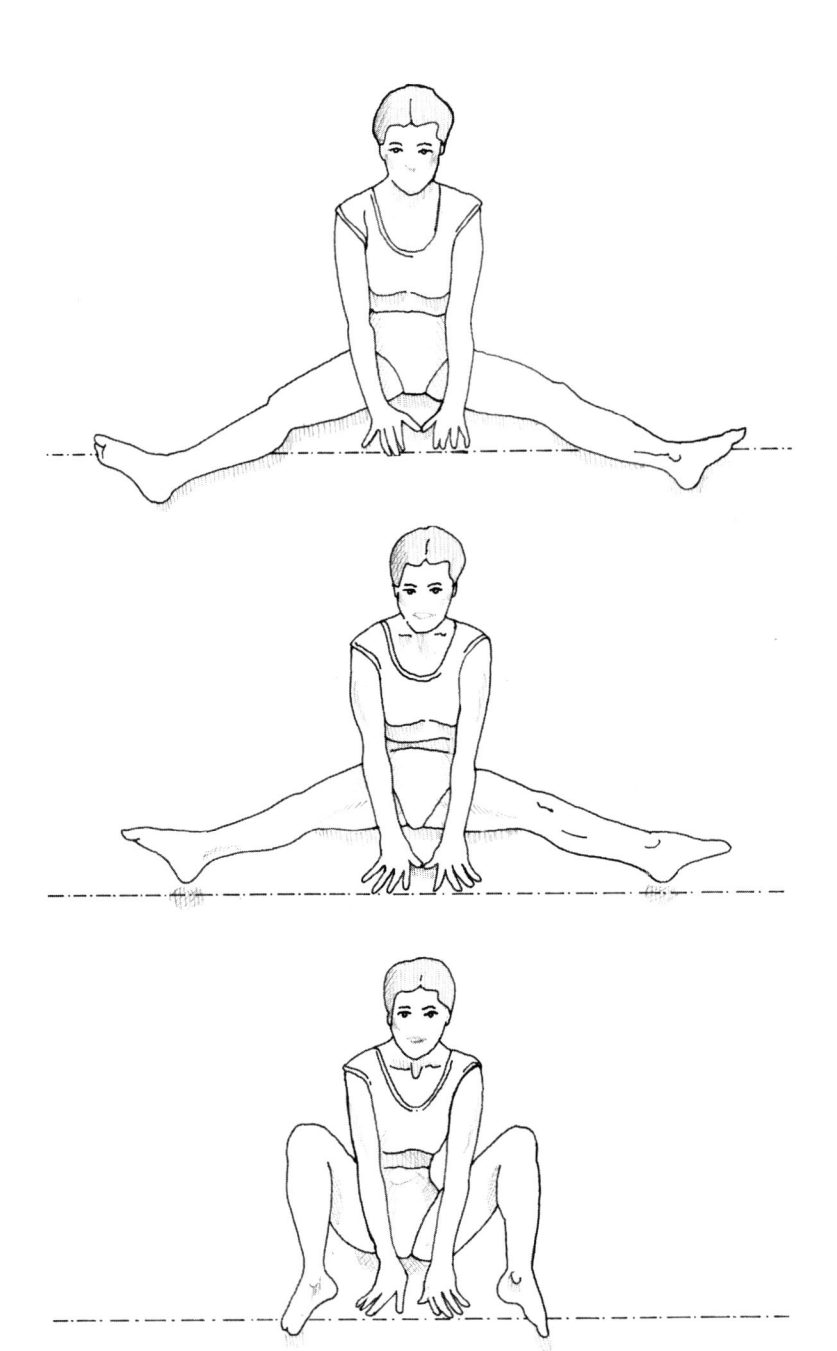

Or . . . Sit on floor with legs wide apart. Rest palms on floor between legs. Keep back straight. Lift legs an inch or two off floor and stretch them straight. Keep weight on hands. Bend legs and continue rhythmically to bend and stretch not letting legs touch floor. Relax, repeat two or three times. Increase with practice.

To Help Back Muscles—and Abdominal Ones, Too

1. Lie flat on back, arms at sides and try to bend knees to chest as far as possible.

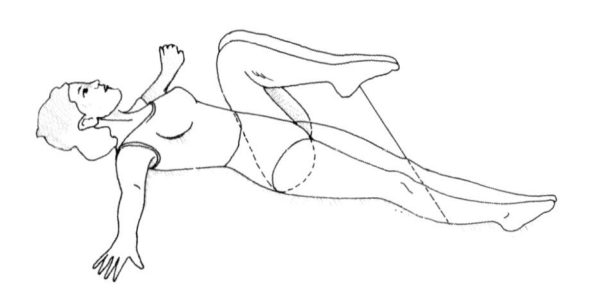

2. Sit on floor and slowly lean back as if sitting in a rocking chair. With arms on hips and knees slightly bent, feet just touching floor, try to rock backward and forward.

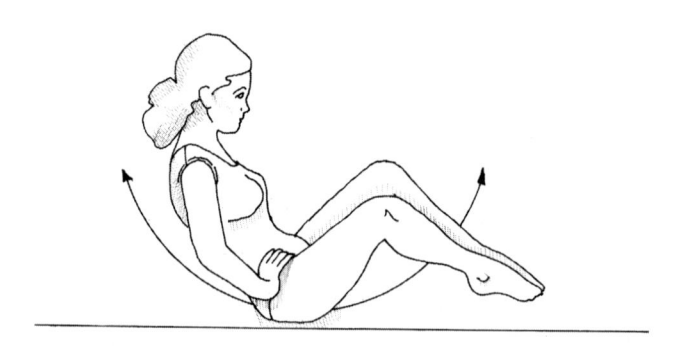

3. Lying flat on floor with arms at sides, raise first one leg as far as it will go, then the other, then both together, returning to floor one at a time and starting again.

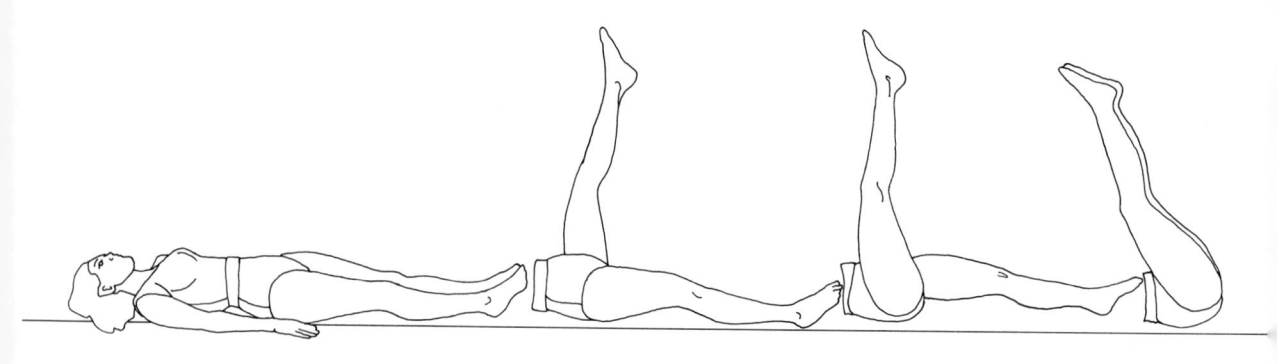

4. Lying on your stomach, reach back to hold ankles with hands. Rock backward and forward twenty times, then relax, breathing in and out deeply. Repeat another twenty times.

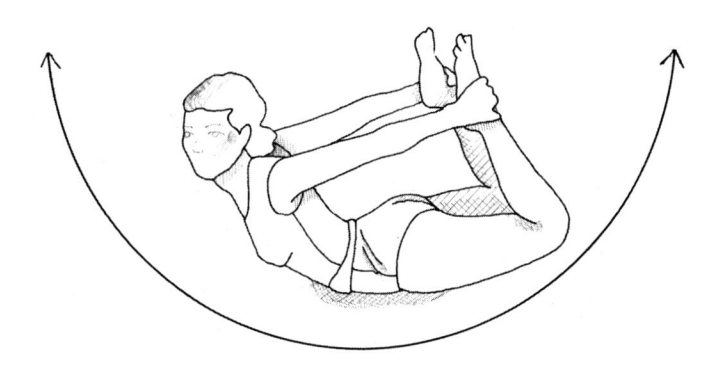

5. Standing upright with feet apart, raise arms over head and hold hands. Bend from side to side, attempting to get as near the waist as possible.

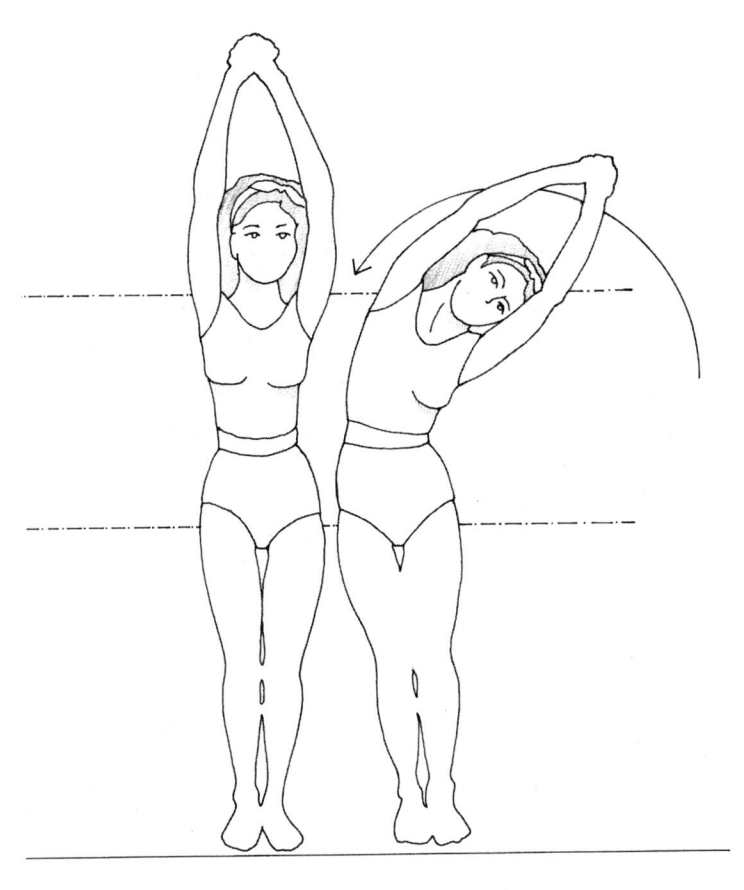

To discover just where your muscles are letting you down—mostly through lack of use—covered up with flab, encouraging more flab, Marvin Hart, shapemaker to the stars (see page 164) devised six simple tests you can try for yourself to assess if and where you need the most help.

1. To test the ability of your *hip muscles:* Lie on your back, hands behind neck, legs straight. Raise both feet at least 10 inches from the floor, holding them still for ten seconds. If you can't do it, you need to concentrate on exercises for your hips.

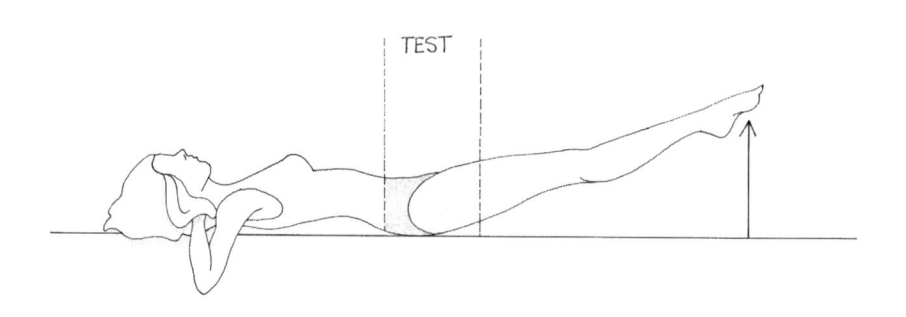

2. To test *hip and abdominal muscles:* Lie on your back, hands clasped behind your neck, legs straight, with your feet under a heavy object, desk, or dressing table. Try to get into a sitting position without moving your hands. If you can't, your stomach and hip muscles need work.

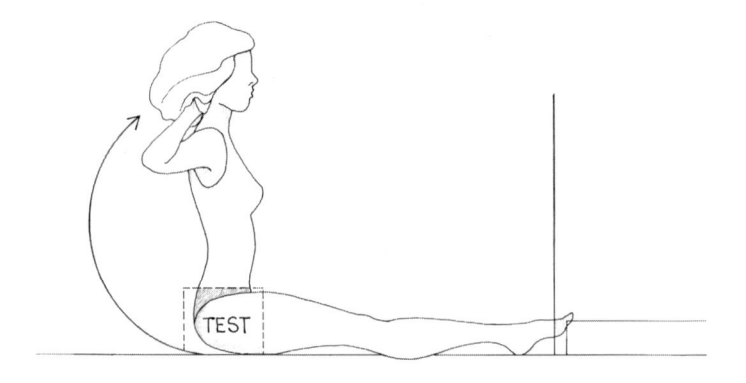

3. To test *stomach and waist muscles:* Lie on your back with hands behind your neck, knees bent with feet under a heavy piece of furniture. Again try to sit up—without the use of your hands. No luck? Get to work on stomach and waist exercises.

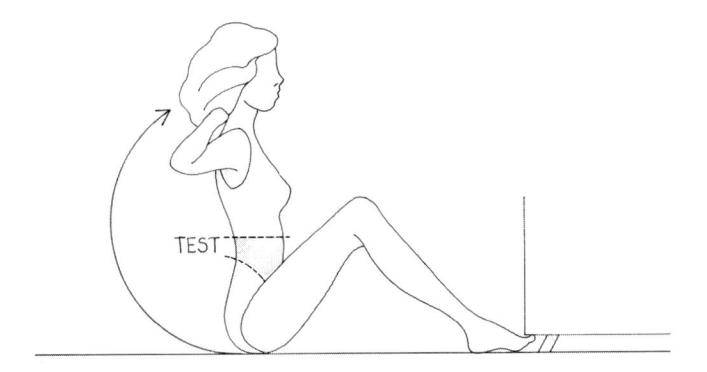

4. To test *upper back muscles* (often where tension ties a knot of pain during a busy working day), lie on your stomach with pillow under your abdomen, hands behind your neck. With someone holding feet and hips down, try to raise your trunk and hold for ten seconds. You should feel your back muscles really working away here. (Marvin Hart frequently acts as the *resistance* against which his pupil has to exert his or her muscles.)

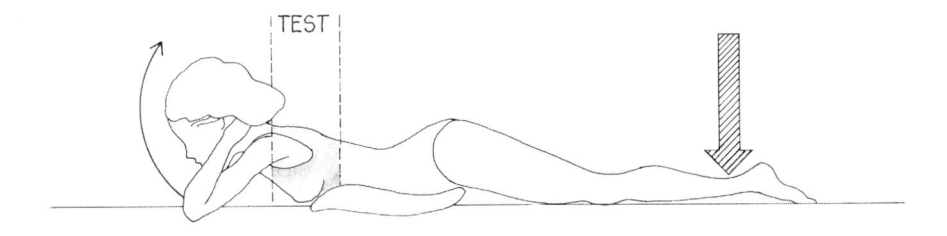

5. Again in the position for the above exercise, this time have someone hold your shoulders and hips down, and try to raise your legs, holding for ten seconds. This is a test for *muscles of the lower back*, where fat loves to accumulate.

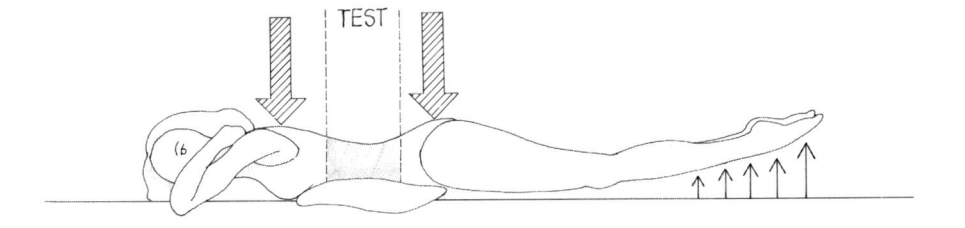

6. For *overall muscle success and flexibility*, test yourself by standing erect with shoes off, feet together, knees stiff, hands at sides. Try to touch floor with fingertips. If you can't do it, try again. Relax, drop head forward and attempt to let your torso "hang" from your hips, keeping knees straight. Chances are you'll do better the second time. If this eludes you, you must think about an exercise program that gives you an overhaul overall.

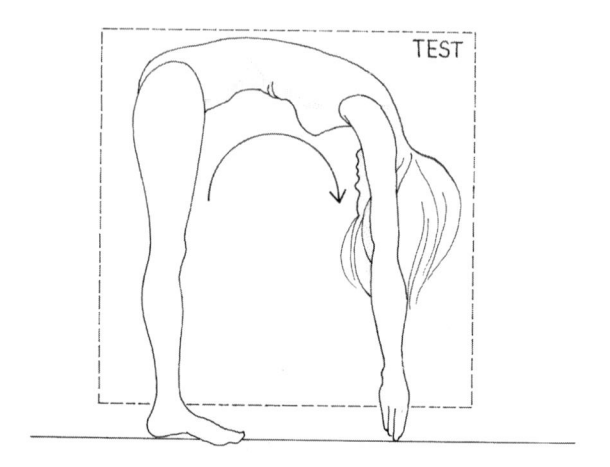

Exercises to Start the Day

One easy exercise you hardly need to think about is a great start to the day as it firms not only the waist, but *the sides of waist*, shoulders, hips, back and front of legs, thighs, plus helping the spine become more flexible:

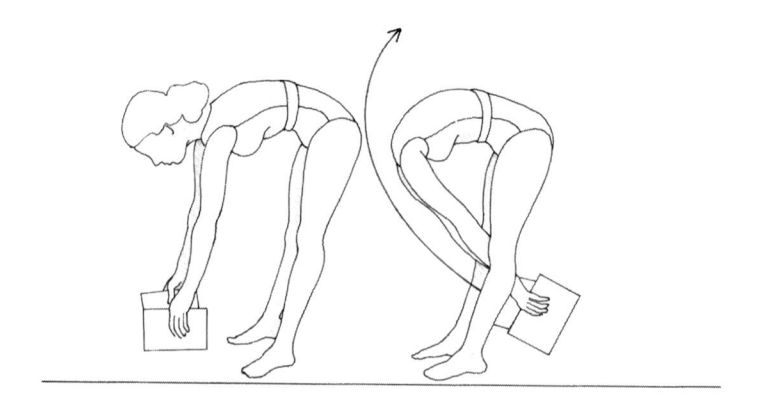

Stand upright, with legs apart, holding a fair-size book in each hand. Swing forward, bending loosely at the waist, then swing your hands through your legs as far as you can go—still holding the books, of course. Swing hands up again over your head and as far back as possible. The most important point: KEEP BREATHING, inhaling through the nose, exhaling loudly through the mouth. Repeat the exercise at least three times at first, working up to ten the first two days, twenty by the end of the week.

Blink your eyes, stretch like a cat from head to toe, throw back the covers over your ankles, bend your knees, and sit up. Lie down again, sit up again—do this several times to get your "motor" on the move.

If you oversleep and have to run for the train, be conscious of your running, and breathe the *right* way as you run, inhaling and exhaling. Once on board, stretch every muscle as you put your bag on the rack or coat on the seat. *Think* shape all the way to work, and don't forget the word if you're sitting in front of a typewriter all day. Occasionally, contract your abdominal muscles, tighten your seat, straighten your shoulders and hold that position as you work for a few minutes. Walk that way to lunch, and if you sit that way at lunch, you'll find you won't eat so much.

The easiest way to start exercising by yourself, following the exercises mentioned here is to *start slowly*—telling yourself you will carry out five exercises every day the first week, increasing the number until it becomes second nature.

The most important thing to remember is that once you *start*, you must *continue* for any results to take place.

Don't find excuses. If the thought bores you, tires you, exhausts you, exercise first thing in the morning before you brush your teeth—as soon as you wake up so that it's out of the way. DON'T leap out of bed to start work. If you need an alarm clock, set it a few minutes early, and before you start thinking what a drag and fall back to sleep, look at an unflattering photograph of yourself you've placed by the clock to remind you what you need to do.

Marvin Hart thinks repetition is the main drag about exercise. For this reason, he has many variations of each shape-making movement to give the body a change and, he thinks, give his obviously delighted clients the interest to keep at it.

The key words are *consistency, breathing, stretching* for your own exercise program to do *you* all the good in the world.

If You're a Jane at Heart, Tarzan or No Tarzan at Home

Apparatus is not the crutch the knee-bend girls think. All over the world—but particularly in the United States—apparatus work is one way certain of the species get their bodies in trim and keep them that way.

A regular date at a gym, run by well-qualified people, is far more exhilarating, they think, than halfhearted attempts at body stretches all by themselves at home.

Larry Lorence, who actually encourages his pupils to fly through the air on a flying trapeze, has a big following in New York, and sensibly gives a program that offers endless variety of movements and *lots of challenge.* You start on the floor and end up as described literally flying through the air.

Some of the basic routines for physical fitness that play a part in the Olympic gymnasts' regime are fitted into these classes—which kept to six at a time—are always full.

In case you think I'm talking only about the natural athlete or super-Amazon type, I'm not. Gym can be for tired old bodies, too—the owners learn how to lose fatigue and stand up straight. As Larry Lorence says, "It's possible to relieve emotional tension *physically,* by recognizing that tension causes a tense person to breathe incorrectly and cramp up. Exercise is one way to correct all this. *We're satisfied when a pupil gets as far as she possibly can considering her age, weight, physical condition, and mental attitude.* Sometimes we wait years before we see a change, but it's always gratifying when it comes."

Typical of most leading gymnasts, Larry suggests two hours a week at the gym with a daily routine of ten minutes of exercise at home, mostly breathing and bending, plus a good helping of sport—always the best introduction to gym work.

A coordination test is one of the first things many gyms insist on before work begins, to discover how soon—if ever—you will be performing. Workouts are devised with light dumbbells to help posture, stretches on specially devised bars, handstands and tumbling with instructors at the ready to hold you up until you hold yourself up.

Mat work trims waists, strengthens backs.

Routines on the bars firm hips.

Work on incline boards and balance beams is good for hips and knees.

Back bends, head stands, and weight lifting are for all-over toning.

Rings are for balance and to increase coordination.

Many gyms have ingeniously devised apparatus that use springs, pulleys, and sliding blocks to provide extra resistance against which students work.

The incentive is the obvious one—better shape for out-of-shape areas, but some gym groups are so anxious for their students to succeed, they offer a magnum of champagne to anyone who can kick a horizontal bar way above their heads ten times. Needless to say, you don't get to the horizontal-bar class until you've worked your way through many dumbbell routines. Not even a glass of beer for that—*especially* not a glass of beer.

Whatever the apparatus work you try, the end of the first lesson is apt to leave you exhausted—so say pupils who've been through it. But when they have the willpower to return for the next class and the next until it becomes a regular part of their lives, they also say they experience an extraordinary new sensation—relaxation with exhilaration. Physical tuning *does* affect psyche.

How Many Calories You Burn Up in One Hour's Activity

Jogging at home	300
Jogging outdoors	500
Ball throwing	200
Flying a kite	30
Ice skating	200–600 (depending on the vigor of your figure eights)
Cycling	200–600 (uphill)
Walking slowly	115
Walking fairly fast	215
Walking as fast as you can	550
Window shopping (for one day)	900
Museum viewing (large)	1,250
(small)	750
Dancing	200–400 (depending on the music)
Rowing	500–900 (depending on how many in the boat)
Tennis	500–700
Skipping rope	300
Horseback riding	150
Trotting	600
Judo	800
Exercise class	250–1,000
Skiing	350–600
Cross-country skiing	650–1,000
Cross-country running	500–700
Cleaning house (scrubbing etc.)	165
Ironing	50
Washing dishes	50
Painting	150–200
Wallpapering	150–200
Mowing	300
Golf with no cart	145
Card playing	
with money involved	100
no money—no emotion	50
Billiards	250
Ping-Pong	180
Standing at cocktail parties	
30 minutes	20
60 minutes	50

Lazy Way to New Shape—Sometimes

Classes, salons, spas, and studios offering *equipment* are not necessarily offering apparatus. The two are far apart, and qualified gymnasts are anxious to have them differentiated. *Apparatus* needs *your* muscles, *your* participation, *your* work for anything to happen. *Equipment* generally means you lean your body against *it* in a certain way, and *it* attempts to do something to you while you could—if you were so inclined—read your horoscope, manicure your nails, and we hope, breathe consciously and correctly as you do during any other body-endeavor program.

In California, where much of the equipment originated, you can find mechanical wonderlands, spine correctors, reformers, towers, wunda-chairs, tensors, pedi-pulls, trapeze tables. Whatever it's called, each piece of equipment usually has to be plugged in to the current, so that with only one turn of the switch parts of the machine wallop away at your posterior or abdomen or stretch your arms and legs. It doesn't do you any *harm*—but unless you're watching your caloric intake and moving your own muscles yourself, it doesn't do much good, either!

In Europe various faradic machines are at work—faradic meaning moving muscles involuntarily with low-frequency current. You lie there counting sheep, and except for a slight tingling sensation, don't feel anything at all—no aches and pains, no strains—although your muscles alternately contract and relax.

Here in the United States, stringent regulations mean the faradic method is by no means widespread. The operator has to have medical qualifications before it can be used, which means it won't appear in every trim-down salon you enter.

The machine using jets of hot air to get at your flab is another popular piece of equipment.

Generally described as a reducing treatment, this type of machine, which looks like a home hair dryer with fat tubes, works by directing jets of hot air under considerable pressure onto your bulges. The hot air produces a rippling effect on the skin as you might expect, stimulates circulation, and generally is soothing and relaxing, but frankly it again cannot have any dramatic results without a lot of other work.

Cellulite—the Truth

Hot-air machines and low-current machines are probably at work right now somewhere in the world on the controversial affliction known currently as *cellulite*.

Does it exist or doesn't it? The French are convinced it does. The Americans—some of them at least—say cellulite is just plain fat that shows up more on some women than others, depending on the thickness of the skin.

In Europe most doctors don't think cellulite is *plain fat* at all, but rather an association of fat, water, and waste created by too much toxin in the body.

Because of this, they say, tissues lack normal elasticity, so you can literally *see* "bubbles" or lumps imprisoned in the flesh—particularly in the thighs—causing a look that has been described variously as chicken skin, orange peel, and in other attractive word pictures.

Whatever it's called, cellulite doesn't look good, can ruin the line of a skirt, and makes some people positively paranoid about going to the beach.

Cellulite appears more in the thigh area than anywhere else, and it usually means that (1) a woman has poor circulation (which can lead to varicose veins); and (2) her pelvic muscles are weak.

Where else is it found, apart from its favorite resting places (the upper exterior side of thighs, inside and back of thighs)? Cellulite likes the inside of the knees, hips and buttocks, the upper arms, ankles, and sometimes the abdomen. And what are the main offenders for this condition? Tension (many people retain extra fluid under emotional stress), air pollution, poor breathing, and poor diet are the main ones, *with lack of exercise backing them all up.*

How to Lose Cellulite

The objective of any cellulite treatment is to rid the body of this trapped mixture of fluid and fat, draining it through the usual elimination points of the body. In Paris, machines stimulate muscles electrically, using sponges impregnated with thyroid base and silicon medicaments. These are applied to the cellulite areas, metal plaques being placed on top, which in turn are plugged into an instrument which shoots through the current causing mild muscle spasm. A series of at least ten treatments is advised but often many more are needed before any difference can be seen.

As cellulite is often found around muscles, hot-air jet machines are used in the United States (often by French operators) to get between skin and muscle and so attack the hated lumps. The hot air can be helpful because it zips up circulation, too.

If you're machine-minded and would back up their use with a definite anticellulite diet, you may well cure or at least improve your problem. You'd have to aim for food containing anticellulite minerals, particularly iodine, which means liberal helpings of seafood—no hardship for most—asparagus, cabbage—a valuable and underestimated food—and bananas, plus at least a quart of water a day to flush the system, and decrease salt intake.

One piece of equipment you can use to help your own shape

along—away from the salon, studio, and/or gym—is the simple garden hose. In the summer aim it at your thighs for a few seconds to create your own "machine"—not using hot air but pleasantly warm water, which can attack the "lumps" in a refreshing way.

Do-it-themselves girls swarm together in the sunny states like California, for instance, where Betsy Bloomingdale, Mrs. Henry Mancini, and Ursula Thiess Taylor, among many others get together to exercise once or twice a week at least with or without apparatus or machines but with exemplary discipline. Ursula has never let once being named the Most Beautiful Girl in the World cramp her realization she is a Beautiful Big Girl, whose figure has to be watched. Mrs. Henry Fonda conducts a yoga class that husband Henry is occasionally allowed to join. Polly Bergen never stops exercising for, although she wavers between size 6 and 8, she still has a giant-size *mental* picture of herself as she once was—a size 14—and this helps her continue and *maintain* her good shape making.

Figure control is easier in the sun, but it's also easy *wherever* you are, if motivation is great enough.

Learn About Massage—It's Good for You

"I know when a body is out of tune," said the lady with the magical hands. "I can retune it as well as my cousin retunes a Stradivarius."

Most good masseurs are large people, which must have something to do with their muscle power, something they never show; their touch, often as light as a feather, working wonders on tired-out, tense bodies.

A $75-million-a-year business in Los Angeles alone, massage is a panacea to many of the pacesetters and people who must follow that pace. Massage is not a medicine as many think, and the masseur who offers it as a cure for arthritis or to banish wrinkles or to help you lose weight *is the masseur to avoid.*

In the hands of a trained and licensed physical therapist, however, massage makes you feel better psychologically and physiologically, for massage helps the body in so many different ways—affecting our complex combination of nerve endings, skin, muscle, and blood circulation.

The best time to have a massage is when you feel worn out—an improvement on rest alone, as from the right hands, it unknots bunched muscles and stimulates the blood flow to cleanse the body faster of waste matters, toxins.

Response from nerve endings revolves around the psychological benefits—important in that the sense of touch conveys a great deal of information to the person being massaged. Indifference or sympathy is relayed via hands—one reason that one pair of hands will relax you

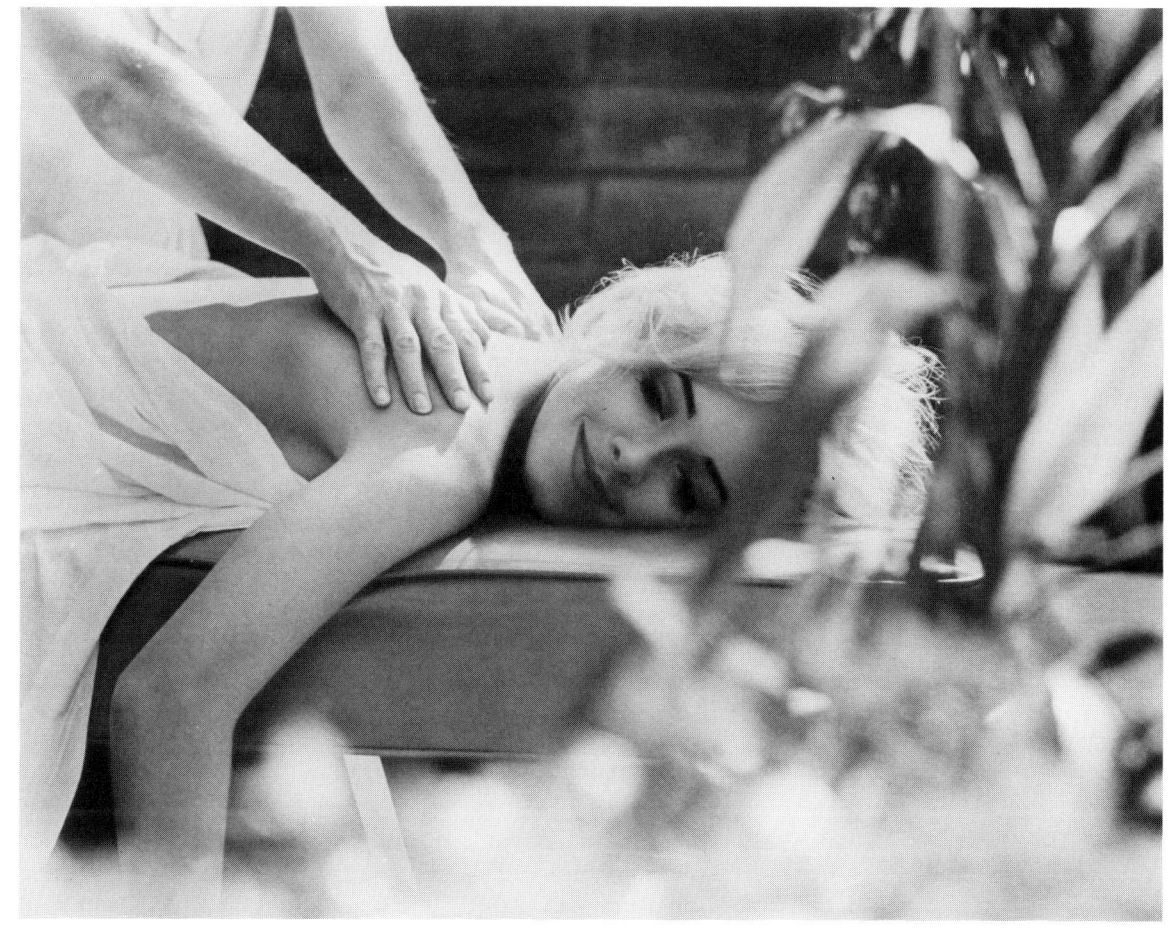

The best time to have a massage is when you feel worn out. It's better than rest alone.

to the point you are lulled to sleep, while another pair will make you wish you'd never come in the first place. When it is, as it should be, tranquilizing, massage works faster than alcohol or drugs—and is obviously much better for you.

The right massage can relax muscles, so that if they're under pressure, contracting with spasms because of too much work through tension, or taking on the work load of other muscles (this can happen in the case of whiplash), the right pressure can reduce the problem, helping them return to normality.

The better the masseur, the more quickly he or she can get a response from skin itself, inhibiting the sensory spots that send messages to the brain, inducing serenity and drowsiness, so that the client can withdraw from the world for at least an hour of tranquility.

At the same time, massage helps blood circulation by accelerating the blood flow in areas where blood vessels may be constricted.

Commercial masseurs are not necessarily physical therapists, (who you can find listed in the yellow pages under *Physical therapy*). But if you find one who *is* at a salon, gym, or spa, he or she will not only be trained in techniques of massage, but should know a great deal about anatomy, pathology, physiology, the muscular and skeletal structures, the nervous and circulatory systems of the body.

Unlike commercial masseurs (who in most states are not allowed to massage the opposite sex), physical therapists can work on both sexes, although males rarely give full body massage to a woman, and vice versa.

Generally in the United States, commercial masseurs use the hundred-year-old Swedish method based on a system from Per Henrik Ling, a Swedish medical gymnast, working from toe to top. This is the opposite of the physical therapist's pattern, who generally works from the top down—although both use strokes *up* toward the heart to move the blood in the veins in that direction. The masseur uses effleurage (stroking), friction (rubbing), petrissage (kneading), and tapotement (tapping) all to increase blood and lymph flow through veins and lymph vessels rather than through the arteries.

Because of the drain on their own energies, the names and telephone numbers of some of the best masseurs in the country are as closely guarded as those of great free-lance French chefs and inexpensive dressmakers who can make a Halston-like style in a week.

George King is one name with an illustrious roster of clients, like Truman Capote, ballet dancer Edward Villella, Charlotte Ford Forstmann, and Candice Bergen. "I can heal so much tension with my hands," he says, and has clients with happy relaxed faces to prove it. When you walk into his studio, you may find it darkly lit, incense filled. Before he begins, he suggests a sauna followed by yoga exercises. Again—as I find over and over again with the experts—he believes *breathing* properly executed is the key to looking and feeling your best. His training also includes channeling *energy* through proper breathing. The finale is what you came for in the first place—a remarkable massage, very gentle with fragrant oils, that undoubtedly induces responses from nerve endings, skin, muscles, and blood flow as it was all intended to do.

Some masseurs prefer to use rubbing alcohol, talcum powder, or even salt, which feels coarse but gives the body an extraordinarily clean, smooth feeling once it's washed off with a fragrant warm cloth.

George King's massage table differs from the pink-toweling–padded variety. It's huge, made of exquisite mahogany with four large legs carved like tree trunks. It seems it's necessary that the table be of such solid proportions, for if he thinks you need it, King massages your back with his toes—which means what it says, he walks on you.

Josef Rottenburger is another name that sends the right sort of spasms through muscles in the know. Boxer, war hero, and masseur for many years to royal families across the world, he describes his massage still as "zone therapy"—working on stiffness and pain often through the feet. Each part of the foot, he believes, can be worked on to affect a different part of the body—which is a belief that is acted upon in many health spas of Europe.

In Paris today the Shiatsu method of massage is as familiar to patrons of salons on the Faubourg St. Honoré as to clients on the Ginza in Tokyo. Shiatsu, now practiced here, is a form of acupressure—a finger massage like acupuncture in that it follows the pressure points of the body but uses thumbs or fingers, not needles. Pressure applied in this expert manner reduces muscle tension, aches, and pains, especially of the head or back. The underlying purpose is to activate organs that are not working correctly, to help them feel younger, more active, and to correct faults in circulation.

Shiatsu devotees believe it helps the condition of their skin as well as their shape. As one Shiatsu masseur says, "Skin is one of the best indicators of intestinal and respiratory health. If it looks drab, the intestinal muscles are tired, but a change in diet won't always help—because the food can't be digested properly. Shiatsu massage can help correct this."

Hindu massage also follows the acupuncture route. Up from the heels along the *sides* of the body, from the base of the neck up into the center of the skull (where a baby has its soft spot) this type of massage is also result-producing—particularly refreshing and relaxing.

A deep hand massage—sometimes worked in concert with low-frequency electrical impulses carried through pads placed on the body—is aimed at starting sluggish muscles working and this was Louise Long's specialty. Louise, a byword in California, used to refuse interviews because she already had to start her day at 5 A.M. and finish at midnight in order to get to all of her top show-business names. She died in 1974 but luckily passed on her special technique to her assistants, who are busy as ever. Louise's secret was deep, strong, *knowing* massage—which is what the business is all about.

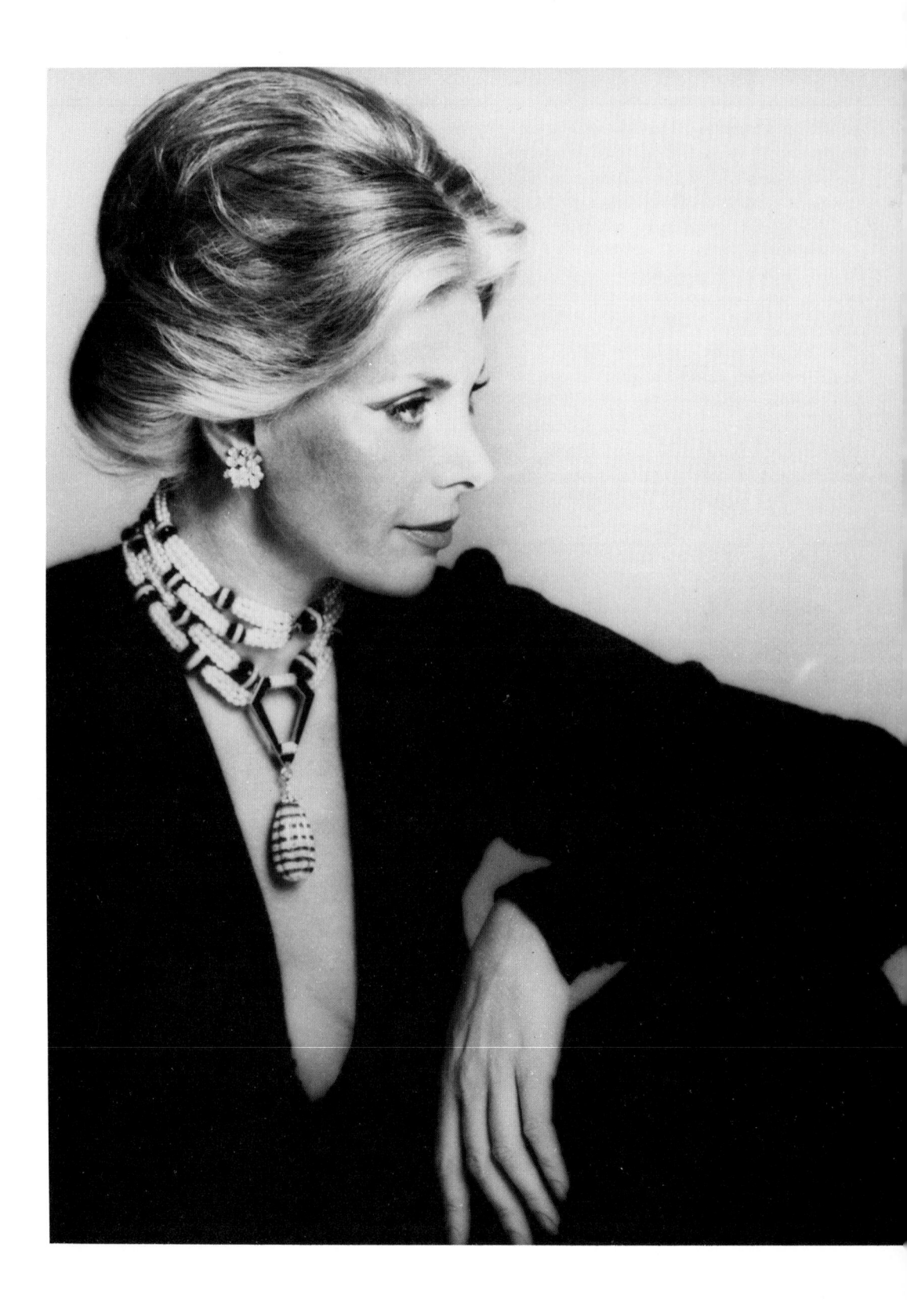

7

Has She or Hasn't She...

*Had Her Face/Bosom/Thighs Lifted?
Had a Nose/Stomach/Chin Job?*

The question is still not asked directly—but the conjecture never stops. More significant, every day all over the world the number of plastic surgery operations taking place grows, while the age of the patient is getting younger.

For those who care, it's London, Miami, and New York for facelifts, Tokyo for nose jobs and eye openers, Moscow for hair transplants, and Rio de Janeiro or Buenos Aires for thigh lifts in particular, body tucks in general—sometimes poetically described as body sculpting, a poetic description but the most painful of all plastic-surgery operations.

All over the world the traffic in clients in search of the right plastic

FACING PAGE
Beautiful Luciana Avedon, one of the first "to tell."

surgeon grows, as the need to look younger becomes more of a necessity. The plastic surgeons say that forty now seems to be the age women begin to want a fresh start.

Once magisterial toward purely cosmetic jobs, more and more plastic surgeons exchange views, and even hold worldwide symposiums to discover how best to correct or improve on nature's imperfections, while in the United States and Europe more and more articles "disclose" facts about the famous and their various lifts.

When Vidal Sassoon revealed he'd had the bags beneath his eyes removed, he told me he thought he had a good reason for having done so: "I go to a gym every day to keep my body in top shape. Why shouldn't my face match up? I may be over forty, but I feel like twenty-five. My body looks it. Now so does my face."

According to the American Society of Plastic and Reconstructive Surgeons, this makes Vidal typical of the million younger men and women who annually undergo some kind of surgery for the sake of their looks alone. Since 1949 the number of operations has skyrocketed—in the last decade, tripling for women, doubling for men, operations all carried out for what the society calls "surgery performed in an attempt to improve the appearance, not necessary for physical health or safety, but desirable for emotional and/or psychological benefit."

A typical plastic surgeon's year, according to the society, will include at least 50 breast operations (mostly to reduce, rather than increase, size), 100 face-lifts, 150 nose operations, 20 chin corrections, and 75 ear-flattening operations.

In London and East Grinstead, Sussex, at the Queen Victoria Plastic Surgery Hospital, disciples of the late, great daddy of plastic surgery, Sir Archibald McIndoe, admit the volume of jobs for vanity's sake alone increases every month.

In France and Switzerland, husbands and wives go to clinics together, with the intention of regaining lost looks, while in Rio de Janeiro, Brazil, the celebrated Dr. Ivo Pitanguy is booked from one year's end to the next for his equally celebrated body-lifts, particularly the operation for removing what he calls "riding breeches"—ridding the thigh area of excess flab, as distressing to women over thirty as is deadly cellulite (see pages 196–197).

As Dr. Pitanguy explained to me, "Where there is a question of life and death, the surgeon has to make the arbitrary decision—to operate or not. In the case of plastic surgery, it is the patient who makes the arbitrary decision, coming to the plastic surgeon with his or her mind made up, often after a lengthy period of worry and indecision, asking perhaps for a nose like Mary Tyler Moore's or a chin like George Hamilton's. It is up to the surgeon to *try* to realize the patient's dreams, if they are within the realms of reality. Sometimes, they are not. The nose or chin they want won't work with the rest of their features. Then the surgeon has a psychological problem on his hands—to help the patient readjust her dream to the "right size," one that *is* possible to fulfill with surgery. It is very important that everyone realize they have to approach plastic surgery with the right size dream. Then they can work with the surgeon toward making it come true."

Lifting the Face

There's more than one kind of face-lift. The basic version takes up only the slack in the cheeks and upper jowls, whereas the radical kind means cutting around the entire hairline to the nape of the neck. Even the average lift takes about four hours, but if all goes well, the patient should be able to face the world happily within three weeks. As far as scars are concerned, the better the surgeon, the fewer the scars, usually concealed in the hairline.

Most surgeons agree a face-lift should give a fresh approach from at least *five to eight years,* but it all depends on the skin. Some skins react better than others, so some last longer.

How old should one be to contemplate a lift? Opinions vary. Princess Luciana Pignatelli (now Mrs. Burt Avedon) was one of the first to "tell it all" about her silicone injections, her nose job, and eye ops. She says, "I prefer not to wait until something drastic has to be done. There's no sense in trying to come out as smooth as a baby when you go in looking like an old topographic map."

Most surgeons would agree with her, although they often try to dissuade the forty-year-old patient from having her first face "job." The best deterrent: the news that the earlier the visit, the more return visits may have to be made.

At Your First Appointment

When you make up your mind that something has to go—whether it's eye bags, cheek droops, or just a baggy old face, you may have different ideas from the surgeon you select.

At your first interview he will examine you, advise, and ask for your medical history, just like any other doctor would do before an operation, because—make no mistake about it— *this is an operation,* not a lark, however frivolous *your* reason for the visit. The surgeon may show you pictures of operations he's carried out, demonstrating his work with before-and-after photographs, and he will certainly photograph you for planning and record purposes.

The surgeon's main challenge in a face-lift is how far he can undermine the skin from the fat and muscle beneath, how much excess can be excised, how far it can be stretched and in which direction. A woman may arrive at the surgery thinking she needs the "works"—a standard face-lift called a *rhytidectomy*—whereas the surgeon may point out with pictures and demonstrations on her own face that only a *blepharoplasty*—removal of eye bags—is needed.

For a full face-lift job, the surgeon usually starts with an incision in the scalp about midway along the forehead—back from the hairline, continuing down on either side to the point where the ears are attached to the head. From there the incision proceeds in front of the ears, curving around them, continuing upward and sharply backward, finishing at the back just above the nape of the neck.

Once the skin is separated from the underlying tissue, the surgeon's most delicate job is to gather the tissue upward and backward on either side toward the ears, suturing it firmly to the fascia (which protects facial muscles), tightening it, so providing a smooth ground over which the aging inelastic skin can be "stretched," any excess being cut off. A local anesthesia, combined with intravenous analgesia, is often used for this op because a general anesthesia tube can obscure the face's overall condition and shape. Some sutures are removed after three to five days; those behind the ears not for ten days. With lines "ironed" out, skin stretched but not too taut, the face in the right surgeon's hands will inevitably look smoother and so younger—for a few years at least.

Away with Baggy Eyes

The older the eyes, the more beautiful they often become with experience showing in their expression. The skin around the eyes is not so pretty. This is where the blepharoplasty—eye-wrinkle job—comes in, one in which fat and excess skin is removed from the upper or lower lids or both.

Rapidly becoming top of the pops in plastic-surgery ops—the number being carried out nowadays approaching that of the number of nose jobs—blepharoplasty is even sought by model girls in their late twenties who want to cover all markets and not lose their lucrative "teen look."

To smooth out bags, the surgeon starts by making an incision just beneath the lower lashes, angling downward at outer corners, drawing the loosened skin upward, trimming, then stitching. To correct a sag on the upper lid, incision is made at the eyelid's crease, when again off comes skin and unwanted fat, followed by a fine seam angled upward. Many operations take place under local anesthesia, as many surgeons like patients to be *awake enough* to cooperate when asked to open or close their eyes. If it sounds simple, it isn't. The surgeon has to be able to measure *exactly* the right amount of skin to be excised. Too little and it would all be a waste of time. Too much—even by a fraction of a millimeter—and the eye will look distorted or—worse—not be able to close properly. The surgeon also has to decide whether the aging look comes from sagging lids or drooping eyebrows. If it's the latter, he elevates the brow by excising skin above the browline, with the suture line buried in the upper hairline.

Step-by-Step Anti Bag

One friend of mine went into a clinic at the beginning of the week for an anti-bags job. The first morning she was given a blood test, coagulation test, and urine analysis and after about 12 o'clock she wasn't allowed to eat or drink anything, not even a glass of water.

About 1:30 the surgeon came by to explain exactly what he was going to do, demonstrating by drawing on her eyelids with an indelible pencil to show her exactly where he intended to make his cuts. She had to look up, down, right, left, smile, frown, and make as many expressions as she regularly made during a day—surprise was one of them—so that he could see where she made her wrinkles. As he explained the idea behind it was essentially practical—he intended to make his incisions wherever there were wrinkles already, so that each tiny scar could be hidden there.

At 4:00 she was given an injection to make her drowsy and an hour later was taken to the operating room for a second injection. The operation took about two hours and in this case (although it doesn't always happen) a nurse sat with her from 8 P.M. to 8 A.M., putting pieces of ice wrapped in little squares of gauze on her eyes all through the night. Later, she told me she thought this was invaluable, as she never did go black and blue, which can happen.

The next morning she felt fine, although the first sight of herself was a shock—tiny black stitches surrounding little slitty eyes, the eyelids very red and swollen. The nurses were helpful as they kept saying what a marvelous job it was, so she wasn't as depressed as she might have been. Two days later she went home under dark glasses, the underneath stitches completely out, the top ones still in.

By the end of the week her eyes were less swollen; her lids and the skin under the eyes were turning slightly yellow and itched. By the end of the weekend her eyes were even less swollen, and all stitches came out.

A week from the day of the op the upper lid looked perfectly normal, the under one a litte red. At the end of the second week—twelve days after the operation—she started to put on normal eye makeup. She'd waited that long, not so much because it would have bothered her eyes, but because the thought of *taking it off* was unbearable. The result? I and many of her friends told her when next we saw her how very healthy and well she looked—which is how I came to hear the story.

Grandma, What a Big Nose You Have

Plastic surgery and nose jobs, in particular, were mentioned in early Sanskrit literature in 600 B.C. Then, when nose-slicing became a regular punishment in the Middle Ages, nose-mending became a lucrative, if rather inept, job.

Rhinoplasty, as it's called today, is now so refined that surgeons can shorten, lengthen, tilt, straighten, and do almost any shaping on a nose.

Surgeons say often the hardest part of the job is to convince the majority who want a new nose that the one they've chosen isn't the right nose for them.

The decision of how much to remove, and how much to leave behind, is what makes rhinoplasty still one of the most delicate, complex, and unpredictable plastic operations despite the enormous advances that have taken place. The reason? The slightest fraction of an inch at nose level can make or break a face. Sometimes a surgeon has to make a patient realize it's not her nose that's at fault, but rather her chin that needs augmenting with a slice of silicone (see page 209), so that her nose no longer appears to protrude like a beak, but instead adds character to her looks.

In recent years Pablo Manzoni, the celebrated makeup artist discovered in the 60s by Elizabeth Arden in Rome, has worked more and more with plastic surgeons on post-plastic-surgery makeup, helping women capitalize on their new looks—for makeup often has to be completely renovated when face shape is changed. Pablo is an advocate of "character in the face," and if it's a Roman nose that puts it there, he likes to point out to a would-be nose diminisher how disappointed she may be when she has a "little nothing nose" like everybody else. In other words, sometimes what the owner considers a fault, Pablo considers to be potentially a great asset, and demonstrates how he proceeds to illustrate it with makeup. Not always—sometimes he agrees a change *is* necessary.

The best surgeons know how to minimize or build up a slightly faulty nose without losing the character, even the ancestral quality, that gives a face its drama. As one famous surgeon was quick to point out, "The nose is a peninsula, not an island. *It makes no sense unless considered in relation to the mainland—the face.*"

What Goes On in a Nose Op

Surgery is performed from inside the nose under local anesthesia to prevent the patient from bleeding as much as he would under general anesthesia, keeping the face as natural-looking as possible while the operation is in progress.

Generally, to make smaller takes about forty-five minutes, with seventy-two hours spent in the hospital and one week in bandages. The black-and-blue eyes generally associated with this operation vary again according to the patient's skin, its healing capacity, and the surgeon's skill. If the object is to narrow the nose, a knowledgeable handling of the delicate bones is vital to avoid bruises and, as nose bones have a good memory, to prevent them from resuming their previous position.

Where there's not enough nose, *profile* is often built up utilizing the body's own resources—a sliver from the hipbone or from the rib cartilage to be used as an implant, or a piece of silicone to shape into place.

Because of the skin's astonishing resilience and elasticity, it will stretch over the new more substantial "nose" with ease. After a few days on antibiotics, five days to a week in hospital, and regular checking of the bandages, in three to four weeks when the incision has healed, the new profile looks as if it had always been in residence.

Chinless Wonders Can Be Built Up— and Some Double Chins Trimmed Down

It's been reported that until Marilyn Monroe had her chin built up, she was known as a chinless wonder and her career was chinless, too.

Silicone is regularly used to build up but, when *reduction* is needed, in the case of the iniquitous double chin for instance, the best solution is still a matter of controversy, for this is a job that can leave noticeable scars on the neck.

Where does the double chin come from? As Ralph Millard, M.D., Ronald W. Pigott, F.R.C.S., and Abdulhamid Hedo, M.D., from the Department of Surgery, University of Miami School of Medicine, explained in a paper, part of a panel discussion on facial rejuvenation: "Increasing age, loss of skin elasticity, and repetitious stretching of the neck finally end up in loose excess. This excess tends to make the jowl sag. *Repeated gains and losses in weight* over the years also affect the stretching of skin. This can be accommodated in youth, but droops in dewlaps in later years." Descriptive and telling.

Bradford Cannon, M.D., and Hytho H. Pantazelos, M.D., of the Harvard Medical School and the Massachusetts General Hospital in Boston, put it another way in a paper they presented in Australia at the Fifth International Congress of Plastic and Reconstructive Surgery: "The loss of youthful profile of the neck is caused by the widening of the cervico-mandibular angle. This presents a puzzling therapeutic enigma. It may be manifested by the double chin, with an accumulation of fat but with little or no excess of skin beneath the neck except that which encompasses the heavy fat pad. Such patients may be obese, have short necks, recessed chins, and an inclination to deposit fat beneath the skin. Due to aging and stretching of the skin and *repeated gains and losses in weight*, the neck may develop a turkey gobbler deformity." Specialists' opinions on what age, the gradual drooping of the skin, and additional fat deposits can produce!

The best method of erasing this age telltale is called *lipectomy;* and it is generally carried out in connection with a face-lift.

As Dr. Millard explains, various techniques have been used to remove fat from beneath the chin, leaving crisscross scars which are often quite noticeable. Lipectomy means only a small incision is made under the chin for removal of fat and muscle; then a face-lift gives access to further removal of fat along the chin line, "lifting" and "tightening" skin all around. Dr. Millard further elaborates by stating that out of one hundred face lifts he carried out, sixty-three had this combined procedure, the majority ending up with a better neckline than they possessed when younger.

The Big Peel

While the face-lift takes care of face sag, it doesn't necessarily remove *all* the wrinkles on the face, the fine kind that corrugate foreheads, the frown lines we make between our eyes, the fine wrinkling often found between nostril and upper lip.

We spend our lives making these wrinkles, through publicizing our emotions in the same way again and again, although we rarely realize it . . . these are the expressions that are our habitual giveaways, ones that secret agents have to learn to iron out before departing disguised on a mission.

If we could see ourselves through the mattress when we sleep on our faces (about 75 percent of us sleep this way during some part of the night), we would *pin* ourselves *down* on our *backs* rather than ever do it again. Think of how you look when you press your face against a window or mirror, and you'll get the general idea of the mattress picture, one that we press in a little more every night of our lives.

Before twenty-five, our natural expressions come and go as swiftly as the emotions that cause them, leaving no trace, the skin's early and lively elasticity snapping the face back into place (see page 10).

Once the subcutaneous fat beneath the epidermis starts to dissipate with age, however, there's nothing there to do the snapping, and so the patterns we've been making for a lifetime start to settle in for good in the form of wrinkles.

As two eminent plastic surgeons from the University of Miami School of Medicine wrote in the *British Journal of Plastic Surgery*, "The disfigurement of the aging face is a triad of *hollow, sag,* and *wrinkle* and should be dealt with as far as possible in all its triplicity. A surgical face-lift in hands experienced in shifting skin is an excellent operation. Only if claims are extravagant is there disappointment . . . usually the basis of dismay lies in the *persistence of fine wrinkles.* For the wrinkle there is the acid peel."

Since this endorsement, peeling with chemicals—called facial chemosurgery by the medical profession—has become generally accepted as the best method for removing the tiny lines that still give the age game away.

Dermabrasion is another form of peeling, carried out with a fast rotating wire brush that literally scrapes skin's top surface away, used by expert dermatologists and plastic surgeons to remove acne pits or traumatic scars rather than the everyday sort of wrinkles.

Controversy still exists about chemosurgery's limitations, although there's general agreement it works well in conjunction with a face-lift, expelling the fine wrinkles commonly left around upper and lower lip and forehead.

Dr. Ralph Millard states that the treatment should be clearly defined as *a chemical burn*, using phenol to destroy the epidermis (skin's top layer), significantly altering the dermis beneath. This "burns out the wrinkle" by changing cellular construction and collapsing vertical age lines to make them horizontal, so tautening the skin. In other words, *wrinkles are straightened out.*

As acne is already taut and fixed in its furrows and mounds, burning with chemicals can increase this immobility, which is also the case with deep scars. As far as fine wrinkles are concerned, however, peeling does seem to produce a relative permanency in dermal changes, and it has been proved with this treatment there's far less tendency for the wrinkle to reoccur.

Fair complexions react better than dark—for following chemosurgery, a certain "pinkness" can persist for some months. It fades in time, but perhaps pinkness is only a small price to pay for a no-wrinkle-all-smooth texture.

The right makeup is adequate camouflage, but one thing to remember is that sunbathing is *absolutely out forever* (see pages 28–31).

What Happens in Chemosurgery?

First, the skin site is cleaned with ether, then a phenol-based solution (phenol, croton oil, liquid soap, and distilled water) is painted on with a cotton applicator until the skin is uniformly white. Particular effort is necessary to get to the bottom of deep crevices, frown lines on the forehead, the network of fine wrinkles between nose and mouth, the lines stretched from mouth to chin.

Application encroaches on the hairline, to avoid a visible margin, and around the lips the acid is painted right up to skin's vermilion border. The face is then divided into natural sections, and on most skins, except the very delicate, each section is immediately covered by tape following the "painting" to increase the action of the acid. After forty-eight hours the tape is gently eased off to expose flaking flesh—the debris of the burn.

Antibiotic dusting powder is applied frequently for the next twenty-four hours; then an ointment is used to help soften the crust which can be removed the next day.

Beneath lies a new skin, pink and shining, and one that can be washed immediately with ordinary cleansing methods, mild soap and water being recommended, followed by a very emollient cream if skin is dry and scaly.

Makeup *is* permissible after a week, but it's more often two, three or four—for a peel job means you're likely to consider yourself unpresentable for at least that length of time.

What Happens in Dermabrasion?

This surgical procedure is also called skin planing, for, as the name suggests, the skin *is* planed mechanically. First, the skin is frozen; then a rotating wire brush is stroked rapidly across to remove the surface layer of skin. Scabs that develop are shed within two weeks, when skin swells and appears more pink than usual.

It takes quite a few weeks for the face to return to normal in terms of swelling and color, but some dermatologists prefer to work with dermabrasion rather than chemosurgery because they feel there's less natural color destruction.

To sum it up, while chemical peeling works by burning, mechanical peeling works by scraping. As one eminent doctor put it, "In nature a scrape among animals heals faster and more accurately than a burn. It's a more natural procedure." It's also a highly skilled one, which means dermabrasion should *only* be contemplated if it's *certain* a doctor with high credentials is behind the brush. In underqualified hands, dermabrasion can be highly dangerous—for the face can be planed to the point of no return—where only the epidermis around the hair and sweat glands remains. If the epidermis were to be destroyed also at those points, there would be nothing left to regenerate the skin. Because the brush works so fast, unless the hands operating it are extremely qualified, it can catch the lip or nose, leaving behind a scar instead of taking one away.

Because of all these horrifying dangers, the American Society of Dermatologic Surgery is as anxious as the American Association of Plastic Surgeons to rid the country of so-called wrinkle-removing salons, where chemical peeling and dermabrasion are carried out by the unqualified. Check, check and check again when choosing the man to do the job.

Peeling or "brushing" can work wonders, but only when the peeler knows his business and has several medical degrees to prove it.

Post P.S. Makeup

The important part makeup plays post face-lift or skin peel is recognized by the American Society of Aesthetic Plastic Surgery, founded in 1967 to discuss new approaches and improved techniques.

One of the most important things to avoid with post-peel makeup is the use of the wrong colors, permanently staining the ultrasensitive new skin. For this reason all gel makeup should be avoided. Instead the more old-fashioned bases with sediment, colored through powder, not pigment, should be used. A light tan to warm beige is the most flattering shade for most skins, *always* worn over a *very* emollient moisturizer.

Pablo Manzoni, who successfully introduced post-plastic–surgery makeup centers across the United States, also introduced many post-plastic–surgery clients to dyed lashes (black), extra eye makeup (blue pencil above lower lashes, brown beneath the brows) plus advocating brush-on rouge on top of cheekbones, bridge of nose, and forehead.

"Once you've had your face lifted, it should stay lifted," he says. "Makeup color helps create this, giving an illusion of brightness and well-being."

As he also constantly reiterates to all clients, "Pat in everything you put on your face. Never, *never* rub."

Body Jobs—Tucks and Trims and Additions, Too

The Bosom and How to Wear a See-through Without Cold Feet

Revolutionary techniques in breast surgery have occurred during the last two decades. This, combined with the acceptance of the no-bra, see-through, OK-streaking era, has sent many under- and over-endowed women scurrying to see a plastic surgeon. Statistics say the age-group centers around fifteen- to thirty-year-olds, without excluding a very interested over-forty group. I know several who have revamped their bosom shapes successfully in the last few years.

When a woman looks down and sees her front is as flat as her ironing board, her confidence begins to crack. Until 1950 if she felt she couldn't go through life without a lovely pair of bosoms, she had to be prepared to relinquish part of her buttocks. It was a difficult and not too successful operation.

"So Flat-Chested I Could Cry"

I have received many readers' letters over the years with the above sad complaint, and I'm happy today to be able to write back to tell the deprived one that breastlines can be filled out with implants of fluid silastic encased in plastic bags, inserted through incisions at the base of each bosom, and tucked neatly behind the mammary glands for life.

Developed by Dr. Thomas Cronin of Baylor University, Houston, the implant is in effect a "falsie," filled with a silicone gel that comes in eight sizes ranging from petite to extra-full. This is not to be confused with the *direct* liquid silicone injections for extra inches, which, thanks to our medical watchdogs, are no longer allowed. Dow-Corning, the first company to manufacture silicone in the United States (and the only one to produce a medical variety) discovered in the mid-60s that it was being used far too generously and haphazardly by certain doctors. Alarming cases came to their attention of the silicone moving about in the body unchecked, disappearing in one place to reappear somewhere else in alarming lumps under the skin. At that time Dow-Corning immediately and voluntarily listed it with the Food and Drug Administration, so that their medical silicone ceased being an "implant material" and became a drug available only under the strictest medical supervision.

The silicone used today is a specially tested gelatinous silicone, always sealed in silicone rubber envelopes shaped like breasts.

There's another type of insertion—sometimes referred to as the "balloon" implant. Again, this implant is slipped behind the mammary glands, but in the form of a balloon-like silicone empty envelope. This is filled with a sterilized saline solution (pumped through the "balloon's" valve), which, when full, is sealed off, the valve packed beneath the balloon to avoid leakage. This method delivers a softer, more mobile-looking breast, and because the liquid can be carefully measured, in cases of breast asymmetry, it's easy to match the two by filling one balloon a little more or less as the case requires.

For the augmentation process, general anesthesia is usually used, with the stitches and brassiere-like bandages removed after about a week, while convalescence lasts about a month to six weeks, during which time the patient wears a special stretch bra.

Top-Heavy and Awkward—What Can I Do?

Breast reduction, alas, is hard work, say the surgeons, who've been working at it in different ways for the last four decades.

Fat deposits can be removed, nipples relocated, but no matter what technique is employed, reduction *mammaplasty* does leave scars. If the patient heals well, scars fade to a discreet pale color and can be partially disguised by the breasts' natural folds, but they are permanent and, depending on the skin, very visible to slightly visible.

Women, however, who have overdeveloped breasts—called macromastia—usually happily trade in this condition (which can cause chronic exhaustion, arthritis, or even a curvature of the spine, let alone embarrassment) for a couple of scars, pale or not.

Body Darts, Seams and Tucks—No Pleats Wanted

With the continual—and sensible—emphasis on dieting, many people's weight fluctuates for years. Even when the right weight and shape is maintained, skin isn't always accommodating, so that flab ruins the effort, bubbling up on the seat, the stomach, thighs, and/or upper arms.

A frequent victim of unattractive fat is the abdomen which resists all attempts with massage and exercise to return to its original taut state. An operation excising excess flab, tightening and realigning the muscle fibers, is the plastic surgeon's way of coping with this problem. One plastic surgeon told me in a recent abdomen-tightening op he removed twenty pounds of skin and fat, then transplanted the navel to its proper position.

Where large flaps of skin are removed, a thin scar will inevitably remain, but the best surgeons make their final sutures to coincide with the pubic-hair line, almost invisible even in the smallest bikini. It means a hospital stay of about four days to a week; sutures are removed after ten days; and the patient is advised not to engage in any hectic sports—or sex—for at least six weeks.

Bottoms "Up"

The celebrated "riding-breeches" operation, pioneered by Dr. Ivo Pitanguy in Brazil, is now on the surgeons' calendar in Buenos Aires and New York, too. "Riding breeches," as Pitanguy calls the fat jutting from the buttocks onto the thighs, spoil the line of shorts and skirts alike, and it's often obstinate fat that won't go away however stringent a diet or rigid an exercise routine.

In the surgeon's operating room, the quantity of tissue to be cut away from the thigh area is measured. Two lines are drawn on the buttocks—the upper line establishing the first incision, the lower indicating the second. When the patient is anesthetized, obviously lying on her stomach, the cuts are made along the tracings to remove the skin and fat tissue. Several pounds of lumpy fat can be removed from each thigh with this operation, so of necessity it's a lengthy job, lasting anywhere from two to four hours. Recovery is also slow. The first few days the patient must stay wrapped in elastic bandages from the waist down to the knees, and although most patients can leave the hospital after eight to ten days, normal activity is impossible for at least two weeks after. Even sitting down is uncomfortable, which makes the plane ride home to New York or Europe almost as bad as having another op. Depending on the patient, normality returns in about six to eight weeks, when I've heard it said, the new silhouette makes everything worthwhile—and memory is short, after all.

Summing Up the Cost of the Knife

Plastic surgery costs money—big money. First, there's the surgeon's fee, the anesthetist, the hospital-room rate—all these have to be taken into consideration—plus the amount of time you'll be out of circulation.

The saddest story I heard was about the woman who found she couldn't live with her new nose and had to have her old one back—expensive, frustrating, time-consuming—but I'd say she wasn't lucky with her surgeon, or else she didn't listen.

The only way to commit yourself to any plastic surgery is, as Dr. Pitanguy advises, to have the right size dream in the first place—then the right surgeon will do everything in his power to make it come true.

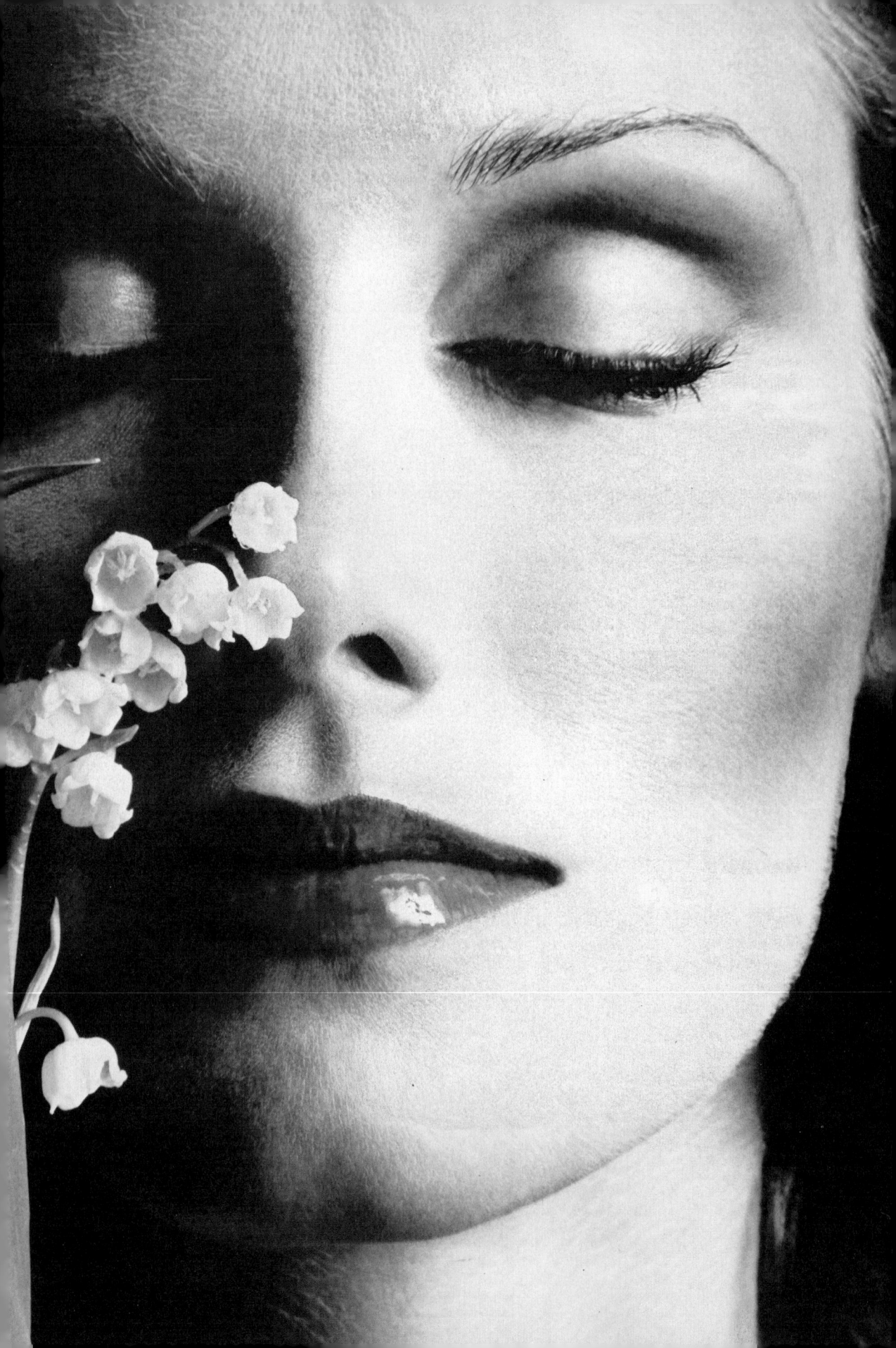

8

Scent and Its Many Implications

There's Much More to It Than Meets the Nose

One of the most important men in the cosmetic industry is crazy about scent. Crazy in the colloquial sense, for he's mad for women to wear it—if it's one of his creations, of course. He's also crazy with frustration that, as yet, he hasn't come up with a scent that's as irresistible as the "chemistry" Mike Todd once described—the invisible attraction that pulls one woman to one man, one man to one woman, as surely as a magnet (often mystifying the onlookers).

Although perfumers have skirted around the fact that sex could be the undercurrent they're after when creating a perfume, this tycoon makes no bones about the fact that to be able to create this "instant chemistry" would be the crowning achievement of his already most successful life.

FACING PAGE
Fragrance and a woman's psyche—intimately related.

The sense of smell plays a greater role in human activity than most people realize. It's at least a thousand times more sensitive than the sense of taste—one reason it can be a penance to sit in a restaurant next to somebody wearing a perfume that acts like gunpowder on the senses, it's so strong. The smell can *annihilate* the taste of anything, even steak au poivre.

A "nose" is another name for a good perfumer, for it's only given to those perfumers who instinctively *know* when a mélange of ingredients have come together to create a great fragrance—usually after years of trial and error.

Time has no effect on a great perfume—it goes throbbing on, as popular one year as the next. Chanel No. 5, Jicky, Emeraude, L'Heure Bleue, and Shalimar are all over fifty years old, while the great Arpège was created in 1927, Joy in 1934—all perfumes that are instantly recognizable. I can spot one friend whenever she's entered the Customs area at the airport. Her aura of Shalimar drifts right through the closed doors to the waiting area.

All of our noses accept, analyze, and identify odors—as different as chocolate from cheese, an onion from an oleander—with a speed that no laboratory instrument can duplicate. A chemist or beauty expert who is labeled a "nose," however, can also immediately pick out the jasmine from the Bulgarian rose in the formula, however deeply it's buried. I'm told some of the most expert can also *smell* the differences in skin and hair color—redheaded women apparently possessing uniquely pleasant-*smelling* skin!

Sexual Urge in a Bottle

Twenty to forty million olfactory receptors are at work in the nose, telegraphing, by electrical impulse, odor information to the brain. Because of this brilliant system, it isn't exaggerated to claim that certain fragrances do send impulses to the part of the brain in charge of sexual urges. The piquancy of this is that what turns one man on will have nil effect on another.

The musklike synthetic called *exaltolide* used frequently in perfume is similar, I'm told, to the *signal* scent produced by the human male. Apparently, it can be smelled most easily by women between the ages of fifteen and forty-five, but although I'm glad to say I fall in that category, I've never been aware of smelling it. That doesn't mean my olfactory system isn't working. I'm told by the experts I could be picking it up without ever realizing it, reacting to his "signal" instead of, say, his dark-brown eyes.

We accept without question the fact that our body chemistry makes the scent we choose smell differently on us than on others. Our *skin* makes the difference to the alchemy in the bottle, not necessarily lessening or increasing its effect but definitely making it *different*.

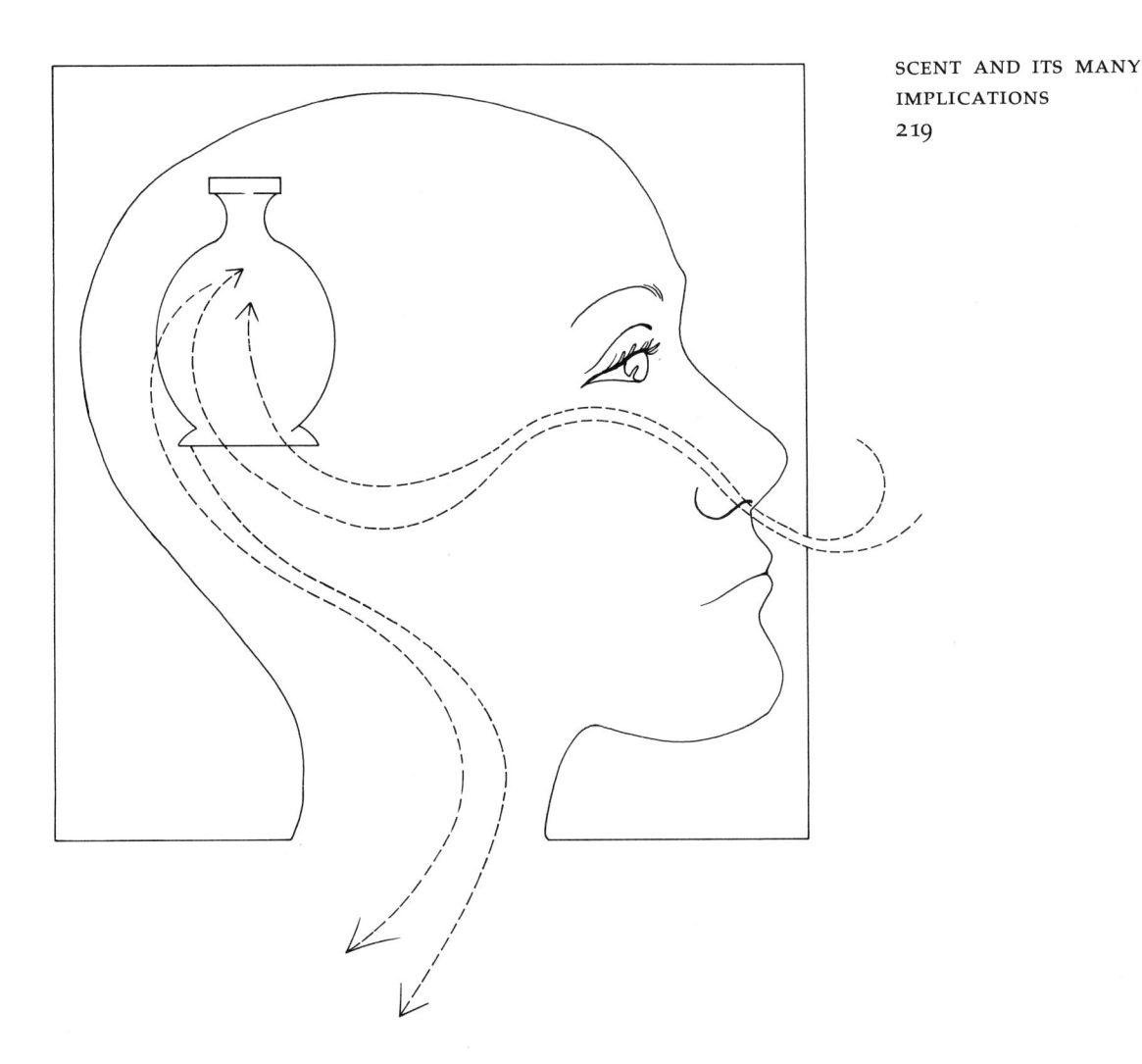

It therefore follows if my body chemistry affects the scent I put on (which it does), it's also going to affect the body chemistry of the person who smells it.

Studies are now going on in this country relating to "chemical substances produced by one individual that affect the behavior or physiology of another." They pose the possibility that marital, social, or even professional discord can be mediated or worsened by people picking up subconsciously irritating or, on the other hand, *provocative* scent signals from another.

Whatever develops with "pheromones" (the term given to these chemical substances), biological phenomena are always there for a REASON. Even if—so far—perfume can't be *proved* to be an aphrodisiac, it's still the most satisfying, extraordinarily mind-boggling booster for a woman's morale, linking her to a past, encouraging her to enjoy the present, and ensuring she has a future. One fact *is* established: fragrance *does* affect psyche—faster than a glass of champagne.

As the chairman of one of the largest flavors and fragrances houses in the world puts it, "The ability of any human being to perceive the environment is directly connected with the five senses, of which smell is one, but we are all divinely different with different odor receptors, so when we see or smell the world around us, we are experiencing something unique. Every fragrance smells differently to different people."

Where Are the Best Places to Put Scent?

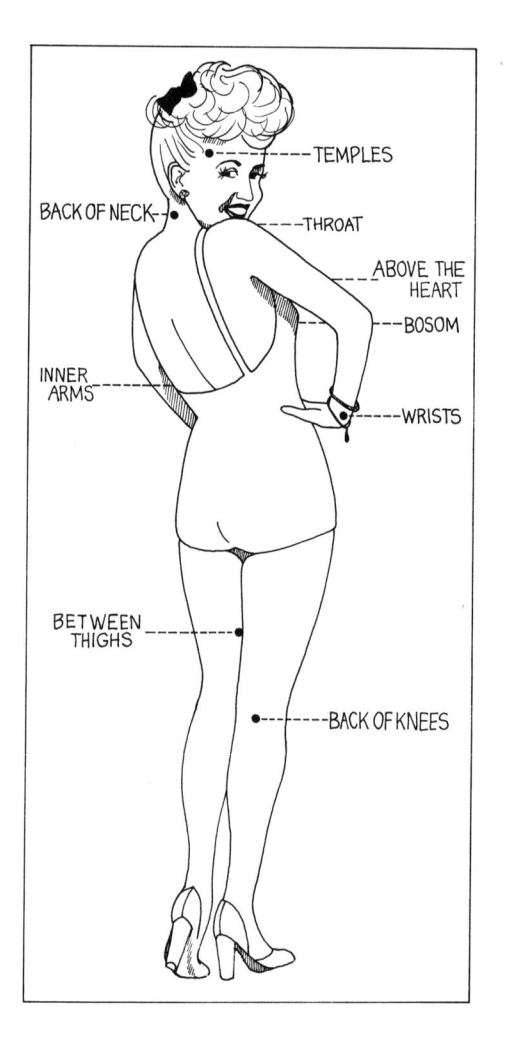

Starting at the toes, hit all the pulse points on the way up—backs of knees, the soft skin between the thighs, above the heart where heartbeat warms it, wrists, inner arms, bosom, throat, back of neck, the temples. Not so much behind the ears, although it isn't a crime if it goes there, but in such a concentrated area, fragrance can mix poorly with perspiration, and so negate its effect. The temples are better scent spots.

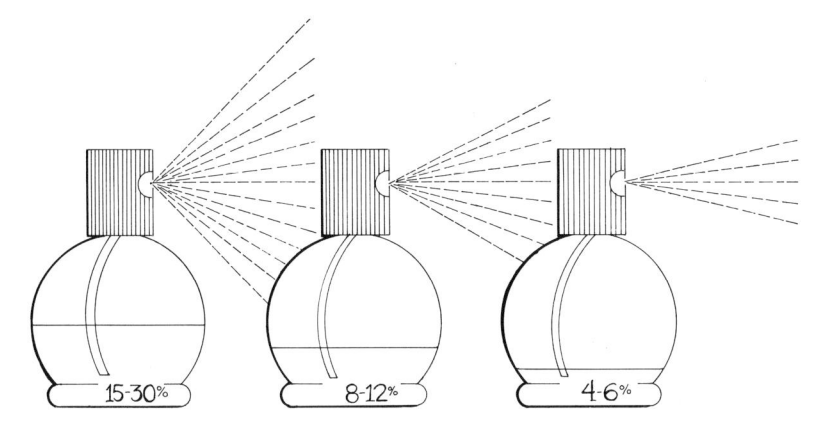

Fragrance application should actually start in the bath—particularly if skin is dry—to ensure it lasts as long as possible. Use bath oil or bath milk that attaches to the skin, the globules getting toweled into the pores. Spray on a cologne or toilet water before dressing, then use a final touch of real perfume before going out—all this ensures fragrance will last at least half a day.

Keep perfume in a dark, cool place, and it will stay in great condition for a long, long time, but *don't hoard it*. The fragrance may change, which is a terrible waste.

Spray cologne on tired feet, it will untire them. *Pour cologne into palms* and inhale for a quick pick-me-up—but *don't drink* it. *Spray cologne over ice cubes*, then saturate a cotton pad in the icy mixture, and place it on your forehead for a few minutes. Instantly refreshing. If perfume refuses to stay put on your skin, choose one without alcohol, in cream or liquid form.

Scent measures like this:

Strongest. The real McCoy is *concentrated perfume*, made of a few hundred ingredients, including flower and plant oils from all over the world—lilac, honeysuckle, lavender, rose, patchouli, fern, jasmine—rare and lovely and part of nature. Apply real perfume via an atomizer to diffuse the alcohol content while the true scent clings to skin. The amount of alcohol added to the formula determines the perfume's strength. Real perfume usually contains 15 to 30 percent of concentrates.

Strong. Eau de toilette, toilet water, eau de parfum, or parfum de toilette—all these contain no other fragrance note than that of the true perfume but have less concentrates of the many ingredients, usually from 8 to 12 percent.

Less strong. Cologne is the lightest form of fragrance, containing only about 4 to 6 percent of concentrates, very beguiling, but so light it can even be used on the hair or the hands to keep them cool and dry. Cologne also relieves aching muscles when used as a rubdown after a strenuous day.

Always apply perfume directly to your skin when choosing a new one—you can't learn the true fragrance in the bottle; it has to work with your skin.

Wait for a few minutes before passing judgment; let the heat of your body develop the scent your way.

Never buy a perfume because you like it on your best friend—or worst enemy. *It won't smell the same,* because—to reiterate—the chemistry of your skin affects it considerably. Test a new one in a bath-form product, less expensive and still effective for you to know if you're going to like the real McCoy.

Don't forget to encourage your man to wear fragrance, increasingly important in this hostile world.

A herbal manual of 1447 advised, "Ye will by smelling learne." That still makes a lot of sense when it comes to choosing your perfume.

Character in Perfume

The sign of a great perfume is its character, one that never gets lost or accidentally mistaken for something else—just like a human being's. That character can be *sultry* (also described as Oriental), blending together ingredients such as musk, ambergris, civet, and other exotica. It can be green and woodsy—clear compositions of sandalwood, rosewood, oakmoss, or ferns. It can be essentially *floral* like an English garden full of roses, lily of the valley, delphiniums, tuberoses, honeysuckle. The newest note is woody, *not* woodsy, and not at all green, but an unusual blending of floral and wood bark notes. Halston was one of the first to use it. *To come:* Unusual perfumes with fruity notes, pineapple particularly making its mark.

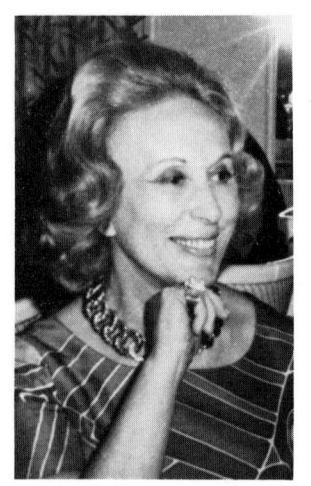

Estée Lauder, creator of great American perfumes.

Who Wears What:

Lauren Hutton likes the musk she bought in Ethiopia, and frankincense from Egypt. She also likes to rub fresh mint over her hands and oil of rosemary through her hair.

Barbara Walters doesn't like to wear scent when she starts work at 5 A.M., starts "revving up" about 2 P.M., with a burst of Ma Griffe on wrists, neck, back of her knees. This scent was much admired by the Chinese when she went on the Presidential trip to China in 1973.

Beverly Sills has used the same perfume for years—Piguet's Fracas. "The men I sing with say it turns them on, and my husband always knows where I am just by sniffing the air."

Lady Sassoon—widow of multimillionaire industrialist, Sir Victor—

is an inveterate traveler. Friends know when she's in customs, about to emerge, for Shalimar is always with her.

Until *Pauline Trigère* created her own products, she wore Shalimar day and night, in the bath, in cologne A.M., perfume after 6 P.M. Now she wears only Trigère by Trigère.

Estée Lauder, the first American lady to create breathtaking American fragrant compositions, still wears the Private Collection she originally created only for herself. Selflessness pays off—more and more American women are in love with her American perfumes.

Mrs. Harold Robbins, wife of the best-selling author, loves Weil's Secret of Venus, but in bath-oil form for maximum impact—buys several colognes for her husband, which he uses when the mood strikes.

Jackie O. changes her own perfume constantly but is faithful to cinnamon sticks in the fireplace, burning with the logs in winter to create a fragrant aroma throughout the house.

Greta Garbo is addicted to Vetiver; *Ali McGraw* to a man's scent, Dior's Eau Sauvage; *Liza Minnnelli* to Vivara by Emilio Pucci—which she sprays on while she's in the shower . . . she knows that "wet skin makes perfume work better"; *Mala Rubinstein,* niece of the great innovator Helena, to the emotive Courant or the happy-go-lucky essence of Heaven Sent.

A to Z of Perfume

(Without ever suggesting the alphabet
can supply all the fragrant answers)

Ambergris stands for grey amber—the odorless *fixative* that sets the ingredients together to ensure they last. It's difficult to find, and so expensive. In actuality ambergris is the spew of the sperm whale that's goaded by indigestion, in the same way that an oyster, maddened by a grain of sand, makes a pearl.

Bergamot is the small fragrant member of the citris family tree that flourishes only in Calabria in southern Italy. The fruit looks like a green orange, but it's inedible, bursting instead with an oil that's essential to making zippy, tangy perfume. Bergamot is tricky, however, because it *can* cause a phototoxic reaction on skin (brown spots) when exposed to too much sun. For this reason a synthetic Bergamot is often used now.

Cologne is the lightest form of scent originating in the eighteenth century.

Divisions are the categories into which the pros grade scent varieties, such as Floral Singles (one-note perfumes such as gardenia, violet, lilac), Floral Bouquets (a medley of flowers), Spicy Bouquets (including cinnamon, ginger, clove), Green Scents (mossy, grassy), Musky Blends (made with musk, amber, sandalwood, civet and patchouli), Citrus and Modern Blends (man-made synthetic departures and innovations).

Erotic. The description given to any scent chemists consider arouses sexual desire, or makes itself *felt* through an appeal to the olfactory senses.

Fixative (see *Ambergris, Musk*). The essential substance that sets or binds the more volatile ingredients together to keep them stable, harmonious, and lasting.

Grasse. The perfume capital of the world, an enchanting eighteenth-century town in France's *Alpes-Maritime*. Flowers grow there in profusion, for no sooner are they plucked and stripped of their perfume-producing petals than more crowd the slopes to take their place. The valuable oils of these—roses, orange blossoms, violets, jonquils, acacias, mimosa, and jasmine, to name only a few—are shipped all over the globe. No well-known perfume is made in Grasse, but it's the chief supplier of the main ingredients to perfumers everywhere.

Herb. This seed plant remains soft and succulent, never develops bark and is used for scent or flavoring. Lavender, rosemary, Clary sage, and costus are the most aromatic and so are most used by makers of perfume.

Incense. The perfume that has been burned through the ages to create a fragrant atmosphere. Offered to the gods in ancient Rome, then as today the most aromatic categories come from China, and to the Chinese perfume *means* incense; they divide it into six types: Tranquil, Recluse, Luxurious, Beautiful, Refined, and Noble, each of which is meant to induce a corresponding mood. In the West we try to make it with perfumed candles.

Jasmine. The most precious and thus the most expensive perfume ingredient—about five thousand dollars a pound! White, and intensely scented, it reaches its peak at dawn, when anyone who can get up in time is rewarded with its full sweetness, even *voluptuousness*. Every classic perfume—like those mentioned that are at least fifty years old—contains at least a pinch. So far, man has not been able to synthesize jasmine.

Kinds of perfume. These are now endless . . . . you don't only get your scent in perfume anymore, but in cologne, toilet water, sachet, soap, bath bubbles, bath gel, oils, powders, soothing lotions, candles, towelettes, shampoo, hair spray—now even in a kissing gloss that dispenses musk mouth to mouth (not recommended for resuscitation), and a felt-tip pen that literally dispenses *fragrant* messages on the skin.

Linger. In pro language, the cling or persistence of a scent. Perfumes that use musk or civet as a fixative are *very* clingy. It's a fact that perfumes linger longer when sprayed on wet skin.

Musk. Used to be used only as a fixative, found in the glands or pods of the male musk deer, smelling strongest during the mating season. The dried pods are nearly odorless, but when moistened, become ambrosial, in fact overpowering.

Nose. Refers to the perfumer, usually a man who possesses an extraordinary and creative sense of smell, and the one to cry "Eureka" sometimes after five or six years when he *knows* with one sniff he has composed a great scent. There are very few *great* noses—and they've all usually had a training stint in Grasse.

Orange Flower. An ardent, sweet ingredient that adds a certain "intoxication" to perfume. It's believed it originated with the Saracens and was brought to Europe by the Crusaders.

Patchouli. Has a wild, haunting odor, possibly the most intense in the whole plant kingdom. It's used mainly in exotic perfumes that seem to carry a touch of the East.

Quasi. What many perfumes really set out to be—in that they are direct copies of a celebrated scent, with just a slight amendment, so it's not so obvious to the sweet-smelling public. In fact, copies lack a lot, as all quasi things must do.

Rose. The all-encompassing scent, created only after at least half a ton of petals has been crushed—to make one pound of rose attar. Again the great perfumes all use at least a trace.

Synthetics. The fragrant inventions of man, born in a laboratory, and often formulated to resemble real flowers. They produce en masse what nature does a drop at a time, so make the perfume operation a more economical one. Synthetics have introduced a more lasting quality to perfume, too, as well as—in a few cases only—introducing a totally new type of smell.

Top Note. The first expression of a perfume, the immediate scent that attacks your senses before you absorb the whole. It has been likened to the excitement of a beautiful solo voice that first carries a musical message, and then recedes to let the orchestra take over.

Unisex. More and more the description is given to new scents, ones that can work wonders on both male and female, a source of pleasure to both.

Vetiver. An essential oil derived from the roots of aromatic grasses, growing in Java, Haiti, and South America. Intense and smoldering, it is a memorable part of many perfumes.

Witchcraft. In the Middle Ages perfume was associated with sorcery, women being persecuted for wearing it to "attract the devil."

X. The unknown element in perfume that relates to *your* skin and your skin alone, adding an intangible note that either makes it special to you or an also-ran you won't buy again.

Ylang Ylang. Meaning "flower of flowers," it has a poignant, ethereal odor. Woven into love-garlands on tropical islands, it makes otherwise overheavy perfumes more subtle.

Zanzibar. An island where the air is thick with the spicy breath of cloves; also an important part of many floral scents.

Index

(Page numbers in italics indicate illustrations.)

acid mantle, 11, 12, 48, 91
acne, 15–17, 18, 47, 210, 211
acupressure, acupuncture, 200, 201
adrenal glands, 18, 149
aging, 5–10, 13, 22, 23, 36, 37, 38, 39, 117, 119, 206, 209, 210
Air Force Diet, 140
alcohol, drinking, 55, 58, 62, 145, 146, 147, 199
Alexandre of Paris, 100, 119
allergies, 18–20, 41, 120
American Association of Plastic Surgeons, 212
American Medical Association, 152
American Psychiatric Association, 152
American Society of Aesthetic Plastic Surgery, 212
American Society of Dermatologic Surgery, 212
American Society of Plastic and Reconstructive Surgeons, 204
amphetamines, 136
androgen, 89, 90
Ann-Margret, 69

anorexia, 149
antibiotics, 17, 209, 211
antiperspirants, 43-46
appetite suppressants, 136, 137
Arden, Elizabeth, 24, *60*, 67, 212
    Maine Chance and, 55, 59, 60, 62
aromatherapy, 22-23
Aslan, Dr. Ana, 37
astringents, 15, 24, 50
Avedon, Luciana (Mrs. Burt), 122, *202*, 205
avocado, 20, 21, 26, 39, 48–49, 143–144
Azzolini, Dina, 104

baldness, 87–92
balsam, 100, 111
Bandy, Way, 65–66, 67
bath oil, 14, 35
bath (*see also* spas), 42
    accessories for, 48–49
    beauty ritual of, 26, 35, 43, 46–52, 221
    oil for, 14, 26, 35, 48, 49
    as pick-me-up, 49
    procedure for, 50

bath (cont.)
   special kinds of, 49, 50, 53, 62–63
   temperature of, 47, 51–52
   types of, 51–52, 62–63
   water for, quality of, 46–47
Beck, Toni, 61
Bell Island, Alaska, 54
Bello, Josef, 61
Bépanthène, 97–98
Bergen, Polly, 198
Berk, Lotte, exercises of, 186–187
Blanchard, Leslie, 116, 124–125
Blank, Dr. Irwin, 13
blepharoplasty, 205, 206
blood:
   circulation of, 23, 41, 95, 97, 98, 135, 198–200
   -sugar levels, 136, 149
Bloomingdale, Betsy, 198
blusher, 72–73
body brush, 48
body odor, 44–46
Brauer, Dr. Earle, 19
breast surgery, 213–214
British Journal of Plastic Surgery, 210
Bucharest Geriatric Institute, 37
Burnett, Carol, 113

cabbage, in diet, 27–28, 197
calories (*see also* diet):
   amount of, used in hour's activity, 195
   calculations for, 140, 142
   chart for counting of, 140–142, 154–159
Cannon, Dr. Bradford, 209
carbohydrates (*see also* diet), 137, 139–140, 150
   food chart for, 154–159
carcinoma, 6, 29
Cella, Dr. John A., 1
cellulite, 60, 196–198
Channing, Carol, 112–113
chemosurgery, 210, 211
Cher, 26, 86
Chiles, Lois, 2–3, *66*
Choudhury, Bikram, 164
circulation, of blood, 23, 41, 95, 97, 98, 135, 198–200
collagen, 10, 37, 92
cologne, 221–222, 223
Cooper, Gloria Vanderbilt, 122, 148
Cormia, Dr. Frank, 88–89
cosmetic industry, 1, 2, 19–22, 23, 66–67
cosmetics, *see* makeup

Craig, Marjorie, exercises of, 179–180
Crawford, Joan, 122
Cronin, Dr. Thomas, 213
cuticle, 40

Dahl, Arlene, *4, 6,* 49, 112, 180
dandruff, 92
Davis, Adelle, 21
deodorant, 43–46
dermabrasion, 210, 212
dermis, 7, 8–9, 10
Diba, Farah, 165
Dick-Read, Dr. Grantley, 154–155
diencephalon, 130–131
diet (*see also* nutrition):
   for acne, 15, 16
   appetite suppressants and, 136, 137
   calorie and carbohydrate food chart for, 154–159
   childhood and, 130–132
   diuretics and, 12, 135–136, 137
   hypnosis and, 150–155, *151*
   and low calories, 134, 140–143, 146–148
   and low carbohydrates, 93, 137–140, 142, 146
   metabolism and, 135
   motivation for, 132, 133, 137, 148, 152, 153
   psychological aids for, 145–146
   for severe obesity, 132–134, 137–139
   at spas, 53–62
   for the underweight, 148–150
   vitamins and, 144, 150
diuretics, 12, 135–136, 137
Dobloug, Lisa, 56
drinking, *see* alcohol, drinking; water
drugs, 44, 89, 199, 214
dry skin, *see* skin, dry
Dudley, Jane, *4, 6*
Duke, Mrs. Angier Biddle, 122
Dunaway, Faye, 121

effleurage, 200
Elizabeth I, of England, 46
Elizabeth II, of England, 13, 86
emollients, 14, 35
emotional outlook, 3, 22, 44–45, 86, 163–164, 197, 199
   effects of, on skin, 6, 15, 16, 18, 36
enzymes, 36, 37, 117
epidermis, 7, 9, 212
estrogen, 17, 18, 89, 90
exaltolide, 218
exercise:
   for abdomen, 179, 186–187, 188–189

INDEX

exercise *(cont.)*
  with apparatus, 193–194, 196
  for back, 188–189
  in the bath, 50
  belly dancing as, 169
  boredom of, 163–164
  breathing and, 166
  as daily routine, 3, 15, 164–165
  dance as, 168–169
  with no equipment, 176–179, 196
  in gym, 193–194
  headstand as, 172
  for hips and waist, 179, 180, 182, 184–187
  importance of, 197
  instructors and, 165–166
  jogging as, 179
  methods of, 167, 196
  as physiotherapy, 173–175
  in the pool, 175–176
  at spas, 53–62
  for spot reducing, 179–189
  to start the day, 192–193
  tests for, 190–192
  for thighs, 180, 181
  for upper arm, 182–183
  yoga as, 169–172
exfoliating cream, 9
eye makeup, 73–78, 90

facials, 16, 24–25, 59
faradic machines, 196
Farrow, Mia, 122, 125, 148
fat *(see also* obesity), 130–131, 134, 136, 149, 197
  surgical removal of, 204, 209, 210, 214–215
Fonda, Mrs. Henry, 198
food, *see* diet; nutrition
Food and Drug Administration (F.D.A.), 19, 36, 37, 213
Ford, Cristina, 49, 122
Ford, Eileen, 62, 178
Forest Mere spa, 173
Forstmann, Charlotte Ford, 200
Fracas, 222
François (hairstylist), 67–68, 86, 104
Fraser, Lady Antonia, 49
friction strap, 48
frostbite, 35–36

Gabor, Eva, 112
Gallant, Ara, 102, 105, 111
Garbo, Greta, 223
gels, 48–49, 68, 72–73, 212
Gerovital H3, 37

Golden Door, 53, 55, 58, 59
  exercises used at, 184–189
Grace, Princess, of Monaco, 61
Graham, Karen, 26, 111
Grapefruit Diet, 140
Greenhouse Spa, 55, 61
  exercises used at, 181
Grey, Aida, 23, 27–28
Guercio, Nicholas, 76–77

hair *(see also* hair coloring), 84
  caring for, 85–99
  comb-out of, 111–112
  conditioners for, 99–100
  cutting of, 87, 95, 97, 100–105, 106, *107*
  damaged, 95–97
  dry, 93–95, 100
  length of, 100–104
  loss of, 87–90, 97
  makeup and, 67–68
  of models, 111
  new image and, 104–105
  nutrition and, 90–91, 92, 93, 94, 95, 97–98, 100
  oily, 92–93
  rules for home care of, 98–99
  self-evaluation of, 105–110
  shampooing of, 91–94, 96, 97, 98, 99, 102, 112, 113, 125, 126
  styling of, 2, 100–110, *107, 108*
  transplanting of, 90, 203
  types of, 92
  vitamin B$_5$ and, 97–98
  wig instead of, 112–116
hair coloring:
  color dictionary, 126–127
  double process of, 120–121
  experts at, 116, 121–123, 125
  frosting, 123–124
  natural color in, 116–117, 118, 119
  one-step process of, 118–119, 120
  patch test for, 119–120, 126–127
  permanent, 118, 119, 120, 125, 126
  peroxide and, 117, 118, 119–120
  salon checkup for, 124–125
  selection of shade for, 118–120, 124–125
  special effects in, 123–124, 126, 127
  types of, 117
  washout of, 117
hairstylists, 2, 100–110, 111, 113, 116
hands, care of, 38–40
Hart, Marvin, 164, 190, 193
health, importance of, 3
Hedo, Dr. Abdulhamid, 209

height-weight tables, 160–161
henna, 93, 125
Hepburn, Audrey, 132, 148
Hoffman, Dr. Joseph, 6, 8
hormones, 16, 17, 18, 44, 89, 90, 134, 135, 137
Horne, Lena, 32
Hot Springs, Virginia, 53
humidity, 32, 35
Hutton, Lauren, 2, 26, 73, 111, 222
hyaluronic acid, 27–28
hydrogen potential, *see* pH
hypnosis, 150–155, *151*
hypoallergenic products, 19

infrared rays, 29
insomnia, 13, 179

Jevons, Professor, 36
Johnson, Beverly, 83
Johnson, Lady Bird, 61

Kelmenson, Mrs. Leo, 6
Kempner, Dr. Walter, 137–139
Kenneth (hair expert), 67, 85, 98, 113, 116
keratin, 9, 120
Khan, Sally, 6
Khanh, Emmanuelle, 102
King, George, 200
Kissinger, Nancy (Mrs. Henry), 178

La Costa spa, 53, 57–58
LaLanne, Jack, 166
Lancet, The, 134, 136–137
Lancôme (makeup artist), 62
Laszlo, Dr. Erno, 3, 13
Lauder, Estée, 222, 223
Lee, Don, 95
Levine, Dr. Rachmiel, 149
Levitt, Simone, 100–101, 104
Ling, Per Henrik, 200
Linter, Sandra, 78
lipectomy, 209–210
lipstick, 79–81
Long, Louise, 201
loofah, 48
Loos, Anita, 117
Lord, Shirley, *viii*, 1, 2, 3, 26, 67, *104*, 114
  Harper's Bazaar editorial of, 66
  rules of Marc Sinclaire for, 111, 112
  skin of, 11–12
Loren, Sophia, 129
Lubowe, Dr. Irwin, 89–90

McGraw, Ali, 223
McIndoe, Sir Archibald, 204

Maine Chance, 55, 59–61, 62
makeup:
  base coat of, *66*, 68–72
  for Black women, 81–83
  contour color of, 72–73
  for eyes, 73–78, 90
  and hair, 67–68
  lips and mouth, 79–81
  medicated, 15
  moisturizers and, 14–15
  natural look in, *64*, 65–67, *70*, *71*
  after plastic surgery, 67, 208, 212–213
  powder as part of, 78–79
Mancini, Mrs. Henry, 198
manicure, 40
Manzoni, Count Pablo Zappi, 67–68, 72, 208, 212–213
Margaret, Princess, 86, 104
Marie Antoinette, 46
mascara, 74
masks, facial, 14, 21, 23–24, 37
massage, 22–25, 60, 95, 198–201
masseurs, 59, 60, 198, 200–201
Maury, Marguerite, 6, 8, 22
Mayo Clinic Diet, 140
Mazzanti, Mrs. Szekely, 59
melanin, 18, 28, 29, 31, 116
menopause, 89
Merrill, Dina, 122
Millard, Dr. Ralph, 209–210
minerals, 144–145
mineral water (*see also* spas), 26
Minnelli, Liza, 24, 223
moisturizers, 13–14, 15, 24, 35, 36, 83
Monroe, Marilyn, 66, 209
Moore, Mary Tyler, 81
mud pack, 23–24, 58, 62
Murrieta Hot Springs, spa at, 58

nails, care of, 39–40
natural look, 1, 66, 67
"natural" beauty products, 19–20
Nevelson, Louise, 49
Nidetch, Jean, 148
Niehans, Dr., 36
nose, size of, 67, 72
  surgery on, 203, 204, 207, 209
nutrition (*see also* diet), 2, 3, 35, 36, 44–45, 93, 95
  calorie and carbohydrate chart for, 154–159
  effect of, on hair, 90, 93, 95

obesity (*see also* diet), 134, 137–139, 147–148, 209
  reasons for, 129–132

O'Brien, Edna, 186
oil, 14, 21, 22–23, 32, 48–49
oil glands, 38
oily skin, *see* skin, oily
Onassis, Jacqueline, 164–165, 223
Orentreich, Dr. Norman, 90
organic beauty preparations, 19–20
oxygen baths, 62

Palm–Aire, Spa at, 55–57
Palm Springs, Spa at, 54
paraffin wax baths, 62
patch test, 119–120, 126–127
pedicure, 40
perfume:
  as aphrodisiac, 217–219, 224
  application of, 220–222
  character of, 222
  definition of terms for, 223–225
  preferences of personalities in, 222–223
  strength of, 221–222
peroxide, 117, 118, 119–120
Peters, Jon, 104
petrissage, 24–25, 200
petroleum jelly, 14, 32
pH (hydrogen potential), 11, 21, 51, 91–92
pheomelanin, 116
physiotherapy, 173–175, 198–200
Pignatelli, Princess Luciana, *see* Avedon, Luciana (Mrs. Bert)
Pigott, Dr. Ronald W., 209
Pill, the, 17–18, 88–89
Pitanguy, Dr. Ivo, 204, 215
pituitary gland, 18, 131
plastic surgery, 10, 67
  for bags under eyes, 204, 206–207
  body tucks, 203, 213–215
  on breast, 203–214
  chemosurgery and, 210, 211
  on chin, 209–210
  cost of, 215
  dermabrasion in, 210, 212
  excess fat removed by, 214–215
  face-lift by, 65, 203, 204, 205–207, 210–212
  hair transplanted by, 90, 203
  makeup after, 67, 207, 208, 212–213
  on nose, 203, 206, 207–209
  use of silicone, 208, 209, 213–214
Poland Springs, Maine, 53
polymers, 39
Pompadour, Madame de, 24
pores, of skin, 14, 15, 17, 26, 39, 47
posture, 163–164

powder, facial, 78–79
protein, 9, 10, 21, 24, 36, 37, 44
  in diet, 90, 93, 95, 138, 141, 142, 143
  for hair, 90, 92, 93, 94, 95, 96, 99, 100, 111, 141–142
psoriasis, 92
pumice stone, 48

Quant, Mary, 102

Radziwill, Lee, 186
Rancho La Puerta, 58–59
Read, Dr. Charles, 130
Redgrave, Vanessa, 69, 178
Régine (nightclub owner), 49
rejuvenation, 36–37
Reti, Rose, 122, 125
Revson, Charles, 37
rhinoplasty, 208
rhythm (of life), 3, 22
rhytidectomy, 205
Rice Diet, 137–139
Rita (hair expert), 98
Robbins, Mrs. Harold, 223
Rosemary (hair colorist), 121
Rothschild, Jeanne de, Baroness, 6
Rottenburger, Josef, 200–201
rouge, 67, 72–73, 213
royal jelly, 36
Rubinstein, Helena, 13, 24, *25,* 62, 91, 223
Rubinstein, Mala, 223
Rykiel, Sonia, 49

Safety Harbor, 54–55
sand bath, 63
Sandieson, Norman, 173
Saratoga, spa at, 53, 54
Sassoon, Lady, 222–223
Sassoon, Vidal, 102, *103,* 204
sauna bath, 63, 200
Savoia, Maria Beatrice de, 148
scent, *see* perfume
seborrhea, 92, 98
sebum and sebaceous glands, 9, 11, 15, 17, 24, 92
Secret of Life and Youth, The (Maury), 6
self-confidence, 2–3, 16
sex, importance of, 3, 6, 135, 167
Shiatsu massage, 201
shampoo, *see* hair, shampooing of
shower, 46, 51
silicone, 143, 208, 209, 213–214
Sills, Beverly, 222
Simeon, Dr. A. T. W., 134, 136–137
Sims, Naomi, 82

Sinatra, Frank, 137
Sinclaire, Marc, 111–112, 116
skin:
   aging of, 5–6, 9–10, 13, 22, 32, 38–39
   allergies and, 18–20
   Black, 31–32, 33
   dry, 11, 12–14, 21, 24
   effect of emotions on, 6, 15, 16, 18, 36
   effect of environment on, 11–12
   effect of Pill on, 17–18
   facial masks for, 14, 23–24, 41
   facial massage for, 24–25, 41
   functions of, 8
   on hands, 38–39
   hydrated, 11, 16
   layers of, 7–9
   on neck, 38–39
   normal, 11, 14–15, 24
   organic products for, 20–22
   oily, 11, 15, 17, 21, 24, 48
   Oriental, 23
   recycling of, 36–37
   rules for general care of, 41
   sun and, 6, 11, 12, 28–31, 36
   tips on care of, 26–27
   types of, 10–12
   winter and, 32, 34, 35–36
   workings of, 8–9
Slepyan, Dr. Albert, 88
soap:
   dry hair and, 94
   dry skin and, 12, 48
   medicated, 17
   normal skin and, 14–15, 48
   oily hair and, 93
   winter and, 35
spas:
   in contemporary America, 53, 54–55
   in Europe, 53, 54, 201
   permissive and nonpermissive, 55–58
   rules of, 59–61
   on shipboard, 61–62
   special baths at, 62–63
Spiegel, Dr. Herbert, 150, 152, 153
Stafford Springs, 53
Steamboat Springs, Colorado, 54
steroids, 90
Streisand, Barbra, 104, 164
subdermis, 7, 8
sun:
   benefits of, 28, 29, 56
   harmful effects of, 6, 11, 12, 28–31, 36, 41, 91, 94
suntan oil, 30, 31

Swanson, Gloria, 13
sweat glands, 44, 212
Szekely, Professor Edmond, 58–59

tapotement, 25, 200
Taylor, Elizabeth, 129
Taylor, Ursula Theiss, 198
tears, 26, 79
testosterone, 17, 18
Theodoracopulos, Betsy, 6, 73, 113, 178
Thyssen, Baroness von, 97
Todd, Mike, 217
toilet water, 221
traction alopecia, 87–88
tranquilizers, 45
Trigère, Pauline, 49, 223
Twiggy, 132

ultraviolet rays, 17, 28, 30–31
Urbach, Dr. Frederick, 30–31

vegetarians, 45, 59
Viera, James, 62
vitamin A, 17, 26–27, 35, 88, 97
vitamin B$_2$, 35
vitamin B$_5$, 97–98
vitamin B complex, 90, 95
vitamin D, 97
vitamin E, 26, 37
vitamins, 17, 20–22, 26–27, 35, 37, 144, 150
Vogue, 1, 2, 3, 26, 66, 67, 104
   eye-makeup tricks from, 77–78

Walden, Barbara, 82
Walters, Barbara, 222
washing, 12, 15, 17
water, 52–53
   amount of, required daily, 15, 41
   for care of skin, 15
   diet and, 136, 197
   hard and soft, 46–47
weight-height tables, 160–161
Weight Watchers, 148
Welch, Raquel, 72
Whitmore, Lady, 186
wig, 112–116, *114, 115*
Wright, Dr. Frederick, 155
wrinkles, 1–2, 198
   facial mask and, 23
   masseurs and, 198
   moisturizer for, 14
   plastic surgery and, 210–212

yoga, as exercise, 55, 58, 169–170, 200

zone therapy, 60, 201